Palliative Care and Nursing

Palliative Care and Nursing

Edited by Lily Bowen

hayle
medical

New York

Hayle Medical,
750 Third Avenue, 9th Floor,
New York, NY 10017, USA

Visit us on the World Wide Web at:
www.haylemedical.com

ISBN: 978-1-63241-814-2

Cataloging-in-Publication Data

Palliative care and nursing / edited by Lily Bowen.
     p. cm.
Includes bibliographical references and index.
ISBN 978-1-63241-814-2
1. Palliative treatment. 2. Nursing. 3. Care of the sick. 4. Medical care. I. Bowen, Lily.
R726.8 .P35 2019
616.029--dc21

Table of Contents

Preface

The field of healthcare concerned with the care of people to help them recover, achieve and maintain optimal health and quality of life is called nursing. A nurse is skilled in assisting patients in performing activities of daily living. The sub-field of nursing dealing with the care of people suffering from life-limiting illnesses is known as palliative care. It is considered effective in providing comfort as it aids in reducing the pain and stress for the patient and the family. The goal of such care is to treat pain and other distressing symptoms, provide relief from suffering and a support system to assist the patient in living as actively as possible. This book elucidates the concepts and innovative models around prospective developments with respect to palliative care. Also included herein is a detailed explanation of the various concepts and applications of palliative nursing. For all those who are interested in this field, this book can prove to be an essential guide.

After months of intensive research and writing, this book is the end result of all who devoted their time and efforts in the initiation and progress of this book. It will surely be a source of reference in enhancing the required knowledge of the new developments in the area. During the course of developing this book, certain measures such as accuracy, authenticity and research focused analytical studies were given preference in order to produce a comprehensive book in the area of study.

This book would not have been possible without the efforts of the authors and the publisher. I extend my sincere thanks to them. Secondly, I express my gratitude to my family and well-wishers. And most importantly, I thank my students for constantly expressing their willingness and curiosity in enhancing their knowledge in the field, which encourages me to take up further research projects for the advancement of the area.

Editor

How can end of life care excellence be normalized in hospitals? Lessons from a qualitative framework study

Christy Noble[1,2,3]* 🆔, Laurie Grealish[4,5], Andrew Teodorczuk[2], Brenton Shanahan[5], Balaji Hiremagular[5], Jodie Morris[6] and Sarah Yardley[7,8]

Abstract

Background: There is a pressing need to improve end-of-life care in acute settings. This requires meeting the learning needs of all acute care healthcare professionals to develop broader clinical expertise and bring about positive change. The UK experience with the Liverpool Care of the Dying Pathway (LCP), also demonstrates a greater focus on implementation processes and daily working practices is necessary.

Methods: This qualitative study, informed by Normalisation Process Theory (NPT), investigates how a tool for end-of-life care was embedded in a large Australian teaching hospital. The study identified contextual barriers and facilitators captured in real time, as the 'Clinical Guidelines for Dying Patients' (CgDp) were implemented. A purposive sample of 28 acute ward (allied health 7 [including occupational therapist, pharmacists, physiotherapist, psychologist, speech pathologist], nursing 10, medical 8) and palliative care (medical 2, nursing 1) staff participated. Interviews ($n = 18$) and focus groups ($n = 2$), were audio-recorded and transcribed verbatim. Data were analysed using an a priori framework of NPT constructs; coherence, cognitive participation, collective action and reflexive monitoring.

Results: The CgDp afforded staff support, but the reality of the clinical process was invariably perceived as more complex than the guidelines suggested. The CgDp 'made sense' to nursing and medical staff, but, because allied health staff were not ward-based, they were not as engaged (coherence). Implementation was challenged by competing concerns in the acute setting where most patients required a different care approach (cognitive participation). The CgDp is designed to start when a patient is dying, yet staff found it difficult to diagnose dying. Staff were concerned that they lacked ready access to experts (collective action) to support this. Participants believed using CgDp improved patient care, but there was an absence of participation in real time monitoring or quality improvement activity.

Conclusions: We propose a model, which addresses the risks and barriers identified, to guide implementation of end-of-life care tools in acute settings. The model promotes interprofessional and interdisciplinary working and learning strategies to develop capabilities for embedding end of life (EOL) care excellence whilst guided by experienced palliative care teams. Further research is needed to determine if this model can be prospectively applied to positively influence EOL practices.

Keywords: Palliative care, Hospital, Qualitative research, Normalisation process theory, Guideline

* Correspondence: c.noble@griffith.edu.au
[1]Medical Education Unit, Gold Coast Health, Level 2 PED Building, 1 Hospital Boulevard, Southport, QLD 4215, Australia
[2]School of Medicine, Griffith University, Griffith, QLD, Australia
Full list of author information is available at the end of the article

Background

Providing high-quality care for dying patients in acute settings is essential to meet changing population needs and societal expectations [1]. Increasingly people live with chronic, potentially life limiting conditions; prognosis is uncertain and inevitably some will spend their final days of life in acute hospital care [2, 3]. In Australia, despite 70% of people wanting to die at home only about 14% do [3, 4]. While healthcare organisations are adopting care pathways to ensure appropriate end of life care, globally, studies report suboptimal care quality in hospitals [5–7].

For many years, the Liverpool Care Pathway (LCP) was considered as a gold standard for care for dying patients, yet it has been withdrawn in the United Kingdom (UK). Significant gaps were identified between the goals of the LCP and its enactment in practice, with criticism focused on failure to have studied the process of implementation, lack of available expertise embedded in acute settings and not addressing the learning needs of non-specialist healthcare professionals [8]. As a result five priorities for improving care for a dying person [9] were identified: a) recognising the possibility of dying; b) sensitive communication with the dying person and loved ones; c) involve dying person and loved ones in treatment and care decision making; d) explore and respect the need of the dying person's loved ones and e) agree and deliver an individualised care plan with compassion [9]. Contrasting with the UK experience, Italian studies suggest that the quality of end of life (EOL) care can be improved using the LCP when implemented with a structured program and clear goals [5–11]. These findings align with emerging evidence suggesting that effective LCP implementation can be aided by a comprehensive understanding of the local context including appreciating and valuing differing professional perspectives and work structures [10, 11].

Achieving high-quality end-of-life care in acute settings is challenging. [6] Acute settings are orientated towards interventional treatment of reversible conditions. Institutions are designed to ensure rapid provision of immediate and urgent care with finite specialist palliative care resources, staff turnover is often high and staff not necessarily experienced in recognising dying, or determining likelihood of reversible causes versus irreversible deterioration [4] despite multiple attempts to educate and improve [5]. Enabling excellence in EOL care in acute care settings is a significant concern, with both national [12] and international [9] strategies being developed to support these provisions of EOL care excellence.

This study aimed to investigate if and how EOL care excellence can be embedded or normalised in acute healthcare settings. Our objectives were to: 1) generate a rich description of individual and contextual barriers and enablers surrounding implementation of the Clinical Guidelines for Dying Patients (CgDp), in an acute setting; 2) identify learning strategies to mitigate barriers and strengthen enablers; 3) integrate our data analysis, using normalization process theory (NPT) (see below), to generate a conceptual model to inform further implementation research.

Methods
Theoretical framework

We adopted a social constructionist research approach [13] to understand the meanings participants generated through interactions when enacting practices related to the CgDp. Normalisation Process Theory (NPT) [14, 15] was used as our theoretical lens as it offers an explanation of processes for implementing, embedding and integrating practices in everyday work [14]. Individual and contextual factors promoting or inhibiting normalisation of practices include coherence, cognitive participation, collective action and reflexive monitoring (see Table 1 for further explanation of each construct). This approach enabled us to develop in-depth descriptions and interpretative explanations for how learning strategies can facilitate the CgDp becoming integrated in practice.

Study design

Given the need to understand local contextual factors for effective implementation [8, 14], an explanatory qualitative interview study, using the framework analytic approach [16], was conducted that aligned to our theoretical stance. Our design facilitated in-depth exploration into the health care professionals' perspective of individual and contextual barriers and enablers to implementing the CgDp. NPT as a sensitising tool for embedding practices [17] enabled us to generate a programme theory and model [18] to inform the development of a complex intervention to normalise end of life care excellence in acute care settings. The study was approved by Gold Coast Health Ethics Committee (HREC/14/QGC/185). To ensure the anonymity of the participants and the practices where they work, all identifiers have been removed. Written consent was obtained.

Table 1 Normalisation process theory constructs - generative mechanisms (From May et al., 2009 [37])

NPT construct	Explanation
Coherence	Work that defines and organises the objects of a practice
Cognitive participation	Work that defines and organises the enrolment of participants in a practice
Collective action	Work that defines and organises the enacting of a practice
Reflexive monitoring	Work that defines and organises the knowledge upon which appraisal of a practice is founded

Setting

This study was conducted in a large acute care tertiary hospital, located in Queensland, Australia with 750 in-patient beds. The study focussed on a 24-bed acute care medical ward, where there were 48 deaths in 2015. In 2009, an EOL care pathway, CgDp, based on LCP was endorsed by Queensland Health for state-wide use within its acute hospitals. [19] (The current version of the CgDp can be found here: https://www.health.qld.gov.au/clinical-practice/guidelines-procedures/patient-safety/end-of-life/guidelines along with further information about the documents and implementation strategy of Queensland Health plus their contact details. The document has undergone minor revisions since the study was conducted). In 2013, acute care providers were charged with providing local education and audits to support implementation of the pathway. However, acute ward hospital staff reported that, from their perspective, the CgDp had 'appeared' on the wards with limited formal training provision. Efforts to address this need provided the opportunity for this study to capture 'real world' acute care clinician challenges as they integrated the CgDp into acute practice settings. Moreover, it offered an opportunity to systematically identify strategies to normalise EOL care excellence in a typical acute care setting.

Participants

Purposive sampling [20] was used to ensure recruitment of a range of perspectives within professional stakeholders, including the nursing, medical and allied health professionals and the palliative care team. Staff were identified through discussion with nursing, medical and allied health staff leaders and participants were recruited in the following ways. For allied health staff, the Directors of each professional group were emailed and asked for the details of the clinician working in the study ward. Seven clinicians were identified and contacted by the study team via email and all agreed to participate in the study. For the medical staff, the researchers presented an overview of the study at their team meeting (*n* = 17) and 8 agreed to participate. For nursing staff, because of shift work, the research team attended two nursing handovers to present an overview of the study and placed posters in the tea room. It is not known how many nursing staff viewed the poster or missed the handover meeting. For palliative care staff consulting to the study ward, we directly contacted, via email and follow up phone call, the consultant, advanced trainee and clinical nurse consultant and all agreed to participate.

Data generation

Qualitative, semi-structured interviews, individual or group, depending on participant availability, were conducted. The interviews, conducted from June to August 2015, explored perceptions, views and experiences of caring for dying patients and how the CgDp was used. Interviews were conducted by the authors who did not work in the study (ward) setting. The interviews occurred face to face in private rooms and were planned so that there was no conflict of interest or perceived hierarchy between interviewer and interviewee. All interviews were audio recorded, transcribed verbatim and rechecked for accuracy. Data collection continued until the research team agreed that theoretical saturation was reached; that is, additional data was not anticipated to produce new perspectives or insights [20].

Data analysis

Data were analysed using a five phase framework method: 1) familiarisation, 2) identifying a thematic framework, 3) indexing, 4) charting and mapping and 5) interpretation [16]. Research team members who conducted the interviews (CN, LG, BS, JM), and led on the analysis (SY, AT) familiarised themselves with raw data and discussed their impressions of the dataset. The NPT constructs provided the a priori thematic framework (See Table 1). Next, the transcripts were divided amongst members of the research team (CN, LG, JM, BS and BH), and each transcript was independently coded or indexed, using the framework, by two researchers who then discussed the coding in pairs and to negotiate agreement. Once the transcripts were coded and the data were charted and mapped in Excel®, themes were agreed upon. This coding and theming was independently reviewed and confirmed by AT and SY. The key themes were presented to the participants, who verified these themes, as part of two usual ward meetings. Patterns and associations between themes were interpreted and used to develop a mid-range theory model to inform further implementation strategies.

Results

Twenty-eight professionals were interviewed, in 18 individual and two group interviews, including allied health (7) (occupational therapist, pharmacists, physiotherapist, psychologist, speech pathologist), nursing (10), medical (8) and palliative care (medical, 2; nursing, 1). The average time for the interviews was 36 min (range: 18–55 min). The results are presented in two parts: 1) based on the NPT constructs, the key barriers and enablers identified (Table 2) 2) implementation and learning model, including accompanying learning strategies (Table 3). A mid-range programme theory, based on these findings, to inform strategies for augmenting EOL care excellence in acute care settings is developed from analysis of the findings (See Fig. 1).

Table 2 Key barriers and enablers

Normalisation Process Theory Construct	Key enablers	Key barriers
Coherence (what is the work)	• CgDp signals a shift to a different type of care • CgDp valued by staff as it supports systematic approach to end of life care • CgDp legitimises caring for the dying in acute setting	• The need for CgDp suggestive of a failure in acute care provision • Lack of education and training in principles of palliative care and care of the dying • Professionals conceptualise CgDp as 'everything' or 'nothing' because challenged by uncertainty posed when variances or individualised care was required
Cognitive participation (who does the work)	• CgDp empowers nursing staff to discuss EOL care with medical staff • Guidance available from palliative care team • Clear lines of responsibilities e.g. medical team lead decision making • Medical profession willing to lead implementation of CgDp intervention • Recognition that effective patient and family communication required	• Lack of genuine multidisciplinary team working • CgDp being enacted without an interprofessional approach • Lack of understanding of roles related to CgDp • Allocation of roles and responsibilities tend to mirror acute practice roles (not recognising that a different approach is required e.g. MDT) • Usual expert guidance structures challenged because EOL care not usual part of practice
Collective action (how does the work get done)	• Familiar with CgDp documentation • Effective collaboration between nursing and medical staff • Established relationships with patients • Nursing staff creating environment conducive to EOL care • Palliative care team provides decision making support e.g. diagnosing dying; symptom management advice • Continuity of care within speciality considered to be important e.g. home-ward • Mentoring and learning occurring through practice	• Challenging to integrate effective EOL care in the context of acute setting (e.g. organisational pressures for discharge) • EOL care provision infrequent activity • Allied health tendency to disengage in and/or excluded from EOL care • Senior medical officers not fully engaged in CgDp intervention e.g. delegate to juniors • Absence of allied health engagement • Documentation considered burdensome and not aligned to technology e.g. electronic medical records • Lack of longitudinal palliative care planning resulting in reactive response to dying patients • Rostering and staffing arrangement hamper allied health and palliative care not able to fully integrate and support
Reflexive monitoring (how is the work understood and changed)	• Desire to integrate/improve EOL decision making processes • Recognition that structured debriefing sessions are required improve quality of CgDp care	• Systematic audit and feedback processes required to inform and improve outcomes • Few opportunities for meaningful clinical supervision to provide emotional support • Staff find it challenging to find ways to meaningfully appraise the effectiveness of CgDp practices and outcomes

Coherence – Making sense of the CgDp

Participants agreed the CgDp's purpose made sense as a support for effective EOL care, yet they experienced tensions when attempting to integrate EOL practice into their daily work. For example, participants indicated that using the CgDp provided evidence to legitimise EOL care provision in acute settings and increased confidence to take action. This was described in the following extract by a nurse who explained:

> … That [the pathway] gives us a bit more reassurance that we can do less [acute care] and focus more on comfort and quality… They just want to cover themselves legally I think. (Nurse-3).

Hence it appeared that the pathway 'gives permission' to shift the focus of care from a more traditional biomedical model to a more holistic approach. Despite this permission, based on their understanding of their role in acute care, other people felt that EOL care lacked alignment with this role:

> I don't want to use them [CgDp]…we are an acute ward…our patients are meant to recover… (Nurse-5).

In this extract, the nurse suggests that using the CgDp is somewhat at odds with her role identity which defines success as cure.

The CgDp did not account for the uncertainties and complexities participants experienced when engaging in EOL care. Participants found recognising dying a particularly challenging aspect. Reasons were multifactorial including a lack of experience and/or guidance; not understanding palliative care principles; experiencing diagnostic uncertainty and avoiding EOL care decision making and/or worrying the wrong decision has been made; wanting to exhaust all treatment options before commencing CgDP and finding the process personally uncomfortable. This is captured in the next extract by an allied health professional:

> I didn't pick up the signs of that last patient that I had that was actually passing away. Ahh! They weren't on a

Table 3 Proposed learning strategies to embed EOL care excellence

Normalisation Process Theory Construct	Proposed learning strategies	Examples
Coherence (what is the work)	• Support development of palliative care knowledge and skills • Facilitate expert guidance for staff in situations of uncertainty e.g. feedback from palliative care on performance	• Regular education programs supporting the development of all acute care staff (including rotational and locum) • Interprofessional team learning, in collaboration with palliative care team where real-life scenarios are explored
Cognitive participation (who does the work)	• Foster an interprofessional approach to EOL decision making and care provision through learning activities • Define duties and responsibilities of health care staff • Promote interprofessional working and learning • Palliative care to provide guidance on interprofessional approaches to EOL care	• Develop and implement interprofessional learning activities to support EOL practices including practice-based or simulation activities
Collective action (how does the work get done)	• Review work structures, rostering and processes to support prioritisation of EOL care • Educate staff on the long trajectory required for effective EOL care • Create learning programs that challenge assumptions about roles and accepted ways of working • Augment opportunities for co-working with palliative care team • Simulated interprofessional learning experiences	• Prioritise dying patients on ward rounds • Integrate EOL practices into outpatient setting e.g. have a checklist; review outpatient list who had multiple admission • Interprofessional case-based discussions – range of contexts e.g. outpatients; acute setting
Reflexive monitoring (how is the work understood and changed)	• Support development of self-regulation on individual practices • Enhance opportunities for audit and feedback • Create opportunities for staff to debrief as a team	• Schedule regular 'after death' care reviews for multidisciplinary team with guidance from palliative care team

care of the dying pathway, so I still treated them actively, which I felt at the time was appropriate. On reflection… maybe I didn't add any benefit to it. I don't think I made it any worse, at least I hope I didn't. (Allied Health-2).

While the CgDp increased awareness of the need for EOL care in acute settings, this was perceived as a challenge rather than empowerment. The CgDp as an artefact introduced into the setting created disruption in routines and consequently staff had to consider the possibility of dying and decide if this might be the case but they found it challenging to do make such a decision. This is reflected in the next extract when two nurses within a focus group outline the difficulty, experienced by doctors, in deciding when a patient is at the point to need transfer to the CgDp:

Nurse-1: It's like they're [doctors] are scared of it.

Nurse-2: …as doctors they're taught to save lives and then when they've got to do this thing [CgDp] where they're basically withdrawing treatment to let somebody die, they worry that they are doing the wrong thing. I think they need to be told that it's okay to do this. This is a good thing for them. (Group interview 1-nursing).

Participants described uncertainty with the duality of aiming to 'reverse the reversible' while holding the

possibility of dying and appropriate CgDp care alongside this. In contrast, participants felt much more comfortable when they could focus solely on one form of practice e.g. active treatment or EOL care:

So to give you an idea, we have had elderly patients who come in with bad pneumonia and are possibly dying, not responding to treatment, and the question is do you continue with full measures, such as antibiotics, fluids et cetera or do you just focus on comfort care? (Medical officer-10).

Participants agreed that the CgDp provided guidance on priorities when caring for dying patients. This was reassuring to staff, especially to novice practitioners:

So, it's more like a guideline. So, it's more of a checklist for everyone making sure that we don't miss things you know. So, it's a cross multidisciplinary thing. (Medical officer-5).

Overall, participants understanding of the purpose of the CgDp in acute care, was that it was to systematise EOL care. However, the key challenges to EOL care excellence were uncertainty when diagnosing dying, appropriately individualising patient care, and difficulties experienced integrating EOL care practices with acute care practices. These findings are presented in Table 2.

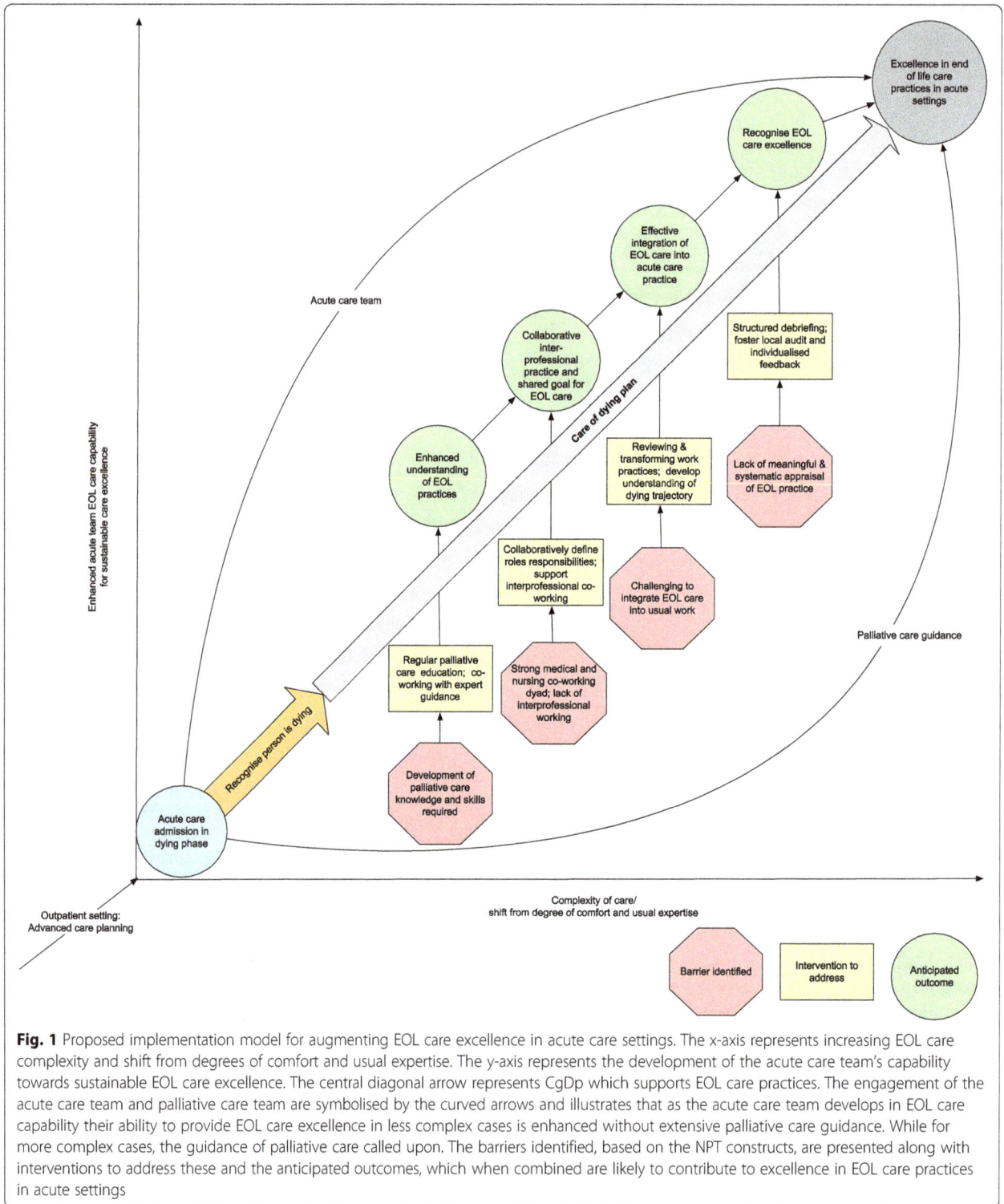

Fig. 1 Proposed implementation model for augmenting EOL care excellence in acute care settings. The x-axis represents increasing EOL care complexity and shift from degrees of comfort and usual expertise. The y-axis represents the development of the acute care team's capability towards sustainable EOL care excellence. The central diagonal arrow represents CgDp which supports EOL care practices. The engagement of the acute care team and palliative care team are symbolised by the curved arrows and illustrates that as the acute care team develops in EOL care capability their ability to provide EOL care excellence in less complex cases is enhanced without extensive palliative care guidance. While for more complex cases, the guidance of palliative care called upon. The barriers identified, based on the NPT constructs, are presented along with interventions to address these and the anticipated outcomes, which when combined are likely to contribute to excellence in EOL care practices in acute settings

Cognitive participation – Getting involved in CgDp

Contrary to the CgDp goal, of providing uniformly good, albeit individualised, care to dying patients, using the guidelines did not disrupt parallel working between professions to achieve fully the integrated multidisciplinary and interprofessional working required. Working in parallel, profession-specific lines meant that some professional groups lacked certainty regarding the legitimacy of their engagement. For example, the decision to commence the CgDp was consultant (senior physician) led, with prompting from nursing staff but little to no engagement from allied health practitioners (AHP). The following extract outlines how AHPs perceived they were potentially excluded from these processes:

> I don't know if I should be doing it [CgDp]. I know there's an allied health section, but I was never really told to or asked to write in the forms, so I never have. (Allied Health-7).

However, using the CgDp promoted certain staff to reflect on and change their existing ways of working. Some nursing staff felt empowered to prompt the medical team to make decisions about EOL care and played a role in reassuring medical staff about their EOL care decision. However, they were often frustrated when waiting for the CgDp paperwork to be completed by medical staff as illustrated in the following extract:

> Interviewee 3: The doctors not filling stuff out.

> Interviewee 4: Sometimes it could take 24 h for a doctor to do it.

> (Group interview 1-nursing)

Nursing staff were concerned this delayed multiprofessional provision of holistic EOL care.

Moreover, some senior nursing staff noted that because patients infrequently died on the ward, they needed to reorient themselves to the practices associated with the CgDp:

> Yes I'm probably a bit shaky on it for myself because I haven't actually used it for quite a long time. (Nurse-3).

This meant usual patterns of co-working e.g. seeking guidance from more senior staff differed for practices associated with the CgDp from usual acute care practices.

The perceptions of medical staff, recognising their need for decision-making reassurance sometimes sought guidance from the palliative care team, usually via telephone consults. Despite this, aspects of EOL care, including completing the CgDp paperwork, were delegated by senior medical staff to their juniors. Thus, some consultants (senior physician) avoided direct engagement with practical complexities required for effective enactment of the CgDp, and did not always appear to have insight into these, as described by a consultant (senior physician):

> I know about it [CgDp] but I don't know ...the details... probably because I'm confident that I know when a patient is near reaching their end stage I don't

need to look for any guidelines to help me. (Medical officer-6).

Additional care strategies were sometimes triggered and adopted instead of the CgDp when complexities became explicit, such as a so-called, 'trial of life' where full treatments were applied for 24 to 48 h to determine if patients might improve. This is described by a consultant below:

> If there's anything that you felt like, oh look, you know, he's not - we'll give him a trial of 24 to 48 h, for example, and there's still no progression and still no improvement and having a chat with the family and things you know say, look if that's not improving I think it's for comfort measures and then that's the time that we'll be looking at the realm of like the Care of the Dying Pathway. (Medical Officer-5).

This suggests an 'either or' conceptualisation of active disease treatment versus palliation remained suggesting that further opportunities for learning about palliative care principles are necessary for effective enactment. In particular, education should include individualised decision-making and the appropriateness of multifaceted approaches when situations are uncertain i.e. using CgDp alongside interventional treatments.

Lastly, the strength of medical and nursing dyad created a barrier to AHP engagement and decision making when the CgDp commenced. All AH participants indicated that they were willing and able to contribute to EOL care. Moreover, they noted that the CgDp specifies the AHP contributions (as above), however, they expressed concern that medical and nursing teams did not understand how they might contribute to EOL care:

> Just someone say, we [nursing and medical staff] want you to do it, because at the moment no one is saying that we need to do it or want us to do it, so we're not going to do something that is going to probably take up more time if we've never been asked to do it...if we sat down and it was said that – a ward says we want everyone to be involved in this, in using this pathway [CgDp], so we work together, then for sure, I wouldn't mind. I'd be more than happy to be involved. (Allied Health-1).

Collective action – Implementing CgDp

Effectively enacting the CgDp in a busy acute setting was challenging and barriers to effective EOL care provision included: 1) an over reactive response to EOL care rather than proactive or long-term i.e. advance care planning and 2) privileging of acute care practices and work. Combined, these two factors created a sense of being overwhelmed faced with the work associated with attending to dying patients' needs as exemplified in the following extract by a medical officer:

> But our days are busy, so I figure there'd almost be a bit of a delay sometimes, because for instance we did one ward round this morning, we finished at 11:00. Then the senior doctors had to go to the radiology meeting until about 12:00. Then comes the next consultant for the next ward round. So, at what point do you have that time to throw that paperwork [CgDp] together as well. It can be quite difficult. (Medical officer 9).

The reactive response, as opposed to proactive (i.e. advance care planning), and lack of prioritisation related to perceptions that CgDp required a complex cascade of actions, many of which fell outside of participants' comfort zone e.g. family meetings, completion of paperwork. This response could also be attributed to complex and busy work practices, staff resourcing and lack of palliative care training. For example, the medical team needing to attend to patients on other wards; allied health work scheduling meant they were not ward-based and therefore not fully integrated into ward practices. Thus, missed opportunities, because some allied health staff were reactively rather than collaboratively invited to participate, existed for appropriate skill mix and building relationship with patients and family members:

> ...it depends on how much rapport you've built with the family I think. I've been thrown in a few where there's such - on the ward with the nursing staff and the doctors it's, he or she is going to pass away, quick, get in there, and the moment you get in there the family is like, who are you. (Allied health-5).

Several system-level issues created barriers to EOL care including: 1) organisational pressure for patient discharges; 2) lack of opportunity for meaningful palliative care team guidance and 3) paper-based CgDp guidelines in the context of electronic medical records. Each of these barriers are explored below. Firstly, the organisational pressures being experienced are described here:

> There is always someone from the top calling you to discharge the patients...and there is not time to go through [the dying conversation] when they are not dying...for example, with chronic obstructive airways disease exacerbation, come in, get steroids and antibiotics, go home... there is no time to talk about dying then. When they come back with acute illness and are dying... all of a sudden someone will ask,

where is their resuscitation plan...there's no plan so you press the panic button ...it's a big mess. (Medical officer-2).

Secondly, participants appreciated palliative care guidance, however, obtaining this guidance was a challenging endeavour due to both teams' busy workloads. Thus, often resorting to telephone conversations rather than face to face collaborations. Palliative care staff were also uncertain if their advice was always sought when needed:

> I think some consultants must have their own views on how the care should be given for a dying patient and I guess they must think that they know. You can't be an expert in every area and I think it's important enough not to think that you could do everything and then blind yourself to the mistakes that you're making. (Palliative care medical officer-4).

Thus, in terms of collective action, some palliative care team members perceived that their contributions were not being acted on.

Thirdly, a further crucial contextual factor was that the hospital uses electronic medical records and the CgDp was paper based. This meant that staff who defaulted to the electronic medical records were not always aware of the decision to commence the CgDp or its progress. Moreover, the CgDp was a large document, which combined with infrequent use became perceived as challenging to complete. These views contrasted with palliative care staff who indicated that despite its size, with practice, the document was relatively easy to engage with.

Reflexive monitoring –embedding and improving CgDp
Embedding EOL care in acute settings requires staff reflection on the implementation of the CgDp and where necessary amending of practices to ensure best outcomes. Despite having the CgDp as a practice guide, the participants indicated further improvements in EOL care were required. Barriers to effective staff reflection and improvement were identified and these included firstly, a lack of structured and meaningful team debriefing to improve EOL care. Secondly, a lack of knowledge and skills to meaningfully appraise EOL care and its outcomes. Finally, a lack of systematic audit and feedback processes to inform and improve EOL care outcomes.

While some staff indicated that they informally debrief after a patient death with peers, there was an absence of interprofessional and structured debriefing. Attempts at changing EOL practices seemed to be largely speculative and participants were not able to describe ways that they were changing or had changed their EOL practices as a team. This meant that important ways to improve EOL care were left unresolved:

I guess the one thing we don't do more of, or I don't do more of, is to actually talk about dying much earlier on. So, we don't have a lot of that. So that discussion sort of comes about in context of Care of the Dying Pathway, which may not be ideal. I'm not sure if it is the right thing to be discussing these things early on. I mean, there's some evidence to say that that's what patients want to know and we probably should do that. But we haven't been, mainly because we don't have a structure for that; who does it and when, do you do it in hospital or clinic? (Medical officer-10).

In these ways, this medical officer recognises the reactive responsive EOL care whilst acknowledging that integrative of EOL care planning had not been addressed.

A key factor hampering staff ability to meaningfully reflect on and improve EOL care was a lack of expertise and experience in palliative care. This meant it was challenging to recognise the features and enact EOL care excellence as evidenced by the next extract:

But we don't know what to compare it [EOL care] to. I don't know if anybody else has worked in a hospice or palliative care where would it be just - could it be not as busy but it could be a lot of noise and trolleys and things trundling up and down and bells going off you know. (Nurse-5).

Since comprehensive audit and feedback processes to inform and improve outcomes related to effective implementation of CgDp were absent, the effectiveness of EOL care was not apparent to participants. As such they were not receiving individualised feedback on the quality of their care nor were they aware of the quality standards to be achieved. Many participants noted that quality EOL care is not being wholly addressed through audit processes:

I mean, we do have deaths in hospital but the kind of deaths we have on our ward are ones that are fairly catastrophic, so where people have had MET calls and had cardiac arrests and gone to ICU [intensive care unit] and then died in ICU. They are few and far between and we review them in our morbidity and mortality meetings and almost always there is nothing that could have prevented that outcome that we can pick up and it's just the natural course of the illness. Then occasionally we have the patients who have come in, not improved with treatment and have just deteriorated and in those situations they are often

patients that we know have severe illness and for them that would seem very appropriate. In fact, you could even argue not starting Care of the Dying Pathway was probably inappropriate and we're just continuing their agony and misery. (Medical officer-10).

Development of a theoretical model for education and implementation

Figure 1, presents a proposed implementation model for augmenting EOL care excellence in acute care settings. The model, presents the key barriers to effectively embedding EOL care in acute settings. In response to these barriers, learning and implementations strategies have been identified which are likely to contribute to EOL care excellence and to sustain these practices [21, 22]. Recognising the complexity of EOL practice, guidance and support from palliative care is recommended [23]. However, as the acute teams' EOL capability is augmented and the key learning outcomes are achieved, guidance is likely to be limited to the most complex cases. This model provides lessons for implementation for acute care settings who are implementing and/or revising their EOL care practices. Additionally, this model presents an EOL learning curriculum for HCP working in acute setting using a range of practice-based pedagogic strategies.

Discussion

This study sought to generate a conceptual model of the realities of embedding an end-of-life-care tool into an Australian acute hospital. Our research team were cognisant of the challenges this presented from international experience. Using the normalisation process theory provided an opportunity to study mechanisms of 'real world' acute care clinician challenges as they integrated the CgDp into acute practice settings and consider if and how these led to desired improvements in end-of-life care. NPT constructs informed the analysis of empirical data collected during the implementation period. NPT was chosen for its resonance with the desired outcomes: behaviour change needs to be normalised to become routine practice. The tensions identified with this ideal and the realities of practice allowed us to generate a model to guide further implementation while drawing attention to barriers and facilitators of success.

The principal findings are that while staff described the CgDp as being intrinsically coherent its use was not in keeping with what they considered to be their primary focus of work, that is, getting patients to recovery. Participants found it challenging to hold the tension created by uncertainty of whether a patient might recover or not in mind, preferring to focus solely on so called 'active management' which they defined as disease focused treatment. The findings confirm other studies for example in intensive care [24] and other areas of the UK health service [10], including hospital doctors [25] and Italian general medicine settings [26]. Additionally, some participants had insight into their difficulties in recognising a dying patient (which is not surprising given the challenges all clinicians experience accurately predicting prognosis [27]). Taken together these factors meant the CgDp would be used late, if at all, as it was only of use once agreement was reached that a person was dying. However, if this point was reached the CgDp was praised for offering a more systematic (and in fact, active) approach to care for the dying patient.

There was evidence of the tool being used as a prompt for collaborative working and in some cases junior medical and nursing staff reported being empowered to raise concerns that a patient might be dying with senior medical staff. In turn, however, senior staff would seek advice and reassurance from the palliative care team and sometimes redelegated the completion and hands-on application of the tool back to junior staff. An unintended consequence of the implementation was that closer working between nursing and medical staff left AHPs to feel excluded and their contributions to EOL care unrecognised. This finding demonstrates a need to further foster effective interprofessional collaboration [28].

Perceptions of extensive paperwork and an expansion of roles, including increased activity outwith professionals' comfort zones, acted as barriers to prospective planning for end of life care and use of the tool was often delayed or incomplete for these reasons. Whilst everyone could contribute, it was possible to opt out from doing so by choosing to focus on other activities and respond to different pressures when prioritising workload. System factors also prevented close working relationships with the palliative care team, and the tool was not integrated into the electronic notes system meaning its use could easily be overlooked. These challenges, the importance of integration of palliative and medical care team working and lack of integration of care of the dying plans with electronic notes, are in keeping with the findings of McConnell et al. [10] and Raijmakers et al. [29], respectively. Thus, for effective implementation and normalisation of EOL care excellence to be achieved, these organisational and systems barriers need to be addressed.

Crucial to the implementation success was the potential for staff to learn from their experiences. Time, opportunities, and lack of skilled facilitation for reflection and case review meant this was not capitalised upon. These experiences need to move beyond provision of education and training, which can be challenging for

practitioners to attend [26], towards generating embedded real time practice-based learning experiences [30].

In summary, implementation occurred but with risks such as the lack of recognition of dying leading to unmet needs, and staff experiences leading to unintended learning. As identified in the UK, there is a risk of the tool taking on a life of its own without professionals learning the foundational principles of good palliative care alongside treating potentially reversible conditions.

Strengths and limitations

This study investigated the real-time perceptions and experiences of interprofessional team members working in an acute medical ward concerning embedding of high quality palliative care. Use of NPT as an analytic framework enabled an understanding of how care of the dying practices were or were not becoming normalized within an acute setting, identification of barriers and enablers to provisions of care excellence and recommendations for learning strategies to support EOL care excellence (see implications section and Table 3). However, the study took place in a single acute care setting within a tertiary hospital which limits the broader applicability of its findings. Potential transferability is enhanced by rich descriptions, using purposive sampling and the findings resonance with existing literature from other settings [20, 31]. The study relied on individual accounts of EOL care practices and engagement with CgDp rather than observations. To increase the study's dependability [31], data were collected until saturation, no new themes, and data were analysed iteratively by an interprofessional team. Further strategies to enhance study credibility included seeking feedback from participants on our data analysis. There would have been value in also having the middle range programme theory model confirmed by further professional validation. This was not practical; however, the model has been informed by NPT and generated through extensive, reflexive discussions within the research team. Finally, to quantify outcomes, there may have been value in conducting a chart audit to determine when the CgDp had been used, and with what effects, however, our goal in the present study was to primarily explore the process of implementation.

Implications for practice and further research

This study provides important empirical evidence from healthcare practitioners working in acute care settings on their experiences of providing EOL care. It is an example of patient focussed theoretically informed medical education research that extends into clinical practice [32]. The findings and conceptual model, could inform and optimise interventions to support practitioners' effective normalisation of EOL care excellence in acute care settings. EOL care excellence requires meaningful collaboration with and specialist support from the palliative care team combined with effective interprofessional co-working [33]. As the acute care team's coherence, collective action, cognitive participation and reflective monitoring are enhanced, the reliance on specialist palliative care may be limited to complex cases.

To achieve these goals in practice, we propose the following learning strategies informed by the NPT constructs and our findings (See Table 3 and Fig. 1). To address coherence, acute care staff need support to develop their palliative care knowledge and skills to recognise dying and the point at which to initiate the pathway whilst developing the ability to hold two approaches to care at the same time during transition [21]. This must also relate to understanding of the importance of integrating care practices and promoting the CgDp as a positive aspect of care rather than a failing (See Fig. 1). Expert and accessible guidance (See Fig. 1) e.g. from palliative care specialist or champions is required to assist acute care staff to navigate such situations of clinical uncertainty e.g. case-based interprofessional and interdisciplinary team learning sessions.

Learning strategies to increase cognitive participation might include harnessing genuine interprofessional working (See Fig. 1) to promote shared understanding of each other's roles (see Table 2) [34]. Furthermore, learning strategies might include creating meaningful interprofessional learning experiences where collaboratively the team work through genuine cases to make decisions on EOL care and to identify team members' roles and responsibilities (See Fig. 1); or learning sessions with palliative care team members who provide guidance on collaborative approaches EOL care (See Table 3).

To address collective action, consideration needs to be given to reviewing work structures, rostering and processes to support the prioritisation of EOL care e.g. prioritising dying patients on ward rounds; ward-based AHPs (See Table 3 and Fig. 1) [22]. In this regard rearranging key documents and pathways within the hospital care processes can help facilitate delivering high quality end of life care. By such so called "textual regulation" [35], the institution can demonstrate that it values end of life care and support workers. Moreover, creation of learning programs challenging assumptions about work practices facilitated by the palliative care team to role model effective interprofessional co-working (See Fig. 1) may further help [21]. A key system factor to support change would be integration of the CgDP into the routine electronic records.

Finally, strategies (also see Table 2) likely to augment acute care staff's ability to reflexively monitor EOL care and recognise EOL care excellence include: 1) local quality improvement processes to assist staff understanding of EOL care and provide local solutions to specific barriers and gaps; 2) foster feedback processes [21, 36] to increase practitioners' ability to self-evaluate EOL care performance and 3) create opportunities for staff to debrief as a team e.g. 'after death' care reviews with support from the palliative care team (See Fig. 1).

Conclusions

Our findings emphasise the importance of in-depth examination of implementation processes and offers strategies for normalising EOL care excellence in acute care setting using guidelines. Further exploration into these experiences will provide insights to how these tensions might be reconciled and/or held to ensure holistic EOL in acute care settings. Finally, research to test and refine our programme theory model is required.

Abbreviations

AHP: Allied health practitioners; CgDp: Clinical Guidelines for Dying Patients; EOL: End of life; LCP: Liverpool Care of the Dying Pathway; NPT: Normalisation Process Theory; UK: United Kingdom

Acknowledgements

The authors would like to thank the study participants and Adele Blissett for her administration support.

Funding

This research was funded by the Gold Cold Hospital Foundation. The views expressed are those of the authors.

Authors' contributions

CN and LG conceived the initial study design and developed the research questions. CN, LG, JM and BS were responsible for data collection. CN, LG, BS, BH and JM contributed to the data analysis. SY and AT contributed to refining the research questions and substantially contributed to the study design, and data analysis and drafting first full draft of the manuscript with CN. All authors commented on draft manuscripts and approved the final manuscript.

Competing interests

The authors declare that they have no competing interests.

Author details

[1]Medical Education Unit, Gold Coast Health, Level 2 PED Building, 1 Hospital Boulevard, Southport, QLD 4215, Australia. [2]School of Medicine, Griffith University, Griffith, QLD, Australia. [3]School of Pharmacy, University of Queensland, Brisbane, QLD, Australia. [4]School of Nursing and Midwifery and

Menzies Health Institute Queensland, Griffith University, Griffith, Queensland, Australia. [5]Gold Coast Health, Griffith, QLD, Australia. [6]Myton Hospices, Coventry, UK. [7]Central and North West London NHS Foundation Trust, London, UK. [8]Marie Curie Research Department, University College London, London, UK.

References

1. Virdun C, et al. Dying in the hospital setting: a systematic review of quantitative studies identifying the elements of end-of-life care that patients and their families rank as being most important. Palliat Med. 2015; 29(9):774–96.

2. Gomes B, Higginson IJ. Where people die (1974—2030): past trends, future projections and implications for care. Palliat Med. 2008;22(1):33–41.

3. Broad JB, et al. Where do people die? An international comparison of the percentage of deaths occurring in hospital and residential aged care settings in 45 populations, using published and available statistics. Int J Public Health. 2013;58(2):257–67.

4. Swerissen, H. and S. Duckett, Dying Well, G. Institute, Editor. 2014, Grattan Institute: Carlton, Victoria p 37.

5. Costantini M, Alquati S, Di Leo S. End-of-life care: pathways and evidence. Curr Opin Support Palliat Care. 2014;8(4):399–404.

6. Australian Commission on Safety and Quality in Health Care, National Consensus Statement: essential elements for safe and high-quality end-of-life care in acute hospitals. 2015, Australian Commission on Safety and Quality in Health Care: Sydney, NSW, Australia.

7. Robinson J, Gott M, Ingleton C. Patient and family experiences of palliative care in hospital: what do we know? An integrative review. Palliat Med. 2014; 28(1):18–33.

8. Department of Health, More care less pathway: a review of the Liverpool Care Pathway. 2013, Crown Copyright.

9. Leadership Alliance for the Care of Dying People. One chance to get it right: improving people's experience of care in the last few days and hours of life. London: Leadership Alliance for the Care of Dying People; 2014. https://assets.publishing.service.gov.uk/government/uploads/system/uploads/attachment_data/file/323188/One_chance_to_get_it_right.pdf

10. McConnell T, et al. Factors affecting the successful implementation and sustainability of the Liverpool care pathway for dying patients: a realist evaluation. BMJ Support Palliat Care. 2014;

11. McConnell T, et al. Systematic realist review of key factors affecting the successful implementation and sustainability of the Liverpool care pathway for the dying patient. Worldviews Evid-Based Nurs. 2013;10(4):218–37.

12. Palliative Care Australia, Standards for Providing Quality Palliative Care for all Australians. 2005, Palliative Care Australia: Deakin West, ACT.

13. Crotty M. The foundations of social research. London: SAGE Publications Ltd.; 1998.

14. May C, Finch T. Implementing, embedding, and integrating practices: an outline of normalization process theory. Sociology. 2009;43(3):535–54.

15. May C, et al. Understanding the implementation of complex interventions in health care: the normalization process model. BMC Health Serv Res. 2007; 7(1):148.

16. Ritchie, J. and L. Spencer, Qualitative data analysis for applied policy research, in Analyzing Qualitative Data, A. Bryman and R. Burgess, editors. 1994, RoutledgeFalmer: London.

17. Murray E, et al. Normalisation process theory: a framework for developing, evaluating and implementing complex interventions. BMC Med. 2010; 8(1):1–11.

18. Davidoff F, Dixon-Woods M, Leviton L, Michie S. Demystifying theory and its use in improvement. BMJ Qual Saf. 2015;24:228–38. https://doi.org/10.1136/bmjqs-2014-003627.

19. Queensland Health. Queensland Health clinical guidelines. 2018 [cited 2018 26/6/18]; Available from: https://www.health.qld.gov.au/clinical-practice/guidelines-procedures/patient-safety/end-of-life/guidelines

20. Creswell JW. Qualitative inquiry and research design: choosing among five approaches. London: SAGE Publications Ltd.; 2013.

21. Johnson MJ, May CR. Promoting professional behaviour change in healthcare: what interventions work, and why? A theory-led overview of systematic reviews. BMJ Open. 2015;5(9):1–13.

22. Cummings A, et al. Implementing communication and decision-making interventions directed at goals of care: a theory-led scoping review. BMJ Open. 2017;7(10):1–17.

23. Billett S, Choy S. Learning through work: emerging perspectives and new challenges. J Work Learn. 2013;25(4):264–76.

24. Sleeman KE, et al. 'It doesn't do the care for you': a qualitative study of health care professionals' perceptions of the benefits and harms of integrated care pathways for end of life care. BMJ Open. 2015;5(9):1–7.

25. Twigger S, Yardley SJ. Hospital doctors' understanding of use and withdrawal of the Liverpool care pathway: a qualitative study of practice-based experiences during times of change. Palliat Med. 2017;31(9):833–41.

26. Di Leo S, et al. 'Less ticking the boxes, more providing support': a qualitative study on health professionals' concerns towards the Liverpool Care of the Dying Pathway. Palliat Med. 2015;29(6):529–37.

27. White N, et al. How accurate is the 'surprise question' at identifying patients at the end of life? A systematic review and meta-analysis. BMC Med. 2017; 15(1):139.

28. Edwards A, Daniels H, Gallagher T, Leadbetter J, Warmington P. Improving inter-professional collaborations: Multi-agency working for children's wellbeing. Oxon: Routledge; 2009.

29. Raijmakers N, et al. Barriers and facilitators to implementation of the Liverpool care pathway in the Netherlands: a qualitative study. BMJ Support Palliat Care. 2015;5(3):259–65.

30. Billett S. Learning through work: workplace affordances and individual engagement. J Work Learn. 2001;13(5/6):209–14.

31. Lincoln, Y. and E. Guba, Naturalistic Inquiry. 1985, Newbury Park, CA: Sage Publications.

32. Teodorczuk A, et al. Medical education research should extend further into clinical practice. Med Educ. 2017;51(11):1098–100.

33. Kilbertus FMDM, Ajjawi RP, Archibald DBP. "You're Not Trying to Save Somebody From Death": Learning as "Becoming" in Palliative Care. Acad Med. 2018;93(6):929–36.

34. Billett S. Securing intersubjectivity through interprofessional workplace learning experiences. J Interprofessional Care. 2014;28(3):206–11.

35. Smith D. Institutional ethnography as practice. Oxford: Rowan and Littlefield; 2006.

36. Boud, D. and E. Molloy, Feedback in Higher and Professional Education: Understanding it and doing it well. 2013, New York: Routledge.

37. May C, et al. Development of a theory of implementation and integration: normalization process theory. Implement Sci. 2009;4(1):29.

2

Towards a public health approach for palliative care: an action-research study focused on engaging a local community and educating teenagers

Sandra Martins Pereira[1,2,3]* [iD], Joana Araújo[1,2,3] and Pablo Hernández-Marrero[1,2,3]

Abstract

Background: Education sessions about palliative care among teenagers are uncommon in developed countries. However, very little is known either about the impact of this type of intervention or about how this age-group perceives its impact. The purpose of this study was therefore to (i) implement an education program about palliative care among teenagers and (ii) to investigate the impact of the program on the participants.

Methods: An action-research study was conducted at a local community parish in Portugal in November 2015. An education programme was purposively built about palliative care, using active educational strategies adapted for teenagers. Quantitative and qualitative techniques and instruments were used for data collection: questionnaire; reflective diaries; interviews and written testimony. The program had three stages: preparation; intervention; and evaluation. Qualitative data were analysed using thematic content analysis; quantitative data were analysed descriptively.

Results: 69 people (47 teenagers) participated in the education program. Findings show that the education program contributed to creating awareness about palliative care. Both the teenagers and other participants assessed the education program positively. At the end of the program, teenagers had a constructive message about palliative care.

Conclusions: The education-intervention contributed to create awareness about palliative care among the participant teenagers, who ended the program with a positive message about palliative care. Based on our findings, the following policy implications can be drawn: (1) Further research is needed to evaluate the effect of education programs about palliative care among younger age groups (teenagers and children), particularly in relation to the changing of attitudes toward palliative care. (2) Education about palliative care should be promoted to local communities, involving all age groups, to foster involvement, participation and empowerment. (3) Compassionate communities should be promoted to enhance the health and wellbeing of all citizens at the end of their life.

Keywords: Public health education, Palliative care, Teenagers, Action research, Compassionate communities, Community-based intervention, Public health policy

* Correspondence: martinspereira.sandra@gmail.com; smpereira@porto.ucp.pt
[1]Instituto de Bioética, Universidade Católica Portuguesa, Rua Diogo Botelho, 1327 4169-005 Porto, Portugal
[2]UNESCO Chair in Bioethics Instituto de Bioética, Universidade Católica Portuguesa, Porto, Portugal
Full list of author information is available at the end of the article

Background

Healthcare education is paramount to ensure citizens' awareness, knowledge and empowerment on any issues related to health. It involves giving information and teaching individuals and communities about how to achieve better health [1–3].

The worldwide trend of ageing populations raises major challenges to health (e.g., increasing number of older people with several co-morbidities, chronic, progressive diseases, among others). Health promotion activities through education become therefore increasingly relevant. Health issues need to be addressed by using a holistic approach that fosters individuals and communities' empowerment to take action both for their health and for the development of inter-sectoral actions to build public policies capable to create and maintain sustainable healthcare systems [1–4]. In this context, palliative care, defined as 'an approach that improves the quality of life of patients and their families facing the problems associated with life-threatening illness, through the prevention and relief of suffering by means of early identification and treatment of other problems, physical, psychosocial and spiritual' [5], has progressively been recognized as an essential ethical responsibility of health systems worldwide [6–11].

Evidence shows that public awareness of the concept of palliative care remains insufficient [12–14], thus showing the need to further implement societal actions and education programs on this matter. This has been identified worldwide as one of the key pillars of a public health strategy for palliative care [15–17].

Health-promoting palliative care activities are aimed at implementing education and information programs, reorienting health education and services toward community partnerships [2, 3, 18]. This may be particularly helpful to develop more compassionate communities, defined as communities that understand that contributing to the care of those living with a life-threatening disease is an intrinsic part of the health and well-being responsibilities of all citizens [18, 20].

To be successful and effective, healthcare education strategies and programs, especially those focusing on sensitive issues like palliative and end-of-life care, should be participatory and involve the wider community [18–20]. Involving schools, workplaces, places of worship, the media or local businesses can help mobilize untapped sources of care and support as well as practical resources [20].

As the health impact of education lasts a lifetime [21–24], it is paramount that healthcare education programs begin during the early stages of human development. These programs should be culturally and educationally appropriate [25] and can foster the development of critical perspectives towards issues and problems with implications for human health [24].

Education activities about palliative care (e.g., short thematic sessions) among teenagers are uncommon practices in developed countries. Therefore, very little is known about how this age group perceives the impact of this type of interventions. Despite a few initiatives, there is limited research available on the process of implementing educational programs about palliative care specifically focused on teenagers. To our best knowledge, only two studies have been developed on this matter [25, 26]. These two pilot-studies aimed at developing and piloting an in-depth intervention on severe illness and palliative care in high schools, assessing students' interest in and knowledge of palliative care, the overall impact of this experience, and the usefulness of the intervention components and procedures in both teachers and students [25, 26]. The findings of these studies suggest that teenage high school students deemed the education program about palliative care to be a helpful and positive experience [25, 26].

Triggered by the abovementioned experiences, the objectives of our study were: (i) to implement an education program about palliative care among teenagers and (ii) to investigate the impact of the program on the participants.

Methods

An action-research study was conducted in a local community parish in the North of Portugal. A mixed-methods approach was used for data collection, combining both quantitative and qualitative techniques and instruments to achieve more comprehensiveness. The triangulation or synthesis of multiple sources of data is a core element of action-research as it is very important to ensure that all available data is used to build rigorous and cohesive conclusions [27, 28].

Action-research seeks to bring together action (the education-intervention program) and reflection (how to make this education-program effective and positive, and how to create knowledge about palliative care among teenagers), theory and practice, in participation with others (teenagers, parents, catechists – i.e., people responsible for the religious education activities at a parish, the community, the educator-researcher) in the pursuit of practical solutions to issues of pressing concern to people [29–31]. This methodological approach is of special relevance in palliative care and education [31–34], particularly in terms of community-based interventions aimed at improving change [34–37]. Following the action-research approach, the education program was tailored to the specific context of its implementation [38].

As a research methodology, action-research focuses on how people's situations can be improved and helps to empower people through the process of constructing and using their own knowledge [30, 39, 40]. Furthermore, action-research helps to transform organizations and/or communities into collaborative and self-reflective contexts, empowering subjects (researchers and participants) as part of the process [39, 40].

The education program and action-research assumed the form of the typical cycle or spiral of action-research [31, 34, 35, 40] and embraced three intertwined stages:

(1) a preparatory stage, during which the participating teenagers were invited to write a sentence and/or question about palliative care;
(2) the education-intervention stage, i.e., an education session rooted and developed using the sentences/questions written by the teenagers during the preparatory stage;
(3) the evaluation stage, during which the participants assessed the overall education program using a questionnaire entailing a set of four dimensions: Organization of the overall education program, Preparatory stage, Education-intervention stage (session), and Evaluation stage (possibility to assess the education program), which were scored on a seven-point Likert scale ranging from 1 = very bad to 7 = very good. This evaluation tool also included two open questions entitled "Additional comments" and "Take-home message" resulting from the education-intervention stage.

All stages were guided and followed by the researcher-educator together with the catechist responsible for the religious education activities of the group of teenagers at the participant parish. It is worth mention that the initial contact was made by the catechist of the parish who approached the researcher-educator with the idea of implementing this type of initiative. The study was conceived as a way of comprehending the impact of the education program for teenagers among the participants. The education program on palliative care for teenagers was structured as follows:

1. Preparatory session:

The preparation session was held approximately one month before the education session. This session was led by the catechist and had a duration of 2 h. The following contents and activities were held during this session:
Concepts of palliative and end of life care.
Brainstorming of ideas and questions on palliative and end of life care.

2. Education session:

The education session was based on the ideas and questions raised by the teenagers during the preparatory session. This session was led by a palliative care nurse and had a duration of 3 h. The following contents were taught using an active and interactive approach:
Clarification of concepts: palliative and end of life care.
Answer to the 'what, why, who, when, where, how' questions in relation to palliative and end of life care.
Ethical and existential issues in palliative and end of life care.

3. Evaluation:

No specific session was designed for the evaluation. The program was evaluated throughout its duration, following the principles and approaches of action-research.

This catechist responsible for the group of teenagers had a relevant role in the implementation of this initiative. The latter was fully supported by the reverend who decided to open the education session to the local community. This is aligned with the principles and practices of action-research where the stakeholder participants have an active role in decision-making [31].

The education program and data collection period occurred from October 2015 to December 2015. The education session happened on November 6, 2015, and had a duration of three hours. Interviews were held in the weeks following the education session. Further details on the data collection are described in the next section.

Instruments for data collection

As aforementioned, a mixed-methods approach was used for data collection as this brings more comprehensiveness and is coherent with action-research. The following data were collected: (1) the complete list of sentences/questions written by the teenagers during the preparatory stage; (2) the field-notes written by the researcher-educator during the overall duration of the education program; (3) the evaluation questionnaire applied to the participants who attended the education session; (4) semi-structured interviews conducted with the catechist responsible for the group of teenagers and two community members (adults) who participated in the education session; and (5) a written testimony about the session written by the reverend at his own initiative and publicly available.

The interview guide for the semi-structured interviews included the following questions:

(1) Could you please share your thoughts about organizing/attending this education program/session about palliative and end of life care?
(2) Do you think that the program was well tailored for teenagers?
(3) Considering the three stages of the education program (i.e., the preparatory stage, the education

session, and the evaluation stage), how would you evaluate each one of them?

(4) What were the main weaknesses and strength of this initiative?

(5) Would you repeat this experience? If so, what suggestions do you have for improvement?

(6) Is there something else that you would like to add or share about this initiative?

The combination of diverse instruments for data collection is an inherent dimension of action-research. It is worth mention that the inclusion of field-notes (also named as reflective diaries) and written testimonies is a common component of palliative and end-of-life care education programs, and of education research, as they allow participants and researchers-educators to revisit their own experience [41].

Figure 1 illustrates the combination and integration of techniques and instruments used for data collection within the action-research spiral.

Participants, data collection and ethics approval

The education-program and research-action on palliative care for teenagers was held at a community parish in the North of Portugal. Participants were a convenience sample of teenagers attending the religious education activities of this parish, the catechists and community members.

A total of 69 persons participated in the education session, 67 (97%) of whom completed the evaluation questionnaire. Although specifically prepared for teenagers (69% of the participants), the education session also included the participation of 8 parents (12% of the participants), 11 catechists (16% of the participants) and 2 members of the local community parish (3% of the participants). The teenagers were aged between 12 and 18 (72% aged between 15 and 18), with the majority being female. The educator-researcher had a clinical background as a nurse and more than ten years of experience in the field of palliative care.

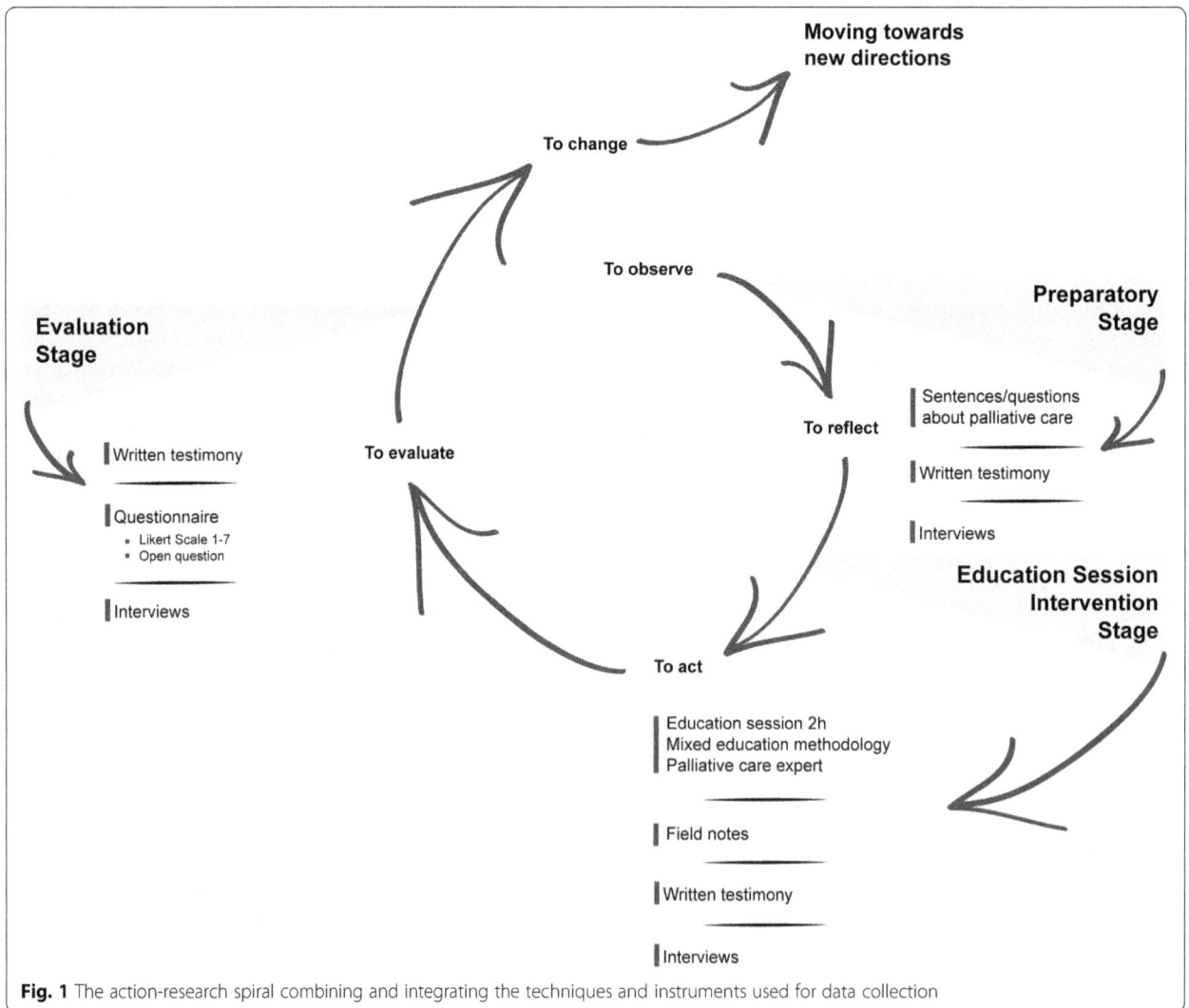

Fig. 1 The action-research spiral combining and integrating the techniques and instruments used for data collection

Ethical approval was obtained from the Ethics Lab: Ethical Analysis, Consultation and Monitoring of Scientific Research Projects and Clinical Trials (former SACE: Serviço de Análise e Consultoria Ética de Projetos de Investigação Científica e Ensaios Clínicos) of the Universidade Católica Portuguesa [Ref.08.2015]. As the study involved minors (i.e., the participant teenagers), a few specific ethical procedures were followed and ensured, namely: (i) Parents and other educators were involved sidelong the education and research process; (ii) parents were informed and consented teenagers to be engaged in the education-research process about palliative care; (iii) verbal parental consent was acquired for participants under 18 years of age for participation in the study; (iv) no confidential data were collected; (v) anonymity was fully ensured; and (vi) no harm was caused to any of the participants. In fact, due to the sensitivity of the topic, researchers and educators were informed upfront if any teenagers were experiencing the process of a life-threatening disease (personally or through a next-to-kin); there was no such situation among the participants. In addition, all data were anonymized, analysed and presented with maximum confidentiality.

Analysis
Data analysis varied as follows:

(1) Qualitative data: Both content and thematic analysis were applied to the sentences and questions written by the teenagers during the preparatory stage, to the field-notes written by the researcher-educator, to the answers given by the participants to the open questions of the questionnaire (i.e., "Additional comments" and "Take-home messages"), to the transcripts of interviews, and to the written testimony. This approach allowed the analysis of multifaceted, important and sensitive phenomena of educating teenagers on palliative and end of life care [42].

(2) Quantitative data: A descriptive analysis was performed on the questions of the evaluation questionnaire. Percentages were calculated for each dimension and item.

Data were analysed independently by two researchers (SMP and PHM).

The triangulation steaming from the use of different instruments, data and researchers ensures the reliability and comprehensiveness of the findings. This type of approach is useful to build meaning from different sources [43, 44]. This is a valuable strategy used in qualitative research, such as this form of action-research, as engaging multiple methods and techniques leads to more valid, reliable and diverse construction of realities [43–49].

Table 1 shows the integration of the education program and research methods.

Results
Results are presented considering the education program on palliative care. Data and information gathered from the different sources are integrated to provide a more comprehensive answer to our research objectives, namely: to implement and understand the impact of an education program about palliative care for teenagers.

Table 1 Integration of the education programme and research methods

Education programme on palliative care for teenagers	Participants	Method for data collection	Analysis
Preparatory stage	Teenagers (n = 48) Catechists (n = 11)	Written sentences/ questions about palliative care	Thematic content analysis
		Interviews	
	Reverend	Written testimony	
	Researcher-educator	Field notes	
Intervention stage 'Education Session'	Teenagers (n = 48) Parents (n = 8) Catechists (n = 11) Community members (n = 2)	Education session materials (PPT) Interviews	Thematic content analysis
	Reverend	Written testimony	
	Researcher-educator	Field-notes	
Evaluation stage	Teenagers (n = 48) Parents (n = 8) Catechists (n = 11) Community members (n = 2)	Questionnaire Interviews	Descriptive (%) Thematic content analysis
	Reverend	Written testimony	
	Researcher-educator	Field-notes	

Note: Although the evaluation stage is described at the end of the process, it focused on all stages of the education programme

The preparatory stage

During the preparatory stage, the teenagers solely wrote questions about palliative care. These questions were organized into eight domains: Definitions of concepts; Articulation (palliative versus curative care); Care beneficiaries; Care timings and timeframe; Organization; Directories; Economic costs; Philosophy, practice and meaning(s) (Table 2).

In the written testimony, the reverend valued the fact that this education-intervention program resulted from the initiative of a community catechist, who organized the overall action and had a major role during its preparatory stage. According to the educator-researcher's field-notes and one of the interviewees (the catechist in charge of the group of teenagers), the questions raised by the teenagers were of relevance and depth. Table 3 illustrates themes and categories emerging from the education-intervention stage.

The education-intervention stage

The education-intervention stage had a three-hour duration and comprised a mixed-strategy. This session was fully developed based on the questions raised by the teenagers and interleaved some more theoretical moments with interactive ones. Field-notes revealed the following dimensions: Openness and positive attitude of the teenagers; teenagers' high participation during the education-intervention session; and positive feature of opening the session to the parents and local community. In his written testimony, the reverend also valued the positive attitude of the teenagers towards the education-intervention about palliative care. The two community members who were interviewed also acknowledged the possibility of attending the education session, as it allowed them to improve their knowledge about palliative care, feeling now more able to further discuss palliative and end of life care issues with other people (Table 2).

The evaluation stage

The questionnaire allowed the evaluation of the following items: "Organization of the education program", "Preparatory stage", "Education-intervention stage/session", and "Possibility to evaluate the education program". 71% of the participants rated the "Organization of the education program", the "Preparatory stage", and the "Possibility to evaluate the education program" with 7 points (Very Good). The "Education-intervention stage/session" was assessed as being very good by 65% of the attendees. Table 4 shows the complete evaluation rates.

From the content analysis performed to the answers given to the open questions, two major dimensions emerged, compelling the following categories: Main take-home messages, namely "Moments of happiness" and "Societal relevance", and Additional comments, explicitly "Excellent", "Exciting" and "Enlightening". In addition, the field-notes and transcripts of interviews showed that the duration of the session was short, highlighting the need for more time in order to ensure a proper discussion of all questions and ideas raised by the participant teenagers. Findings from the written testimony also show the gratitude of the community parish and reverend for having had the opportunity to host and participate in this education-intervention program about palliative care (Table 5).

Table 2 Themes and categories emerging from the preparatory stage

Dimensions	Categories	Examples of text units
Definition of concepts	–	*"What is palliative care?"* (WQS12)
Articulation	Palliative care versus curative care	*"Does palliative care prevent patients from receiving medical drugs or treatments?"* (WQS2)
Care beneficiaries	–	*"Does palliative care act on patients in vegetative condition?"* (WQS 4)
Care timings and timeframe	–	*"Are patients in palliative care cared by these teams until death or is there a timeframe?"* (WQS 3)
Organization	–	*"How is a palliative care team compounded?"* (WQS 1)
Directories	–	*"How is it possible to find palliative care resources?"* (WQS13)
Economic costs	–	*"(…) is palliative care cost-free for patients?"* (WQS 6)
Philosophy, practice and meaning(s)	Philosophy and ethics	*"Do we have the right to end the life of a person who is between life and death?"* (WQS11)
	Meaning(s)	*"Is there happiness (…) in palliative care?"* (WQS10)
Relevance and depth of questions	–	*"The questions raised by the teenagers are very interesting, relevant and show some in-depth reflection about palliative care"* (RFN1)
Role of the community catechist	–	*"Mr. X, catechist of our community parish, was the inspirer of this education initiative…"* (WT)

WQS Written Questions/Sentences by teenagers. *RFN* Researcher Field Notes. *WT* Written Testimony

Table 3 Themes and categories emerging from the education-intervention stage

Categories	Examples of text units
Openness and positive attitude of the teenagers	*"(…) teenagers were very attentive, paying attention to the answers given to the questions they raised during the preparatory stage… They also looked very open, interested and willing to learn more about palliative care"* (RFN) *"I must acknowledge the clear interest shown by all participants, especially our teenagers, to this bioethical dialogue"* (WT)
Teenagers' high participation during the education-intervention session	*"(…) teenagers wanted to participate more…"* (RFN) *"It was quite positive to see how many questions the teenagers raised during the session"* (RFN)
Positive feature of opening the session to the parents and local community	*"It is really important and positive that parents and other members from the local community attended the education session!"* (RFN) *"I am very grateful that our priest wanted to open this session for anybody willing to attend it. I feel now more confident and prepared to further discuss these issues with my family and friends"* (I2)

RFN Researcher Field Notes. *WT* Written Testimony. *I* Interviewee

Discussion

Our findings show the positive impact of implementing an education-intervention strategy and program aimed at increasing awareness about palliative care among teenagers. It highlights the openness of both teenagers and their parents to this topic, as well as the relevance of engaging the community in this type of initiatives. This is aligned with the two previous studies identified in our literature review, suggesting that educating teenagers and high school students about palliative care is not only appreciated by them, but also improves their attitudes toward dying, death and loss [25, 26].

As suggested by Becarro et al. [25, 26], our education-intervention program was appreciated by the teenagers. This was shown by the high level of attention and participation during both the preparatory stage and education-intervention session, and by the feedback given during the evaluation stage. The majority of the participant teenagers asked for more time to allow a more thorough discussion of more sensitive topics. This was reinforced by the two community members (adults) who also attended the session.

The in-depth and quality of the questions raised during the preparatory stage show the openness and interest teenagers have about palliative care. Moreover, it suggests the societal impact of education programs on this matter, specifically when targeted and tailored for teenagers. In contrast to traditional and wide-spread sources of health information (e.g., flyers and conventional education program), interactive and interpersonal health communication and health education strategies offer the potential for more individually tailored messages. This may have contributed to the positive evaluation of our action-research program as the participants, particularly the teenagers, had an active role throughout the overall set of activities and phases.

It is worth mention that some of the questions raised by the teenagers focused on ethical issues, such as euthanasia and assisted suicide, equity in the access to palliative care, organizational aspects and integrative care approaches. While a previous study published elsewhere showed that end-of-life decisions were accepted by adolescents under certain circumstances [50], our findings suggest that the participant teenagers were more interested in discussing these ethical issues rather than on having a clear position or attitude towards them. This is in line with a study conducted about teaching bioethics in high schools, which indicated that teenage students were enthusiastic and willing to discuss ethical issues [24]. In our study, this preference to discuss rather than assuming a position may have occurred for two main reasons. On the one hand, our study and education-program was implemented in a religious context. This may have prevented teenagers from assuming publicly their positions and needs further clarification. On the other hand, another possible explanation for the interest in discussing these topics may have been because of the current public and legal debate on the legalization of euthanasia and physician assisted suicide in Portugal.

Another interesting finding of our study was the involvement shown by parents, catechists and other members from the local community. In fact, considering that the education-intervention session was held on a Sunday morning, it is remarkable that about 30% of the participants did not belong to the teenage group who regularly have their meetings on this day. This shows the local potential of this specific community in terms of awareness about palliative care, fostering the potential of the participant teenagers to further discuss some of the topics developed during the education-intervention session. The participation of adult members of the community in the education-intervention session is also a sign of the possibility to develop a compassionate community, more able to contribute to the actual care of those in need of palliative care [19, 20]. Previous studies have shown that community-based educational initiatives promote knowledge and awareness of palliative care [13, 20], which can promote empowerment [2, 3, 36] and foster the implementation of initiatives to improve care provision at

Table 4 Evaluation rates of the education session

Stage of the Education Program	Qualitative assessment	Scoring in the Likert Scale	N = 67%
Organization of the overall education program	Very Good	7	71%
		6	15%
		5	8%
		4	6%
		3	0%
		2	0%
	Very Bad	1	0%
	Total	–	100%
Preparatory stage	Very Good	7	71%
		6	15%
		5	7%
		4	7%
		3	0%
		2	0%
	Very Bad	1	0%
	Total	–	100%
Education-intervention stage (session)	Very Good	7	65%
		6	22%
		5	5%
		4	8%
		3	0%
		2	0%
	Very Bad	1	0%
	Total	–	100%
Evaluation stage (possibility to assess the education program)	Very Good	7	71%
		6	22%
		5	6%
		4	1%
		3	0%
		2	0%
	Very Bad	1	0%
	Total	–	100%

Table 5 Themes and categories emerging from the evaluation stage

Dimensions	Categories	Examples of text units
Take-home messages	Moments of happiness	*"Happiness can exist during a bad disease"* (AWT2) *"… nurturing the value of life in order to experience happiness"* (WT)
	Societal relevance	*"Palliative care is crucial for the population"* (AWT48)
Additional comments	Excellent	*"Excellent session!"* (AWE7)
	Exciting	*"Exciting"* (AWT38)
	Enlightening	*"(…) enlightening and with very clear and relevant information"* (AWE66)
	Revolutionary	*"(…) revolutionary education session"* (WT)
	Thank you	*"(…) the gratitude we feel for having had this education programme. Thank you!"* (WT)
Education session: Need for more time		*"it would have been good to have more time to further discuss some of the issues and give a more complete and comprehensive answer to the questions raised by the teenagers"* (RFN) *"We really need more sessions like this one! This one was great, but we needed more time to deepen some discussions."* (I1)

AWT Answers written by teenagers. *AWE* Answers written by catechists. *RFN* Researcher Field Notes. *WT* Written Testimony. *I* Interviewee

the end of life for all citizens. Direct engagement with communities can indeed improve a multicultural understanding of populations' cultural and health needs about palliative and end of life care [51].

Finally, it is remarkable how the education-session contributed to spread a positive and constructive message about palliative care among the participant teenagers. Based on the "Take-home messages" written by these teenagers, at the end of the education session/program, they perceived palliative care as having the potential to contributing to "moments of happiness" for those suffering from a life-threatening disease. These findings suggest that although it is challenging to engage people in education about palliative care [52], active and participatory strategies as those implemented in this action-research study can be useful and have a positive impact. The societal relevance of palliative care was also highlighted and the participants considered the education session and program as being revolutionary, excellent, exciting and enlightening.

Strengths, limitations and further research

A major strength of our study is its originality and relevance to a wide audience. In fact, although specifically focused on a group of teenagers, our action-research study allowed the implementation of an education program about palliative care to parents and other citizens of the local community. Furthermore, our study used an action-research approach, which is considered both to be a relevant approach in palliative care research and in health education and promotion [27–29, 31–34, 53]. The inclusion of a wide range of instruments and techniques for data collection ensures the validity and reliability of our findings [40–49]. Nevertheless, a few limitations need to be considered. First, as the education program was developed in a parish, some religious bias needs to be reflected and findings cannot be widespread to other settings. Second, as this is a single-centre study, some caution is needed in the interpretation and generalization of the findings. Further research (including the replication of this study on other contexts) and other education-program specifically focused on teenagers and local communities, and using other educational approaches (e.g., web-based ones) [54] need therefore to be promoted. For instance, health education programs about pressing issues, such as palliative and end-of-life care, and using multi-centred designed interventions could be designed as part of high school education, requiring further attention and study.

Conclusions

The education program about palliative care was deemed to be excellent, exciting and enlightening by the teenagers to whom it was specifically designed. Positive feedback was given by the teenagers, parents and other participants. The findings of this action-research study show that the education program and education-intervention contributed to create awareness about palliative care among the participant teenagers, who ended the program with a positive message about palliative care.

Implications of this study

The societal challenges of ageing populations have been recognized worldwide. Moreover, the relevance of community involvement and the active participation of citizens are seen as making a valuable contribution to the development of palliative care [17]. Nevertheless, although attention to palliative care is increasing, further developments and policy initiatives are needed to improve access to and quality of palliative care for all citizens who are in need of this type of care. The following policy implications can be drawn based on our findings. First, while our study highlights the positive impact of education initiatives about palliative care in early ages, further research is needed to assess the actual impact of education about palliative care in the acquisition of specific knowledge, development of competences and change of attitudes among teenagers and younger age groups (e.g., children). Second, education about palliative and end of life care should be promoted at local communities, for instance in primary and secondary schools, to foster community involvement, participation and empowerment. Finally, compassionate communities, described as networks that could encourage people to take some active responsibility for care and recognize that ageing and dying, death and bereavement are part of everyday life and happen to everyone [18–20], could and should be promoted to enhance the health and wellbeing of all citizens at the end of their life.

Acknowledgments
The authors would like to thank the local community priest of the parish where the study was conducted, the catechists who promoted this initiative locally, and the teenagers, parents and community members who actively participated in the education program about palliative care.

Authors' contribution
SMP: study concept and design; implementation of the action-research; data collection; analysis and interpretation of the data and writing of the manuscript. PHM: study concept and design; implementation of the action-research; analysis and interpretation of the data and writing of the manuscript. JA revised and commented the manuscript. All authors (SMP, JA, and PHM) approved the final version of the manuscript before submission. SMP and PHM contributed equally to the manuscript. All authors read and approved the final manuscript.

Funding
The authors declare that no funding was obtained to conduct this research. This manuscript was written during the duration of Projects InPalIn "Integrating Palliative Care in Intensive Care" and Subproject ETHICS II of Project ENSURE "Enhancing the Informed Consent Process: Supported Decision-Making and Capacity Assessment in Clinical Dementia Research". Therefore, SMP and PHM would like to thank Fundação Merck, Sharp & Dohme and Fundação Grünenthal for their financial support to Project InPalIn and ERA-NET NEURON II, ELSA 2015, European Comission, and Fundação para a Ciência e a Tecnologia (FCT), Ministério da Ciência, Tecnologia e Ensino Superior, Portugal, for their financial support to the Subproject ETHICS II of Project ENSURE. The funders had no role in the design of the study, collection, analysis, and interpretation of data, and in writing the manuscript.

Competing interest
The authors declare that they have no competing interests.

Ethics approval and consent to participate
Ethical approval was obtained from the Ethics Lab: Ethical Analysis, Consultation and Monitoring of Scientific Research Projects and Clinical Trials (former SACE: Serviço de Análise e Consultoria Ética de Projetos de Investigação Científica e Ensaios Clínicos) of the Universidade Católica Portuguesa [Ref.08.2015]. As the study involved minors (i.e., the participant teenagers), a few specific ethical procedures were followed and ensured. Parents were informed and consented teenagers to be engaged in the education-research process about palliative care. Verbal parental consent was acquired for participants under 18 years of age for participation in the study. Further ethics procedures are thoroughly described in the methods section.

Author details
[1]Instituto de Bioética, Universidade Católica Portuguesa, Rua Diogo Botelho, 1327 4169-005 Porto, Portugal. [2]UNESCO Chair in Bioethics Instituto de Bioética, Universidade Católica Portuguesa, Porto, Portugal. [3]CEGE: Centro de Estudos em Gestão e Economia [Research Centre in Management and Economics Católica Porto Business School, Universidade Católica Portuguesa, Porto, Portugal.

References

1. Zimmerman EB, Woolf SH, Haley A. Understanding the relationship between education and health: a review of the evidence and an examination of community perspectives. In: Kaplan R, Spittel M, David D, editors. Population health: behavioral and social science insights. AHRQ publication no. 15–0002. Rockville: Agency for Healthcare Research and Quality and Office of Behavioral and Social Sciences Research, National Institutes of Health; 2015. p. 347–84.

2. Wallerstein N, Bernstein E. Empowerment education: Freire's ideas adapted to health education. Health Educ Q. 1988 Winter;15(4):379–94.

3. Thompson B, Molina Y, Viswanath K, Warnecke R, Prelip ML. Strategies to empower communities to reduce health disparities. Health affairs (Project Hope). 2016;35(8):1424–8. https://doi.org/10.1377/hlthaff.2015.1364.

4. Kumar S, Preetha G. Health promotion: an effective tool for Global Health. Indian J Community Med. 2012;37(1):5–12. https://doi.org/10.4103/0970-0218.94009.

5. Council of Europe. Recommendation rec (2003) 24 of the Committee of Ministers to member states on the organisation of. palliative care. 2003;

6. World Health Organization. Strengthening of palliative care as a component of integrated treatment throughout the life course. EB134/28. 134th session; 2013.

7. Davies E, Higginson IJ. Better palliative care for older people. Copenhagen: World Health Organization; 2004.

8. Hall S, Petkova H, Tsouros AD, Costantini M, Higginson IJ. Palliative care for older people: better practices. Copenhagen: World Health Organization; 2011.

9. Kite S. Palliative care for older people. Age Ageing. 2006;35(5):459–60. https://doi.org/10.1093/ageing/afl069.

10. Bone AE, Gomes B, Etkind SN, Verne J, Murtagh FE, Evans CJ, Higginson IJ. What is the impact of population ageing on the future provision of end-of-life care? Population-based projections of place of death. Palliat Med. 2018; 32(2):329–36. https://doi.org/10.1177/0269216317734435.

11. Currow DC, Phillips J, Agar M. Population-based models of planning for palliative care in older people. Curr Opin Support Palliat Care. 2017;11(4): 310–4. https://doi.org/10.1097/SPC.0000000000000304.

12. McIlfatrick S, Noble H, McCorry N, et al. Exploring public awareness and perceptions of palliative care. Palliat Medicine. 2013;28(3):273–80. https://doi.org/10.1177/0269216313502372.

13. McIlfatrick S, Hasson F, McLaughlin D, et al. Public awareness and attitudes toward palliative care in Northern Ireland. BMC Palliat Care. 2013;12:34. https://doi.org/10.1186/1472-684X-12-34.

14. Benini F, Fabris M, Pace DS, et al. Awareness, understanding and attitudes of Italians regarding palliative care. Ann Ist Super Sanità. 2011;47(3):253–9. https://doi.org/10.4415/ANN_11_03_03.

15. Stjernswärd J, Foley K, Ferris FD. The public health strategy for palliative care. J Pain Symptom Manag. 2007;33(5):486–93. https://doi.org/10.1016/j.jpainsymman.2007.02.016.

16. Pillemer K, Chen EK, Riffin C, Prigerson H, Reid MC. Practice-based research priorities for palliative care: results from a research-to-practice consensus workshop. Am J Public Health. 2015;105(11):2237–44. https://doi.org/10.2105/AJPH.2015.302675.

17. Martins Pereira S, Albers G, Pasman R, et al. A public health approach to improving palliative care for older people. In: Van den Block L, Albers G, Martins Pereira S, et al., editors. Palliative care for older people. A public health perspective. Oxford: Oxford University Press; 2015. p. 275–91.

18. Kellehear A. Health promotion and palliative care. In: Mitchell G, editor. *Palliative Care: A Patient-Centred Approach*. Oxford: Radcliffe publishing; 2008. p. 139–56.

19. Kellehear A. Compassionate communities: caring for older people towards the end of life. In: Van den Block L, Albers G, Martins Pereira S, et al., editors. Palliative care for older people. A public health perspective. Oxford: Oxford University Press; 2015. p. 193–9.

20. Kellehear A. Compassionate communities: end-of-life care as everyone's responsibility. Q J Med. 2013;106:1071–5. https://doi.org/10.1093/qjmed/hct200.

21. Wilkinson R, Marmot M, editors. *Social Determinants of Health. The solid facts*. Denmark: World Health Organization; 2003.

22. Paul S, Cree VE, Murray SA. Integrating palliative care into the community: the role of hospices and schools. *BMJ Support Palliat Care*. 2017. First published on April. 2017:16. https://doi.org/10.1136/bmjspcare-2015-001092.

23. Kelly MP, Morgan A, Bonnefoy J, et al. *The social determinants of health: Developing an evidence base for political action Final Report to World Health Organization, Commission on the Social Determinants of Health and the Measurement and Evidence Knowledge Network*. United Kingdom: National Institute for Health and Clinical Excellence and Chile: Universidad del Desarollo; 2007.

24. Araújo J, Costa Gomes C, Jácomo A, Martins Pereira S. Teaching bioethics in high schools. Health Educ J. 2017;76(4):507–13. https://doi.org/10.1177/0017896917690566.

25. Beccaro M, Gollo G, Giordano M, et al. The Ligurian high-school educational project on palliative care: development and piloting of a school-based intervention on bereavement and severe illness. Am J Hosp Palliat Med. 2014;31(7):756–64. https://doi.org/10.1177/1049909113503394.

26. Beccaro M, Gollo G, Ceccon S, et al. Students, severe illness, and palliative care: results from a pilot study on a school-based intervention. Am J Hosp Palliat Med. 2015;32(7):715–24. https://doi.org/10.1177/1049909114539187.

27. Ivankova NV. Mixed methods applications in action research. From methods to community action. London: SAGE; 2015.

28. James EA, Milenkiewicz MT, Bucknam A. Participatory action research for educational leadership. Using data-driven decision making to improve schools. London: SAGE; 2008.

29. Reason P, Bradbury H. Handbook of action research: participative inquiry and practice. London: Sage; 2008.

30. Waterman H. Action research and health. In: Saks M, Allsop J, editors. Researching health. Qualitative, quantitative and mixed methods. London: Sage; 2013. p. 148–67.

31. Sealey M, O'Connor M, Aoun SM, Breen LJ. Exploring barriers to assessment of bereavement risk in palliative care: perspectives of key stakeholders. BMC Palliat Care. 2015;14:49. https://doi.org/10.1186/s12904-015-0046-7.

32. Hockley J, Froggatt K, Heimerl K, editors. Palliative care and participatory research: actions and reflections. Oxford: OUP; 2012.

33. Froggatt K, Hockley J. Action research in palliative care: defining an evaluation methodology. Palliat Med. 2011;25(8):782–7. https://doi.org/10.1177/0269216311420483.

34. Cooper J, Hewison A. Implementing audit in palliative care: an action research approach. J Adv Nurs. 2002;39(4):360–9.

35. Sandoval JUA, Lucero J, Oetzel J, et al. Process and outcome constructs for evaluating community-based participatory research projects: a matrix of existing measures. Health Educ Res. 2012;27(4):680–90. https://doi.org/10.1093/her/cyr087.

36. Brown DR, Hernández A, Saint-Jean G, Evans S, Tafari I, Brewster LG, Celestin MJ, Gómez-Estefan C, Regalado F, Akal S, Nierenberg B, Kauschinger ED, Schwartz R, Page JB. A participatory action research pilot study of urban health disparities using rapid assessment response and evaluation. Am J Public Health. 2008;98(1):28–38. https://doi.org/10.2105/AJPH.2006.091363.

37. Seymour J, Almack K, Kennedy S. Implementing advance care planning: a qualitative study of community nurses' views and experiences. BMC Palliat Care. 2010;9:4. https://doi.org/10.1186/1472-684X-9-4.

38. van de Geer J, Veeger N, Groot M, Zock H, Leget C, Prins J, Vissers K. Multidisciplinary training on spiritual Care for Patients in palliative care trajectories improves the attitudes and competencies of hospital medical staff. Am J Hosp Palliat Care. 2017; https://doi.org/10.1177/1049909117692959.

39. Learmonth AM. Utilizing research in practice and generating evidence from practice. Health Educ Res. 2000;15(6):743–56. https://doi.org/10.1093/her/15.6.743.

40. Carr W, Kemmis S. *Becoming critical: Education, knowledge and action research*. Geelong: Deakin: University Press; 1986.

41. Germain A, Nolan K, Doyle R, et al. The use of reflective diaries in end of life training programmes: a study exploring the impact of self-reflection on the participants in a volunteer training programme. BMC Palliat Care. 2015; 15(28) https://doi.org/10.1186/s12904-016-0096-5.

42. Vaismoradi M, Turunen H, Bondas T. Content analysis and thematic analysis: implications for conducting a qualitative descriptive study. Nurs Health Sci. 2013;15(3):398–405. https://doi.org/10.1111/nhs.12048.

43. Mertens DM, Hesse-Biber S. Triangulation and mixed methods research: provocative positions. Journal of Mixed Methods Research. 2012;6(2):75–9. https://doi.org/10.1177/1558689812437100.

44. Creswell J. Research design: qualitative, quantitative and mixed methods approaches. Thousand Oaks: SAGE; 2003.

45. Golafshani N. Understanding reliability and validity in qualitative research. Qual Rep. 2003;8(4):597–607.

46. Shenton AK. Strategies for ensuring trustworthiness in qualitative research projects. Educ Inform. 2004;22:63–75.

47. Zohrabi M. Mixed method research: instruments, validity, reliability and reporting findings. TPLC. 2013;3(2):254–62.
48. Noble H, Smith J. Issues of validity and reliability in qualitative research. Evid Based Nurs. 2015;18(2):34–5. https://doi.org/10.1136/eb-2015-102054.
49. Leung L. Validity, reliability, and generalizability in qualitative research. J Family Med Prim Care. 2015;4(3):324–7. https://doi.org/10.4103/2249-4863.161306.
50. Pousset G, Bilsen J, De Wilde J, et al. Attitudes of Flemish secondary school students towards euthanasia and other end-of-life decisions in minors. Child Care Health Dev. 2009;35(3):349–56. https://doi.org/10.1111/j.1365-2214.2008.00933.x.
51. Boucher NA. Direct engagement with communities and Interprofessional learning to factor culture into end-of-life health care delivery. Am J Public Health. 2016;106(6):996–1001. https://doi.org/10.2105/AJPH.2016.303073.
52. O'Connor M, Abbott J-A, Recoche K. Getting the message across: does the use of drama aid education in palliative care? Adv Health Sci Educ. 2012;17:195–201. https://doi.org/10.1007/s10459-010-9228-5.
53. Marsh P, Gartrell G, Egg G, et al. End-of-life care in a community garden: findings from a participatory action research project in regional Australia. Health Place. 2017;45:110–6. https://doi.org/10.1016/j.healthplace.2017.03.006.
54. Paul CL, Carey ML, Sanson-Fisher RW, et al. The impact of web-based approaches on psychosocial health in chronic physical and mental health conditions. Health Educ Res. 2013;28(3):450–71. https://doi.org/10.1093/her/cyt053.

3

Palliative care for homeless people: a systematic review of the concerns, care needs and preferences, and the barriers and facilitators for providing palliative care

Hanna T. Klop[1]*(iD), Anke J.E. de Veer[2], Sophie I. van Dongen[3], Anneke L. Francke[1,2], Judith A.C. Rietjens[3] and Bregje D. Onwuteaka-Philipsen[1]

Abstract

Background: Homeless people often suffer from complex and chronic comorbidities, have high rates of morbidity and die at much younger ages than the general population. Due to a complex combination of physical, psychosocial and addiction problems at the end of life, they often have limited access to palliative care. Both the homeless and healthcare providers experience a lot of barriers. Therefore, providing palliative care that fits the needs and concerns of the homeless is a challenge to healthcare providers. This systematic review aims to summarize evidence about the concerns, palliative care needs and preferences of homeless people, as well as barriers and facilitators for delivering high quality palliative care.

Methods: PubMed, Embase, PsycINFO, CINAHL and Web of Science were searched up to 10 May 2016. Included were studies about homeless people with a short life expectancy, their palliative care needs and the palliative care provided, that were conducted in Western countries. Data were independently extracted by two researchers using a predefined extraction form. Quality was assessed using a Critical Appraisal instrument. The systematic literature review was based on the PRISMA statement.

Results: Twenty-seven publications from 23 different studies met the inclusion criteria; 15 studies were qualitative and eight were quantitative. Concerns of the homeless often related to end-of-life care not being a priority, drug dependence hindering adequate care, limited insight into their condition and little support from family and relatives. Barriers and facilitators often concerned the attitude of healthcare professionals towards homeless people. A respectful approach and respect for dignity proved to be important in good quality palliative care.

Conclusions: A patient-centred, flexible and low-threshold approach embodying awareness of the concerns of homeless people is needed so that appropriate palliative care can be provided timely. Training, education and experience of professionals can help to accomplish this.

Keywords: Palliative care, End-of-life, Homeless people, Systematic review, Concerns, Needs, Barriers, Facilitators

* Correspondence: klophanna@gmail.com
[1]Amsterdam Public Health Research Institute (APH), Department of Public and Occupational Health, Expertise Centre for Palliative Care, VU University Medical Center, P.O. Box 7057, 1007 MB Amsterdam, The Netherlands
Full list of author information is available at the end of the article

Background

Homeless people are those without permanent housing, e.g. living in sheltered housing or on the streets [1, 2]. It is known that homeless people often have substance abuse problems, high rates of mental illness and serious physical illness, lack of social support, and lack of health insurance [3–8]. Many of them suffer from complex and often chronic comorbidities, such as liver cirrhosis, cancer and HIV [6, 9, 10]. In addition, they die at much younger ages than the general population [7, 11–14].

It is therefore evident that a large proportion of homeless people can benefit from palliative care. According to the widely accepted definition of the World Health Organization (WHO), "palliative care is an approach that improves the quality of life of patients and their families facing the problems associated with life-threatening illness, through the prevention and relief of suffering by means of early identification and impeccable assessment and treatment of pain and other problems, physical, psychosocial and spiritual" [15]. The definition shows that palliative care covers a broad range of domains and can start in an early phase of a life-threatening illness. Given the multiple problems homeless people have, it is apparent that providing good and accessible palliative care to homeless people a challenge.

Until now, research conducted on this topic has been addressed in three reviews [10, 16, 17]. First, Sumalinog et al. reviewed the effectiveness of three interventions during homeless people's final stage of life, including: an intervention encouraging the completion of advance directives, a shelter-based palliative care programme, and an intervention aiming to improve cooperation between palliative care services and social services for the homeless. They tentatively conclude that there is some evidence that the interventions lead to the completion of more advance care directives and better access to palliative care [10]. In addition, a review by Hubbell also focused on the completion of advance care planning, concluding that clinician-guided interventions with homeless individuals were effective in getting advance directives completed and in obtaining surrogate decision-makers. Hubbell also found that homeless people had several concerns at the end of life, such as a fear of dying alone and concerns regarding burial and notification of family [17]. Furthermore, Hudson et al. summarized the findings in qualitative studies on palliative care among homeless people to get a better understanding of the challenges for palliative care access and delivery [16]. In the review by Hudson et al., three types of challenges were identified, which they described as challenges related to chaotic lifestyles, challenges concerning the delivery of end-of-life care in hostels, and the challenges of caring for homeless people in mainstream palliative care settings.

While the three reviews provide valuable information, they do not provide a complete overview of the existing literature on palliative care for homeless people. First of all, the reviews of Sumalinog et al. and Hubbell focus exclusively on the terminal phase of life, excluding earlier stages of the palliative care trajectory. Additionally, both reviews of Sumalinog et al. and Hubbell are mainly concerned with structure (such as cooperation), ethical decisions (such as advance directives) and homeless people's attitudes towards dying. These two reviews do not look at the care needs of homeless people and how to meet these needs. Furthermore, Hudson's review limits itself to qualitative studies and only focuses on challenges concerning the access and delivery of palliative care, without looking at possibilities for improvements. Given the relatively narrow focus of each of the three previous reviews, we found the need for a more comprehensive review providing a broader overview of relevant literature on palliative care for homeless people. In this review we offer such a comprehensive overview by using the broad definition of palliative care as defined by the WHO, which emphasizes care in four domains - somatic, psychological, social and spiritual - and also recognizes that care can start before the terminal phase. Besides this, by looking at the possibilities available for providing good palliative care (barriers and facilitators), and by including both qualitative, quantitative and mixed-method studies, this review contributes to the existing literature.

In order to provide palliative care tailored to the needs of homeless people, the objective of this systematic review is to summarize what evidence already exists about concerns and healthcare needs, as well as the conditions for delivering good quality palliative care for the target group. The research questions are therefore:

1. What is known from previous research about the concerns, care needs and preferences of homeless people regarding palliative care?
2. What is known from previous research about what barriers and facilitators are found in the delivery of palliative care for homeless people?
3. What is known from previous research about recommendations for practice regarding palliative care to homeless people?

Methods
Design and eligibility criteria
A systematic review of the research literature was carried out to identify studies that examined the concerns and needs in palliative care for homeless people, and/or provided care to seriously ill homeless people. A review protocol was developed based on the Preferred Reporting Items for Systematic Reviews and Meta-Analysis (PRISMA) statement [18].

Studies eligible for inclusion had to meet the following criteria:

1. The study concerns homeless people who provided information about their views, wishes, and/or preferences towards the end of life, including homeless people having a life limiting condition.
2. The study includes data derived from homeless people themselves, from their healthcare professionals or data from registration, medical files or cohorts (either qualitative or quantitative).
3. The study concerns the palliative care provided (somatic, psychological, social and/or spiritual), factors influencing that care, palliative care needs and/or care interventions or innovations for palliative care.

Commentaries, editorials, abstracts, posters for conferences and non-empirical studies were excluded. In addition, studies conducted outside the Western World (outside Northern, Eastern, Southern and Western Europe or Anglo Saxon countries) were excluded. Since Western countries already differ in the way care for homeless people is organized within the health and welfare system, we did however want to ensure comparability in terms of living conditions and welfare levels. There were no restrictions on the setting, year of publication and language of the publication.

Searches
The following sources were searched from inception: Embase.com and Ebsco/PsycInfo (up to 1 April 2016), Ebsco/CINAHL (up to 5 April 2016), Thomson Reuters/ Web of Science (up to 3 May 2016) and PubMed (up to 10 May 2016). To identify studies about homelessness and palliative care, we used a pre-defined search strategy. The string for PubMed is shown in Fig. 1, detailed information for all search strings is shown in Additional file 1.

References listed in review articles and references in papers which were excluded in the full text round were also checked. In order to find grey literature, relevant websites of organizations that are involved in palliative care for homeless people or research into it were consulted by searching for relevant keywords using Google (e.g. Simon Communities Ireland – Homeless Charity and St. Mungo Community Housing Association). Duplicate articles were excluded.

Study identification and data extraction
All the references obtained by searching databases as mentioned above were independently reviewed by two researchers, using Covidence online software (a primary screening and data extraction tool) [19]. Firstly, titles and abstracts were screened in order to determine whether studies met the eligibility criteria. The exclusion criteria were (1) homeless people could not be distinguished as a separate subgroup (2) study was not about somatically ill homeless adults with a short-life expectancy (3) search outcomes included: comments, editorials, abstracts and posters (4) study was not conducted in N-E-W Europe or Anglo-Saxon countries, and (5) study was not about palliative/end-of-life care. Cohen's kappa for the first selection of titles and abstracts was 0. 92 (unweighted), which is almost perfect according to Landis & Koch [20]. In the second round, the remaining full text papers were independently assessed by two reviewers against inclusion criteria. Cohen's kappa for the second round was 0.81 (unweighted), thus also reflecting almost perfect agreement according to Landis & Koch [20]. Disagreements about whether or not the criteria were met were solved by discussion and a third researcher was consulted in the event of disagreement. There was disagreement in 8 of the 91 studies (8.8%).

For data extraction and analyses we followed the assumptions for an integrated design of a systematic review, which indicate that qualitative, quantitative and mixed-method studies can be jointly analysed and synthesized [21]. The extraction form was developed by two researchers, discussed by the research group and adjusted in response to comments. Extracted data included information about the country of the research, the research aims and questions, methods and data collection, characteristics

"Homeless persons"[Mesh:NoExp] OR homeless*[tiab] OR street people*[tiab]

"Terminal Care"[Mesh] OR "Palliative Care"[Mesh] OR "Palliative Medicine"[Mesh] OR Hospice and Palliative Care Nursing"[Mesh] OR "Death"[Mesh:NoExp] OR "mortality"[Subheading] OR terminal*[tiab]OR end of life[tiab] OR life care end[tiab] OR hospice*[tiab] OR bereavement car*[tiab] OR palliati*[tiab] OR limited life*[tiab] OR death*[tiab] OR dying*[tiab] OR die[tiab] OR "Advance Care Planning"[Mesh] OR "Attitude to death"[Mesh] OR mortal*[tiab] OR advanced car*[tiab] OR advance car*[tiab]

Fig. 1 Search string PubMed

of participants, setting, perspective of the publication (homeless people, healthcare providers, relatives/friends, open answer questionnaire), results, strengths and limitations of the study design and key conclusions. The results were extracted with a focus on the research questions; with regard to recommendations for practice we limited ourselves to recommendations given by the authors that were related to the results found in that study. For the first five publications, two researchers extracted the data independently, without any extraction software. When necessary, adjustments were made and conflicts were resolved. For the other papers, data was extracted by one reviewer and checked by a second.

Analysis
Because our aims were 'to summarize evidence about the concerns, palliative care needs and preferences of homeless people, as well as barriers and facilitators for delivering high quality palliative care', we used the findings from the selected studies mainly to describe common themes. Thus, data was analysed using the meta-summary method [21] to identify common themes. The extracted data was classified manually into categories by sorting according to common themes, carried out by one researcher until no new categories came up. These themes were then discussed with a second researcher before discussion in the project team. In the tables the common themes are shown, indicating in which studies they occurred.

Critical appraisal of the methodological quality
The methodological quality of the studies that met the inclusion criteria was assessed the General Appraisal instrument of Hawker et al. [22]. The instrument, which is applicable to quantitative as well as qualitative studies, consists of nine elements (abstract, background, methodology, sampling, data analysis, ethics, results, transferability and implications). Each element is scored on a four-point scale (ranging from very poor to good). Scores for the various are added to give a total score. Total scores range from 9 to 36; scores less than or equal to 18 are rated as 'poor methodological quality', scores from 19 to 27 as 'moderate' and above 27 as 'good quality'. All methodological assessments were done by two reviewers independently. If there was a mismatch of more than five points, disagreements were solved by discussion. The scores of assessment can be found in Table 1, more details of the assessments can be found in Additional file 2.

Results
Review selection
The review process is shown in Fig. 2. We identified 3245 records through database searches, seven additional records were found through websites of organizations. After removing 1656 duplicates, 1596 papers were screened on title and abstract. Of these, the full texts of 91 were checked, resulting in 27 papers meeting our inclusion criteria (Table 1). No additional papers were found by contacting project members.

General characteristics of studies
Table 1 shows the characteristics of all the studies included. A number of authors, namely Ko et al. [23, 24], McNeil et al. [25–27] and Song et al. [28, 29] discussed their own same study in several papers; each paper discussed various aspects of the study. The 27 papers that were included cover 23 different studies. All studies were published in the period 1986–2016 and published in English. Most studies were conducted in the USA ($n = 15$) or Canada ($n = 7$).

Fifteen studies had qualitative designs, generally using semi-structured individual interviews and focus groups. Eight studies had quantitative designs using a variety of methods, such as an e-mail survey and a review of medical records. Of these quantitative studies, five studies evaluated an intervention. The methodological quality was assessed as good for fifteen papers, moderate for nine and poor for three (Table 1).

Setting and participants
Of all 23 studies, 12 derived data from homeless participants, nine studies from healthcare professionals engaged in caring for homeless people (including review or analysis of medical records) and two studies from both homeless participants and healthcare professionals (Additional file 3). Of the 12 studies that derived their data from homeless people and the two studies with both homeless participants and healthcare professionals, the homeless people were terminally ill in three studies (Table 1) [30–32].

Homeless people in the studies stayed or lived in a variety of settings. The most frequently mentioned were various types of shelters, e.g. drop-in shelters and homeless shelters. Other settings mentioned were support homes, housing facilities, hospitals and medical centres, healthcare programmes, palliative care services and hospices, hostels, social service agencies and sites or communities for homeless people (Table 1). Additional file 3 shows more information about the characteristics of the study populations. Most studies stated the age, sex and ethnicity of homeless participants. A large proportion of homeless participants were male, with percentages ranging between 60% and 100% of the study population. The average age of homeless participants varied between 43 and 65. In the studies that provided information about ethnicity, homeless people of several ethnic groups participated. The educational level of homeless participants, health status of homeless

Table 1 Characteristics of the papers included

Reference	Aim	Country	Setting	Method	Participants	N	Information on 1,2, 3,[b]	Critical appraisal score[c]
[31]	To know more about the content of advance directives completed by homeless people who participated in a guided intervention arm	USA	Homeless drop-in shelter	Qualitative analysis of participants' responses to individual items in an advance directive[a]	Homeless people with a terminal illness	Homeless people (n = 17)	1, 2, 3	24/20 Moderate
[32]	To identify the observed changes in general condition or behaviour of homeless people with advanced liver disease who may be in deteriorating health and approaching the end of life in order to better recognize an increased likelihood of death and to explore staff's experiences of death of residents	UK	Homeless shelter	Case note review, focus groups (qualitative)	Case notes about homeless people with advanced liver disease, staff members of a supporting home for homeless people	Case notes (n = 27) staff members (n = 13)	1, 2, 3	22/21 Moderate
[37]	To explore the staff members' experiences of and reasoning about the palliative care they provided	Sweden	Support home for homeless	Paired and individual conversations (qualitative)	Staff members of a support and housing home for homeless	Staff members (n = 12)	1, 2, 3	34/31 Good
[49]	To describe challenges of caring for homeless veterans at end of life as perceived by Veterans Affairs Medical Centre (VAMC) homeless and EOL care staff	USA	Veterans Affairs Medical Centres (VAMC) with programmes for homeless veterans with a short life expectancy	E-mail survey (quantitative)	Care staff of homeless and EOL programmes	50 VAMCs	2	28/23 Moderate
[43]	To assess the extent to which homeless persons may underuse healthcare services even when they are at a high risk of death and to examine potential opportunities for intervention in this population	USA	Boston Health Care for the Homeless Program	Review of medical records (quantitative)	Deceased homeless adults	Medical records (n = 558)	2, 3	27/25 Moderate
[23]	To explore the views, concerns, and needs regarding advance care planning among older homeless adults	USA	Transitional housing facility	Semi-structured face-to-face interviews (qualitative)	Homeless adults aged 60 and older	Homeless (n = 21)	1, 2, 3	30/29 Good

Table 1 Characteristics of the papers included (Continued)

Reference	Aim	Country	Setting	Method	Participants	N	Information on 1,2, 3,[b]	Critical appraisal score[c]
[24]	To explore older homeless adults' perspectives toward good and bad deaths and their concerns regarding their EOL care needs	USA	Transitional housing facility	Semi-structured face-to-face interviews (qualitative)	Homeless adults aged 60 and older	Homeless (n = 21)	1, 2, 3	30/33 Good
[36]	To explore how access to Toronto's palliative services can be improved to better serve the city's homeless	Canada	Providers of care for the homeless	Semi-structured interviews (qualitative)	Homeless care providers with extensive experience and experience dealing with death and dying	Registered nurses (n = 3) outreach workers (n = 4)	1, 2, 3	19/18 Poor
[41]	To determine the rate of advance directive completion using a one-on-one counsellor-guided intervention	Canada	Shelter for homeless men	Counsellor-guided intervention (quantitative)[a]	Chronically homeless individuals in a managed alcohol harm reduction program[a]	Shelter residents (n = 205)	1, 2	31/33 Good
[47]	To identify best practice for managing the palliative care needs of clients experiencing homelessness in a community setting and to guide the development of policies for a community-based palliative care service working with these clients	Australia	Community-based palliative care service	Semi-structured individual interviews (qualitative)	Workers from hospital and community organizations	Staff members (n = 6)	2, 3	27/24 Moderate
[30]	To explore and describe aspects of social networks that have a potential for caregiving during the terminal phase of a disease	USA	Patients of two medical centres, living in single room buildings	Semi-structured individual interviews (qualitative)	Homeless who had been diagnosed with unresectable lung cancer	Homeless (n = 8)	2	21/19 Moderate
[26]	To identify challenges health and social service providers face in facilitating and delivering end-of-life care services to homeless illicit drug users	Canada	Health and social care services	Semi-structured individual interviews (qualitative)	Health and social services professionals involved in end-of-life care services delivery to homeless persons	Healthcare professionals and managers (n = 50)	2, 3	29/31 Good
[27]	To identify barriers to the end-of-life care system for homeless populations and generate recommendations to improve their access to end-of-life care	Canada	Health and social services	Semi-structured individual interviews (qualitative)	Health and social services professionals involved in end-of-life care services delivery to homeless p ersons	Healthcare professionals and managers (n = 54)	2, 3	32/35 Good

Table 1 Characteristics of the papers included (Continued)

Reference	Aim	Country	Setting	Method	Participants	N	Information on 1,2, 3,[b]	Critical appraisal score[c]
[25]	To explore the role of harm reduction services in end-of-life care services delivery to homeless and marginally housed persons with problematic use of alcohol and/or illicit drugs	Canada	Health and social services	Semi-structured individual interviews (qualitative)	Health and social services professionals involved in end-of-life care services delivery to homeless persons	Healthcare professionals and managers (n = 54)	2, 3	32/33 Good
[45]	To determine the benefits and barriers of in-shelter palliative care and possible enablers to future implementation in Toronto	Canada	Three shelters	Semi-structured individual interviews (qualitative)	Shelter-based social service providers	Case workers, social support workers, shelter managers (n = 5)	2, 3	23/19 Moderate
[40]	To examine the treatment preferences of homeless (in comparison with preferences of physicians likely to be providing care for homeless persons and patients with oxygen-dependent COPD)	USA	Homeless shelters, hospitals	Cross-sectional survey (quantitative)	Visitors of homeless shelters, physicians providing care to homeless persons, patients with COPD	Homeless (n = 229), physicians (n = 236), COPD-patients (n = 111)	1, 3	31/32 Good
[44]	To improve the understanding of elderly homeless persons and to describe the living circumstances of the group, especially housing	USA	Multidisciplinary Street Team of Boston	Analysis of an intervention[a] (quantitative)	Elderly homeless individuals (> 50)	Homeless (n = 30)	2, 3	15/13 Poor
[48]	To explore if effective shelter-based palliative care could be provided to terminally ill homeless individuals at substantial cost savings	Canada	Shelter-based palliative care hospice	Analysis of records of a cohort and a five-member panel (quantitative)	Terminally ill homeless	Records of homeless (n = 28)	2, 3	32/30 Good
[38]	To explore the importance of end-of-life care for homeless people and the type of concerns	USA	Sites for homeless in Minnesota	Focus groups (qualitative)	Homeless individuals	Homeless (n = 57)	1, 2, 3	18 Poor
[33]	To understand the viewpoints of people who are homeless regarding end-of-life issues, to elucidate the barriers to good end-of-life care, and to offer insight into the most basic needs and wishes.	USA	Homeless shelter, two service organizations for homeless	Focus groups (qualitative)	Homeless individuals and social workers	Homeless (n = 11) service providers (n = 9)	1, 2, 3	23/24 Moderate

Table 1 Characteristics of the papers included (Continued)

Reference	Aim	Country	Setting	Method	Participants	N	Information on 1,2, 3,[b]	Critical appraisal score[c]
[29]	To explore the experiences and attitudes toward death and dying among homeless persons.	USA	Social service agencies which serve homeless	Focus groups (qualitative)	Homeless individuals	Homeless (n = 53)	1, 2, 3	30/35 Good
[28]	To examine how homelessness influences concerns and desires about care at the time of death.	USA	Social service agencies which serve homeless people	Focus groups (qualitative)	Homeless individuals	Homeless (n = 53)	1, 2, 3	29/32 Good
[46]	To improve the EOL decision-making process for homeless persons by facilitating ACP	USA	Drop-in centre	RCT comparing two types of interventions[a] (quantitative)	Homeless individuals	Homeless (n = 59)	2, 3	32/35 Good
[42]	To determine whether homeless persons will complete a counselling session on advance care planning and fill out a legal advance directive designed to assess care preferences and preserve the dignity of marginalized persons	USA	Sites serving homeless persons	RCT comparing two type of interventions[a] (quantitative)	Homeless individuals	Homeless (n = 262)	1, 2, 3	31/35 Good
[39]	To increase healthcare providers understanding and insight into how to better provide EOL care for homeless people.	USA	Free urban healthcare clinic for homeless individuals	Focus groups (qualitative)	Homeless individuals	Homeless (n = 20)	1, 2, 3	31/28 Good
[34]	To identify and examine the needs of older people who are homeless or who have previously experienced homelessness as they age and are faced with the issues of serious ill health, dying and death.	Ireland	Community where care, accommodation and support are being provided for people experiencing homelessness and those at risk	Interviews (qualitative)	Homeless individuals	Homeless (n = 16)	1, 2, 3	22 Moderate
[35]	To explore the views of hostel staff regarding palliative and end-of-life care for the homeless population	UK	Intermediate or long stay hostels	Semi-structured individual interviews (qualitative)	Hostel workers	Hostel workers (n = 7)	1, 2, 3	28/33 Good

[a]Method includes an intervention
[b]1 = Concerns, care needs and future preferences for care and treatment of seriously ill homeless people needs; 2 = the care provided: barriers and facilitators; 3 = recommendations for practice
[c]Score 1 = HTK, score 2 = AJEV

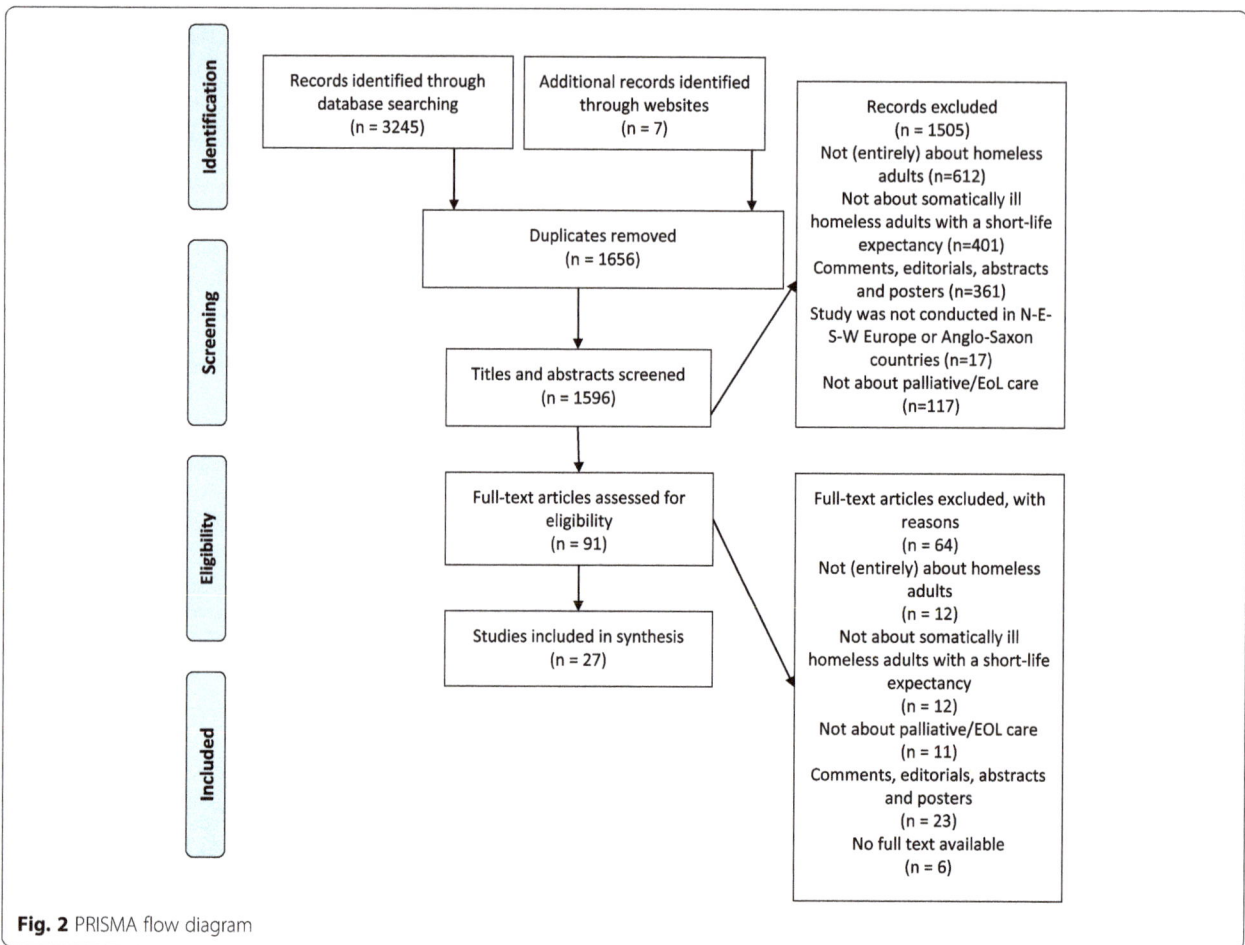

Fig. 2 PRISMA flow diagram

participants and characteristics of healthcare providers were reported less often.

Concerns, care needs and future preferences for care and treatment of seriously ill homeless people

Table 2 shows the main results we extracted from the publications regarding concerns, care needs and future preferences of seriously ill homeless people about the end of life. The 'concerns' considered problems that homeless people had or issues they worried about. Concerns in the physical domain often were about serious illnesses and physical distress [29–31]. Psychological concerns were mostly related to fear of death and dying [24, 28, 29, 32–35]. Social concerns were mostly about being a burden to others [24, 28, 31, 35]. Spiritual concerns were hardly mentioned and were regularly described as consisting of fear of the unknown [31, 33]. Frequently mentioned concerns about care included homeless people expecting end-of-life care to be poor [23, 29, 36, 37].

Care needs concerned topics about the care (including palliative care) that homeless people preferred or expected. Attitudes and behaviour of healthcare

professionals was a theme that was often mentioned, in which treatment with respect and dignity was stated most often [28, 31, 38]. Needs concerning involvement of the family appeared to be somewhat variable. Some of the homeless want family nearby, others do not want to burden their families [28, 38] and some request some type of social contact with family and friends before dying even if they are estranged [24, 32]. Needs for treatment and care appeared to be an important theme; the most frequently mentioned were spirituality and religion [23, 24, 33, 34]. Although few spiritual concerns were mentioned in included studies, spirituality and religion appear to be important encouraging factors for homeless people when it comes needs for treatment and care. In addition, most mentioned was the possibility of expressing various concerns, such as anonymity, estrangement and maintaining control: advance care planning or documentation can help express these concerns [28, 29, 33, 39]. Only one study looked at the domain 'after death', showing an explicit and detailed desire that homeless people's bodies be laid to rest in a personally and culturally acceptable manner [28]. 'Preferences for future care and treatment,' was where we grouped the preferences

Table 2 Concerns, care needs and future preferences for care and treatment among seriously ill homeless people

Concerns	Care needs	Preferences for future care and treatment
Physical domain • Concerns about serious illnesses and physical distress related to specific illnesses, e.g. heart disease, open heart surgery, multiple broken bones [28, 29, 31] • Fear of inappropriate and/or prolonged medical care and heroic treatments [28, 33] • Concerns about losing control over basic physical functions [24] • Concerns about being off medication [31] Psychological domain • Fear of death and dying, partly due to bad and lonely deaths of other homeless people [24, 28, 29, 32–34, 37] • Concerns about psychiatric disorders, in particular schizophrenia, mental illness, depression, affective disorder, anxiety, hearing voices, PTSD, bipolarity, uncontrolled anger [24, 31] • Fear of experiencing death by accident or violence [24, 33] Social domain • Concerns about being a burden on others [24, 28, 31, 35] • Fear of losing independence [24, 31, 33] • Concerns about dying alone [24, 31, 33] • Worries about relationships with friends and family, e.g. family not being notified, leaving a wife and children behind, lack of resources to cover burial costs, being alone, family may not show up [31, 33] • Fear of dying anonymously and no-one will be there to view their body [28, 33] • Fear that family may not know wishes, peers might help to a certain extent, but no assumptions of this help [33] • Concerns about being homeless [31] Spiritual domain • Fear of the unknown [31] • Fear that the death rituals for their culture may not take place [33] Care domain • Many patients had bad experiences from previous healthcare and social service encounters, homeless persons believe that care will be poor at the end of life [23, 29, 36, 37] • Concerns about lack of insurance and receiving sub-optimal treatment due to discrimination by HCP's/insurance companies [31, 39] • Concerns about what will happen to the body after death, fear that their body will not be respected or taken care of [28, 33] • Homeless people who completed an advance direction worry more about the care they would receive if seriously ill or dying [36] • Fear of what will happen if no-one can speak for them [33] • Fear of being transferred to a nursing home [34]	Attitudes/behaviour of healthcare professionals • Homeless patients want to be treated with respect and dignity, e.g. treat patients like others, no judging/labelling, accept patients for who they are [28, 31, 38] • Physicians are preferred as decision-makers regarding end-of-life care treatment [23, 40] • Wish for companionship at the end of life, seeking relationship-centred, compassionate care [28, 39] • Acknowledging emotions; many homeless people have experienced tremendous losses in life. Intensifying of emotions could interfere with participants' future decision-making process [39] • Providers who tell the truth [31] • Providers who respect privacy [31] • Providers should recognize cultural differences, this will serve as the basis for increasing sensitivity and trust [23] • Death and dying are perceived to be temporary matters, and many thought dwelling on the end of life situation was undesirable [23] • Patients prefer to use a GP who specializes in the care of the homeless [32] Involvement of family • Some of the homeless persons want family nearby, others (often a majority) do not want to burden their families [28, 38] • Requests for some form of social contact with family and friends and resolving remaining issues and disagreements before dying even if they were estranged [24, 32] • Participants who are not in contact with their family desire to be placed in a familiar environment where they could be surrounded by a social support network [24] Treatment/care options • Spirituality and religion are important components in defining life and death [23, 24, 33, 34] • Desire for advance care planning/ documentation; this relates to several concerns (anonymity, estrangement, maintaining control, discussion with significant others), with trust as an important condition [28, 29, 33, 39] • Requests for detoxification [32] • Patients predominantly interact with GPS for prescriptions [32] • End-of-life care focus on pain control [28] • Asking how they would like to be remembered, including post-death wishes [31] After death • Explicit and detailed desires that homeless people's bodies be laid to rest in a personally and culturally acceptable manner (due to the misconceptions and fears about body disposal) [28]	Treatment preferences • *Resuscitation:* - Almost all homeless persons expressed a preferences to receive cardiopulmonary resuscitation (CPR) in the event of cardiorespiratory arrest if there was a chance of returning to their current state of health[a] [41] - Homeless people want resuscitation more than physicians and patients with COPD [40] - Homeless men are more likely to want resuscitation than homeless women [40] - Non-white homeless people are more likely to want resuscitation or life-sustaining treatment than white homeless people [40, 42] • *Life sustaining treatment:* - Nearly half of the homeless participants (8/17) indicated that they would want all measures taken, a smaller proportion (7/8) would prefer limited treatment [31] - Between 20% and 37% want life-sustaining treatment depending on condition (lowest in case of dependence, highest for unconsciousness [42] - 31% desired no life-sustaining treatment if dying [42] - In the scenario of a permanent coma or severe dementia, homeless people are more likely to want CPR or mechanical ventilation than physicians [40] Wishes for the dying process • A natural death (dying in sleep, no artificial medical interventions to prolong life, avoiding heroic measures such as prolonged life support without hope of functional recovery) [24, 33, 38] • Homeless people want to have their wishes represented when they become incompetent and/or dying [23, 39] • Dying peacefully, taking care of inner conflicts, being able to express love, apologizing to family and others [24] • Death without suffering [24] Proxy decision-makers • A significant proportion of homeless people named a proxy decision-maker[a] [41] • Nearly all chosen surrogate decision-makers were not related; most often they were service providers, friends or (occasionally) romantic partners [28] • 29% to 34% of homeless participants showed a (written) preference for surrogate decision-making [42] • 87% of homeless participants named a family member as a surrogate decision-maker in their completed advance directives [42]

[a]When completing an advance directive

homeless people had in advance for the end of life; we grouped them into three domains, namely treatment preferences, the dying process and surrogate-decision making. Regarding the first domain 'treatment preferences', a lot of studies mentioned resuscitation and life-sustaining treatments, preferences were found to vary among subgroups of homeless people [31, 40–42]. In terms of the wishes for the dying process, a natural death was mentioned most often [24, 33, 38], e.g. no prolonged life support without hope of functional recovery. Lastly, surrogate decision-making appeared to be an important theme for homeless people at the end of life, in particular the naming of proxy to make decisions [28, 41, 42].

The care provided: barriers and facilitators

Tables 3 and 4 show the results in terms of the barriers and facilitators for providing care to seriously ill homeless people. To give an overview of those barriers and facilitators, we identified and described three perspectives. The perspective called 'barriers and facilitators relating to the homeless person' revealed a lot of barriers and some facilitators. The most commonly mentioned barriers were themes related to receiving healthcare, such as end-of-life care not being a priority and living on a day-to-day basis [23, 26, 34, 39, 43], themes regarding social relationships such as the absence of support from family members and only having small networks [30, 33, 37], and themes about health-related and other behaviour, such as the limited insights homeless people have into their own health [32, 44]. Although studies reported more barriers than facilitators within this theme, a widely mentioned facilitator for homeless people was the importance of religious beliefs and spiritual experience [24, 28, 39].

Contrasting with the previous theme, a lot of studies in the theme 'relating to the interaction between homeless people and healthcare professionals' described facilitators and substantially fewer studies described barriers between homeless people and professionals. The attitudes of healthcare providers towards homeless persons proved to be a major theme, e.g. building and establishing relationships of trust [25, 32, 35, 37]. The treatment of homeless people was also reported to be an important theme as facilitator, e.g. a pragmatic and flexible approach from staff [25, 37, 45]. Furthermore, providing activities and therapies was also often mentioned as facilitator for the interaction between homeless people and healthcare professionals, e.g. counsellor-guided advance directive completion [41, 42, 46]. Feelings of being ignored, discriminated against and disrespected by healthcare providers and a lack of trust were often mentioned as barriers [26, 33, 35–38, 45]. For barriers and facilitators in the third theme, 'relating to healthcare professionals', substantially more barriers than facilitators were mentioned. The most frequently mentioned barriers were lack of knowledge and skills of professionals, e.g. the difficulty for staff in determining when a patient is nearing the dying phase and meeting the palliative care needs [32, 33, 35, 37]. Another barrier mentioned relating to healthcare professionals was the organization of care, e.g. minimal access to palliative care [26–28, 32, 36, 38, 47]. On the other hand, facilitators relating to the knowledge and skills of professionals such as optimizing management of pain, symptoms and functional decline were often mentioned [48, 49]. Facilitators regarding the overall organization of palliative care for homeless people were not found in many papers; one facilitator mentioned in a Canadian study by Podymow et al. was in-shelter hospice care, which also substantially lowers the costs [48].

Recommendations for practice

A significant number of studies made evidence-based recommendations for practice regarding (palliative) care for seriously ill homeless people, themes are shown in Table 5 and more detailed information on the themes is shown in Additional file 4. Training, education and knowledge; delivering care, and overall organization appeared to be the comprehensive themes. A very often mentioned recommendation relating to training, education and knowledge was training for staff working with homeless people to provide palliative care as health deteriorates and death approaches [26, 27, 34, 36, 45]. Related to recommendations on delivering care, addressing themes related to a patient-centered approach concerning dignity and asking questions about death and dying in advance directive formats were most often mentioned [24, 31, 35–37, 42, 46]. Trustful and respectful relationships were also mentioned as a recommendation for delivering care; as well as attention for different domain of concerns of homeless people compared to healthcare providers, flexible programs and availability and support after death. Recommendations concerning overall organization of palliative care to homeless people concerned mostly the availability of accommodation, involved persons and coordination, policies and guidelines and partnering and exchange of knowledge between organizations. This included partnering social communities with the end-of-life care system, such as accessibility and availability of palliative care beds [34, 45].

Discussion

This systematic review summarizes 23 relevant studies: 15 qualitative and eight quantitative studies. The concerns, needs, preferences and the barriers and facilitators described in these studies often concern the attitudes and behaviour of healthcare professionals. In particular, a respectful approach and respect for dignity proved to be important to homeless people for good quality palliative care.

Table 3 The care provided care: barriers relating to homeless people, interaction between homeless people and healthcare professionals, and healthcare professionals

Relating to the homeless people	Relating to the interaction between homeless people and healthcare professionals	Relating to the healthcare professionals
In relation to receiving healthcare • End-of-life care is not a priority; to obtain the basic necessities of survival and living on a day-to-day basis takes precedence over efforts to obtain health and/or end-of-life care [23, 26, 34, 38, 43] • Drug and/or alcohol dependence and non-disclosure of illicit drug use may lead to decreased opportunities for persons to remain in their usual abode or to receive and/or adhere to treatment at traditional end-of-life services due to anti-drug policies [26, 27, 34, 47] • Planning care activities and attending for hospital appointments is often difficult: patients frequently do not adhere to expected routines, arrangements for health service activities, GP and hospital appointments and often have to be reminded about their condition, homeless people are reluctant due to a long waiting time and/or they self-discharge [32, 34, 37] • Very late stage of seeking help and thus medical problems that are difficult to handle and multiple admissions before death [37, 43, 47] • A lot of homeless people are unwilling to accept the recommended treatment [44, 47] • Pain and symptom management of homeless persons who use illicit drugs (high levels of opioid tolerance) and specialists who are unable or unwilling due to fears that they would be liable for adverse reactions [26] • Lack of health insurance [43] In relation to social relationship • No support from family members or relatives and small networks and many without trusted peers [30, 33, 37] • A lot of homeless people who have psychiatric illness and are paranoia, refuse multiple offers of housing [44] • Travel and access to transport when living in a rural area [34] • Relationships between healthier and sicker patients are complex and sometimes manipulative to gain access to further alcohol [32] • Death and dying does affect other homeless patients [32] In relation to (health) behaviour • Limited insight into their condition or unable to acknowledge illnesses [32, 44] • Problems relating to alcohol and/or drug addiction, such as denial of addiction, bingeing, ignoring of risks of overdose [32] • Aggressive or changing behavior [32] • Unwillingness to pay attention to their personal hygiene [32]	• Feelings of being ignored, discriminated and disrespected by healthcare providers and a lack of trust and suspicion (e.g. shown disrespect, withholding of pain medication, inappropriately short hospital stays, not respecting wishes) that initially has to be overcome before any treatment could be started [26, 33, 35–38, 45] • End of life is an uncomfortable topic; some homeless persons do not want to know about their own diagnoses, do not want to talk about their health concerns or are incapable of talking comfortably about death and dying [23, 35, 36] • Barriers to achieving the level of communication and connections homeless people desired, e.g. too little time to chat with staff and volunteers because they were busy [34, 39] • Patients engage with internal services such as key and substance misuse workers but rarely with mental health or social workers [32] • Homeless people express many misperceptions and uncertainties about surrogate decision-making [28] • Homeless persons often describe their problems in a jumbled manner, understanding the most prioritized needs is thus not always easy [37]	Knowledge and skills • It is difficult for staff to determine when a patient is nearing the dying phase and to establish palliative care needs; staff members' notions of palliative care vary and opportunities to prevent deaths are being missed [32, 33, 35, 37, 43] • Deaths of homeless patients are often sudden, staff were often upset [32, 33] • Hostel staff are often not able to plan for end-of-life care with patients [32] • Medical intake personnel (in hospital) do not know how to deal with a homeless person [47] • Little opportunity for funding or training shelter staff in palliative care [45] • Working with limited medical information [35] • Staff of healthcare services not being knowledgeable about the unique issues facing the homeless [36] • Often difficult to interpret reaction of patients suffering from mental illness and/or illicit drug use [37] • Trying to solve all of a patient's problems at once is seldom successful [37] Organization • Access to palliative care, primary care and/or preventive services is minimal (due to competing priorities, attitude of healthcare professionals, anti-drug policies, not conforming to procedures, healthcare system's nonadherence to harm reduction strategies, a lack of caregiver support and/or financial resources) and a significant proportion of homeless persons may be underusing healthcare [25, 27, 28, 32, 36, 38, 43, 47] • Lack of appropriate housing, beds, respite or hospice facilities and programmes and care sites for homeless people at the end of life and limited resources for providing end-of-life care [25, 28, 44, 45, 49] • Poor coordination and/or communication between secondary care and hostel staff or homeless programmes and end-of-life programmes [32, 35, 49] • Setting treatment goals according to routine guidelines were often regarded as unrealistic in this context [37] • In-shelter palliative care means more work for staff and a greater burden for a workforce already thinly stretched [45] • Cost of medications that was not covered by the benefits and had to be paid for in cash [30]

In addition, the limited knowledge and skills of professionals turned out to be important barriers in palliative care for homeless people. Related to that, recommendations in the studies included often concern a need for training, education and broadening of knowledge. This emphasis on change of attitudes and behaviour of healthcare

Table 4 The care provided care: facilitators relating to homeless people, interaction between homeless people and healthcare professionals, and healthcare professionals

Relating to the homeless people	Relating to the interaction between homeless people and healthcare professionals	Relating to the healthcare professionals
• Primacy of religious beliefs and spiritual experience or connection; religious beliefs are a core component of homeless people's end-of-life beliefs and experiences; it provides comfort and solace through spirituality/religion [24, 28, 39] • Allow for patients to have "unscheduled" space to share their life stories and to acknowledge those stories [37] • Freedom is essential to homeless people [33] • Other homeless patients could become involved in the care of fellow residents who are unwilling to work with services [32] • Among homeless people who filled out an AD, there were increasing in plans to write down end-of-life wishes, plans to talk about these wishes with someone and less worrying about death [46]	Attitude towards homeless people • Building and establishing trusting and/or family-like relationships and contact by interacting with patients in everyday situations and staff taking a supportive and/or advocating role in encounters with other health providers [25, 32, 35, 37] • Upholding homeless residents' dignity and maintaining pride by showing human kindness, respect, love, comfort and to name accomplishments and elements of character [29, 31, 35, 37] • Staff must never judge a homeless person as impossible, or in terms of failure, and always patiently give them a new chance [37] • Persistence to engage the patient and to keep them engaged, with a constant effort required for effective follow-up [47] Treatment of homeless people • A pragmatic approach by staff, facilitating flexible care solutions, such as the choice where to die and accepting that planned activities may not happen or need to be cancelled [25, 37, 45] • Compassionate healthcare providers who are present (e.g. not leaving the individual alone during or after death [25, 28, 37] • Staff can respect individual's habits and needs (also if rather unconventional, friends and preferred surroundings (e.g. stay in the hostel) when they are at the end of life [32, 36] • Staff only contacting family members at the end of life if the patients so request [37] • Formulating simple messages towards patients about death and dying [37] Activities/therapies • Advance directive completion rate is higher when counsellor guided that compared to no counsellor guidance [41, 42, 46] • Low-threshold strategies have an increased capacity to deliver end-of-life care services [26, 27] • Harm reduction services (e.g. clean needle exchange, medically prescribed alcohol) are a critical point of entry to and source of end-of-life care and support for homeless people who use alcohol and/or illicit drugs and are unable to access services [25, 48] • Physical contact can enable feelings of safety and appreciation in patients (not all patients) [37] • Memorial services held by staff to give staff members and other patients or visitors a moment to remember and say farewell [37]	Knowledge and skills • Optimizing management of pain, symptoms and functional decline, e.g. by palliative care consultations [48, 49] • End-of-life care and addiction training [26] • To preserve integrity in being close to patients [37] • Treatment for symptoms and distress is often provided simultaneously with the use of illicit drugs and/or alcohol, this necessitates special skills for identification of signs and symptoms and treatment regimens [37] Organization In-shelter hospice care; without it, a large part of homeless patients might not have sought care or received services and died homeless with no pain and symptom management [48] • Costs of in-shelter hospice care are substantially less than the estimated costs of traditional care for the same patients [48]

professionals so that the needs of homeless people can be met was less apparent in the three other reviews that also concerned palliative care for homeless people [10, 16, 17].

Furthermore, many of the barriers we found in the studies proved to be related to the homeless people themselves. End-of-life care is often not a priority for them. Besides this, homeless people are often dependent on drugs, have limited insight into their condition and little support from family and relatives, which all make good palliative care extra challenging. Moreover, the

Table 5 Themes regarding recommendations for practice

Training, education and knowledge	Delivering care	Overall organization
• Training regarding providing palliative care for (older) homeless people and their specific needs • Education about addressing preferences, advance directives, after death wishes and surrogate decision-makers	• Patient-centred approach • Trustful and respectful relationships • Reliability, experience, sensitivity and commitment of healthcare professionals • Attention to various areas of concern of homeless people • Flexible programmes and availability • Support after death	• Availability of accommodation • People involved and coordination • Hospital discharge policies • Policies and guidelines • Partnering and exchange of knowledge between organizations

views of homeless people about what is needed for good palliative care might differ from the views of healthcare providers. Hence, palliative care for homeless people needs a tailored approach and dialogue between healthcare providers and homeless people, as recently mentioned by Tobey et al. [7]. These outcomes are in line with the findings of the three other reviews [10, 16, 17].

As this review included relatively many studies and the methodological quality of the majority of studies was rated as good, it provides good insights into what is presently known with regard to palliative care for homeless people. At the same time, the review also sheds light on gaps in that knowledge. A large majority of the studies were conducted in the USA and Canada. More studies from other countries are needed as it is very well possible that differences in culture, the organization of homeless care and the organization of healthcare could lead to different results for different countries. It remains for instance to be seen whether spirituality and religion – which proved very important to homeless people in this study – will be as important in more secular countries such as the Netherlands. Furthermore, the studies that had qualitative designs often provide important insights into the experiences and ideas of homeless people and their care providers that are helpful in initiatives aimed at improving the care. Although this review mentioned that homeless people get minimal access to palliative care, primary care and/or preventive services, no details are known about homeless people who completely avoid care. If healthcare providers want to provide tailored palliative care to the entire target group, more research is needed into palliative care for homeless people who avoid care. Because the homeless people who avoid care are hard to reach, it is advisable to do participatory observation or to interview people who use successful methods to reach them, such as street pastors. Finally, more information is needed about healthcare providers who provide palliative care to homeless people. The studies included mostly concerned characteristics of homeless people, but little is known about the background characteristics in terms of the experience and preferences of healthcare providers. Future studies can study the healthcare professionals. This can help provide tailored training, education and knowledge for healthcare providers.

Our review also included intervention studies that provide information about interventions for tailoring palliative care to the needs of homeless people. Several studies indicated advance care planning and documentation as a potentially effective way of encountering the concerns and needs of homeless people, such as a fear of death, anonymity, estrangement, maintaining control and discussions with significant others. These studies were also included in the review by Sumalinog et al. that focused on interventions [10]. In that review, the methodology of these studies was rated at between poor and fair, which is lower than our methodological ratings. This can be explained by the fact that we used an assessment tool that can be used for various types of studies, while Sumalinog et al. used a tool that was appropriate for assessing whether intervention studies provide strong evidence for the intervention being effective. While this shows that there is no strong evidence for the interventions being effective, the results of these studies can provide pointers to help develop new interventions and study them thoroughly.

Strengths and limitations
One strength of this systematic review is that it looks at the concerns, care needs and preferences, barriers and facilitators and recommendations for practice, thereby providing a broad overview of topics that are relevant to palliative care for homeless people. In addition, the broad inclusion criteria resulted in a large number of studies being included (given the limited size of the field being researched). Moreover, this review combines both qualitative and quantitative studies. Finally, another strength of this systematic review is that doing a grey literature search meant that we also included studies by organizations working in the field, such as Simon Communities and St. Mungo's.

An initial limitation of this study is that the definition and terminology of palliative and/or end-of-life care differ according to the study. Studies may therefore include other aspects of palliative or end-of-life care while using the same definition and terminology. A second limitation is that both studies of seriously ill homeless people and studies of homeless people who expressed their expectations about being seriously ill have been included. Expectations about the end of life in advance may differ from the reality later. Another limitation was that, although we aimed only to summarize the recommendations from the studies' results, it is was not always certain that the recommendations were not also reflections of the author's opinions. As a fourth limitation, this systematic review lacks studies in published in languages other than English. Finally, a methodological limitation was that in some studies it was difficult to assess the methodological quality because some information was missing. It is possible that in those cases the actual study was conducted in a more thorough way than reported on in the article.

Conclusions

Homeless people at the end of life experience a range of problems and barriers concerning access to palliative care. A tailored, flexible and low-threshold approach consisting of awareness about the fear of death among homeless people (as well as priorities and needs of homeless people other than those assessed by healthcare professionals) can be used to help provide appropriate care in good time. This tailored, flexible and low-threshold approach should at least involve awareness of the concerns of homeless people (fear of death and negative experiences with healthcare providers). This requires sensitivity and patience of healthcare professionals. In addition, awareness about the meaning of dignity and respect to the homeless patient is important when it comes to understanding the needs of homeless people, as well as recognizing important components such as religiosity and documentation of future preferences. Finally, healthcare professionals need to be aware that future preferences may be different for homeless patients compared to a non-homeless patient, and therefore ask specific questions about it. Training, education and experience of healthcare providers can accomplish this.

Additional files

Additional file 1: Search strategies. (DOCX 28 kb)

Additional file 2: Details of assessments of studies by using the Critical Appraisal Tool. (DOCX 22 kb)

Additional file 3: Characteristics of study populations. (DOCX 29 kb)

Additional file 4: Recommendations for practice. (DOCX 30 kb)

Abbreviations

AIDS: Acquired immune deficiency syndrome; COPD: Chronic obstructive pulmonary disease; PRISMA: Preferred reporting items for systematic reviews and meta-analysis; WHO: World Health Organization; ZonMw: The Netherlands Organisation for Health Research and Development

Acknowledgements

The authors wish to thank Johannes C. F. Ket (Medical Library, Vrije Universiteit, Amsterdam, The Netherlands) for his assistance in designing and conducting the literature searches.

Funding

The author(s) received a grant of The Netherlands Organisation for Health Research and Development (ZonMw, grant number 844001205) for doing this systematic review. The authors declare no conflict of interest.

Authors' contributions

HTK planned, conducted and prepared the manuscript for publication. HTK conducted and performed the literature searches with the help of JCFK. HTK and SID screened the papers to be eligible for the full text screening. BDO was consulted in the event of disagreement. HTK and AJEC developed the extraction form, extracted the data of the first five studies and performed the methodological assessments. HTK extracted the data of the other papers, which was checked by AJEV. HTK classified the data into categories, which were first discussed with BDO. Then, categories and classifications were discussed with ALF, JACR, AJEV and SID. All authors read and approved the final manuscript.

Competing interests

The authors declare that they have no competing interests with respect to the research, authorship, and/or publication of this article.

Author details

[1]Amsterdam Public Health Research Institute (APH), Department of Public and Occupational Health, Expertise Centre for Palliative Care, VU University Medical Center, P.O. Box 7057, 1007 MB Amsterdam, The Netherlands. [2]Netherlands Institute for Health Services Research (NIVEL), P.O. Box 1568, 3500 BN Utrecht, Netherlands. [3]Department of Public Health, Erasmus University Medical Center, P.O. Box 2040, 3000 CA Rotterdam, Netherlands.

References

1. National Health Care for the Homeless Council. Official definition of homelessness. https://www.nhchc.org/faq/official-definition-homelessness/. Accessed on March 21, 2018.
2. Department for Communities and Local Government. Statutory homelessness: October to December quarter 2015, in 26 homelessness statistical release 2016. London: Stationery Office; 2016.
3. Kushel MB, Miaskowski C. End-of-life care for homeless patients: "she says she is there to help me in any situation". JAMA. 2006;296:2959–66.
4. Hwang S. Mental illness and mortality among homeless people. Acta Psychiatr Scand. 2001;103:81–2.
5. van Laere I, de Wit M, Klazinga N. Shelter-based convalescence for homeless adults in Amsterdam: a descriptive study. BMC Health Serv Res. 2009;9:208.
6. Slockers MT, Nusselder WJ, Rietjens J, van Beeck EF. Unnatural death: a major but largely preventable cause-of-death among homeless people? Eur J Pub Health. 2018; https://doi.org/10.1093/eurpub/cky002.
7. Tobey M, Manasson J, Decarlo K, Ciraldo-Maryniuk K, Gaeta JM, Wilson E. Homeless individuals approaching the end of life: symptoms and attitudes. J Pain Symptom Manag. 2017;53:738–44.
8. Davis-Behrman J. Serious illness and end-of-life care in the homeless: examining a service system and a call for action for social work. Soc Work Soc. 2016;14:1–11.
9. Garibaldi B, Conde-Martel A, O'Toole TP. Self-reported comorbidities, perceived needs, and sources for usual care for older and younger homeless adults. J Gen Intern Med. 2005;20:726–30.
10. Sumalinog R, Harrington K, Dosani N, Hwang SW. Advance care planning, palliative care, and end-of-life care interventions for homeless people: a systematic review. Palliat Med. 2016;31:109–19.

Palliative care for homeless people: a systematic review of the concerns, care needs and preferences...

39

11. Hwang SW, Orav EJ, O'Connell JJ, Lebow JM, Brennan TA. Causes of death in homeless adults in Boston. Ann Intern Med. 1997;126:625–8.

12. Barrow SM, Herman DB, Cordova P, Struening EL. Mortality among homeless shelter residents in new York City. Am J Public Health. 1999;89:529–34.

13. Vuillermoz C, Aouba A, Grout L, Vandentorren S, Tassin F, Moreno-Betancur M, et al. Mortality among homeless people in France, 2008-10. Eur J Pub Health. 2016;26:1028–33.

14. Hwang SW. Mortality among men using homeless shelters in Toronto, Ontario. JAMA. 2000;283:2152–7.

15. WHO. Global atlas of palliative care at the end of life. http://www.who.int/nmh/Global_Atlas_of_Palliative_Care.pdf. Accessed 9 June 2017.

16. Hudson BF, Flemming K, Shulman C, Candy B. Challenges to access and provision of palliative care for people who are homeless: a systematic review of qualitative research. BMC Palliat Care. 2016;15:1–18.

17. Hubbell SA. Advance care planning with individuals experiencing homelessness: literature review and recommendations for public health practice. Public Health Nurs. 2017; https://doi.org/10.1111/phn.12333.

18. Preferred Reporting Items for Systematic Reviews and Meta-Analysis (PRISMA). www.prisma-statement.org. Accessed 24 Mar 2016.

19. Covidence Online Software. www.covidence.org. Accessed 6 June 2016.

20. Landis G, Koch CG. The measurement of observer agreement for categorical data. Biometrics. 1977;33:159–74.

21. Sandelowski M, Voils CI, Barosso J. Defining and designing mixed research synthesis studies. Res Sch. 2006;13:29.

22. Hawker S, Payne S, Kerr C, Hardey M, Powell J. Appraising the evidence: reviewing disparate data systematically. Qual Health Res. 2002;12:1284–99.

23. Ko E, Nelson-Becker H. Does end-of-life decision making matter? Perspectives of older homeless adults. Am J Hosp Palliat Care. 2014;31:183–8.

24. Ko E, Kwak J, Nelson-Becker H. What constitutes a good and bad death?: Perspectives of homeless older adults. Death Stud. 2015;39:422–32.

25. McNeil R, Guirguis-Yonger M, Dilley LB, Aubry TD, Turnbull J, Hwang SW. Harm reduction services as a point-of-entry to and source of end-of-life care and support for homeless and marginally housed persons who use alcohol and/or illicit drugs: a qualitative analysis. BMC Public Health. 2012;12:312.

26. McNeil R, Guirguis-Younger M. Illicit drug use as a challenge to the delivery of end-of-life care services to homeless persons: perceptions of health and social services professionals. Palliat Med. 2012;26:350–9.

27. McNeil R, Guirguis-Younger M, Dilley LB. Recommendations for improving the end-of-life care system for homeless populations: a qualitative study of the views of Canadian health and social services professionals. BMC Palliat Care. 2012;11:14.

28. Song J, Bartels DM, Ratner ER, Alderton L, Hudson B, Ahluwalia JS. Dying on the streets: homeless persons' concerns and desires about end of life care. J Gen Intern Med. 2007;22:435–41.

29. Song J, Ratner ER, Bartels DM, Alderton L, Hudson B, Ahluwalia JS. Experiences with and attitudes toward death and dying among homeless persons. J Gen Intern Med. 2007;22:427–34.

30. McGrath BB. The social networks of terminally ill skid road residents: an analysis. Public Health Nurs. 1986;3:192–205.

31. Bartels DM, Ulvestad N, Ratner E, Wall M, Uutala MM, Song J. Dignity matters: advance care planning for people experiencing homelessness. J Clin Ethics. 2008;19:214–22.

32. Davis S, Kennedy P, Greenish W, Jones L. Supporting homeless people with advanced liver disease approaching the end of life. 2011. https://www.mariecurie.org.uk/globalassets/media/documents/commissioning-our-services/current-partnerships/st-mungos-supporting-homeless-may-11.pdf. Accessed 8 May 2016.

33. Song J, Ratner ER, Bartels DM. Dying while homeless: is it a concern when life itself is such a struggle? J Clin Ethics. 2005;16:251–61.

34. Walsh K. Homeless, ageing and dying. 2013. http://www.drugsandalcohol.ie/21659/1/Homelessness_Ageing_and_Dying.pdf. Accessed 10 May 2016.

35. Webb WA. When dying at home is not an option: exploration of hostel staff views on palliative care for homeless people. Int J Palliat Nurs. 2015;21:236–44.

36. Krakowsky Y, Gofine M, Brown P, Danziger J, Knowles H. Increasing access-a qualitative study of homelessness and palliative care in a Major Urban Center. Am J Hosp Palliat Care. 2013;30:268–70.

37. Hakanson C, Sandberg J, Ekstedt M, Kenne Sarnmalm E, Christiansen M, Ohlén J. Providing palliative Care in a Swedish Support Home for people who are homeless. Qual Health Res. 2016;26:1252–62.

38. Ratner D, Bartels D, Song JA. Perspective on homelessness, ethics, and medical care. Minn Med. 2004;87:50–2.

39. Tarzian AJ, Neal MT, O'Neil JA. Attitudes, experiences, and beliefs affecting end-of-life decision-making among homeless individuals. J Palliat Med. 2005;8:36–48.

40. Norris WM, Nielsen EL, Engelberg RA, Curtis JR. Treatment preferences for resuscitation and critical care among homeless persons. Chest. 2005;127:2180–7.

41. Leung AK, Nayyar D, Sachdeva M, Song J, Hwang SW. Chronically homeless persons' participation in an advance directive intervention: a cohort study. Palliat Med. 2015;28:746–55.

42. Song J, Ratner ER, Wall MM, Bartels DM, Ulvestad N, Petroskas D, et al. Effect of an end-of-life planning intervention on the completion of advance directives in homeless persons: a randomized trial. Ann Intern Med. 2010;153:76–84.

43. Hwang SW, O'Connell JJ, Lebow JM, Bierer MF, Orav EJ, Brennan TA. Health care utilization among homeless adults prior to death. J Health Care Poor Underserved. 2001;12:50–8.

44. O'Connell JJ, Roncarati JS, Reilly EC, Kane CA, Morrison SK, Swain SE, et al. Old and sleeping rough: elderly homeless persons on the streets of Boston. Care Manag J. 2004;5:101–6.

45. Nikouline A, Dosani N. Benefits and barriers to the homeless by in-shelter palliative care: a qualitative study. 2016 http://www.virtualhospice.ca/en_US/Main+Site+Navigation/Home/For+Professionals/For+Professionals/The+Exchange/Current/Benefits+and+Barriers+to+the+Homeless+by+In_Shelter+Palliative+Care_+A+Qualitative+Study.aspx. Accessed 5 May 2016.

46. Song J, Wall MM, Ratner ER, Bartels DM, Ulvestad N, Gelberg L. Engaging homeless persons in end of life preparations. J Gen Intern Med. 2008;23:2031–6.

47. Mac Williams J, Bramwell M, Brown S, O'Connor M. Reaching out to ray: delivering palliative care services to a homeless person in Melbourne, Australia. Int J Palliat Nurs. 2014;20:83–8.

48. Podymow T, Turnbull J, Doyle C. Shelter-based palliative care for the homeless terminally ill. Palliat Med. 2006;20:81–6.

49. Hutt E, Whitfield E, Min SJ, Jones J, Weber M, Albright K, et al. Challenges of providing end-of-life care for homeless veterans. Am J Hosp Palliat Care. 2016;33:381–9.

4

Advance care planning in dementia: recommendations for healthcare professionals

Ruth Piers[1,2], Gwenda Albers[3], Joni Gilissen[2,9*], Jan De Lepeleire[4], Jan Steyaert[5,6], Wouter Van Mechelen[4], Els Steeman[7], Let Dillen[8], Paul Vanden Berghe[3] and Lieve Van den Block[2,9*]

Abstract

Background: Advance care planning (ACP) is a continuous, dynamic process of reflection and dialogue between an individual, those close to them and their healthcare professionals, concerning the individual's preferences and values concerning future treatment and care, including end-of-life care. Despite universal recognition of the importance of ACP for people with dementia, who gradually lose their ability to make informed decisions themselves, ACP still only happens infrequently, and evidence-based recommendations on when and how to perform this complex process are lacking. We aimed to develop evidence-based clinical recommendations to guide professionals across settings in the practical application of ACP in dementia care.

Methods: Following the Belgian Centre for Evidence-Based Medicine's procedures, we 1) performed an extensive literature search to identify international guidelines, articles reporting heterogeneous study designs and grey literature, 2) developed recommendations based on the available evidence and expert opinion of the author group, and 3) performed a validation process using written feedback from experts, a survey for end users (healthcare professionals across settings), and two peer-review groups (with geriatricians and general practitioners).

Results: Based on 67 publications and validation from ten experts, 51 end users and two peer-review groups (24 participants) we developed 32 recommendations covering eight domains: initiation of ACP, evaluation of mental capacity, holding ACP conversations, the role and importance of those close to the person with dementia, ACP with people who find it difficult or impossible to communicate verbally, documentation of wishes and preferences, including information transfer, end-of-life decision-making, and preconditions for optimal implementation of ACP. Almost all recommendations received a grading representing low to very low-quality evidence.

Conclusion: No high-quality guidelines are available for ACP in dementia care. By combining evidence with expert and user opinions, we have defined a unique set of recommendations for ACP in people living with dementia. These recommendations form a valuable tool for educating healthcare professionals on how to perform ACP across settings.

Keywords: Advance care planning, Alzheimer's disease, Dementia, Elderly care, Guideline, Recommendations

* Correspondence: Joni.Gilissen@vub.ac.be; Lvdblock@vub.ac.be
[2]End-of-life Care Research Group, Vrije Universiteit Brussel (VUB) and Ghent University, Laarbeeklaan 103, 1090 Brussels, Belgium
Full list of author information is available at the end of the article

Background

Due to the aging population, the number of people with dementia is increasing. In 2015, the World Health Organization (WHO) estimated the number of people living with dementia at 35.6 million. This is expected to double by 2030 and even triple by 2050 [1].

To enable caregivers to improve the quality of life of people with dementia, they need to know what is important to them, what specific concerns they are facing and how and where they want to receive care. However, people living with dementia gradually lose their ability to make informed decisions themselves [2]. Therefore it may be necessary to have these discussions in the earlier stages of dementia, when the person is still able to make decisions and express their values and preferences [3].

Providing high-quality care for people with dementia requires advance care planning (ACP) [4]. ACP is a continuous, dynamic process of early reflection and dialogue between a person with dementia, those close to them and the relevant healthcare professionals concerning the person's preferences and values when it comes to future treatment and care, including end-of-life care [5]. If they wish, the contents of these conversations can be recorded in the form of an advance directive, and a proxy decision-maker can be appointed or a permanent power of attorney can be granted in anticipation of future deterioration [6, 7].

Despite the widespread recognition of the importance of ACP for people living with dementia [1–3, 8–10], the reality is different, and only a minority of people with dementia get the opportunity to engage in ACP [11]. For example, studies show that a minority of deceased nursing home residents with dementia had an advance directive [12–14] and that general practitioners (GPs) had communicated infrequently about future end-of-life care options. For example, only 22% of deceased nursing home residents in Belgium had an ACP conversation [13]. Even among a representative sample of non-sudden deaths in Belgium and the Netherlands, only 34% of patients had engaged in ACP with their GP [15]. People with dementia are often a disadvantaged group when it comes to being invited for ACP conversations at an appropriate time and cognitive decline is often seen as a barrier to initiate ACP [16–26].

Although several organisations and professionals have called for guidance on when and how to perform ACP in this specific population [1–3], guidelines that have been developed in a systematic way using the best evidence available are lacking. In an attempt to improve the prevalence, quality and consistency of ACP in people with dementia, we aimed to develop clinical recommendations for applying and conducting ACP in practice, to provide support for healthcare staff (physicians, including GPs, nurses, allied health and care workers) who

work with people living with dementia in the community, residential and hospital settings.

Methods

No informed consent was needed for this study. The procedure developed by the Belgian Centre for Evidence-Based Medicine (CEBAM) (in close cooperation with the Belgian Federal Public Service Health, Food Chain Safety and Environment and the two professional Belgian GP organisations Domus Medica and Société Scientifique de Médecin General or SSMG) was used as methodology to develop a guideline. The procedure entails: 1) a literature search to identify what is already known about ACP in people living with dementia, 2) the development of recommendations based on the existing evidence and expert opinion of the author group, and 3) a validation process to provide feedback on the clarity, acceptability and importance and to discuss possible barriers to implement the recommendations.

1) Literature search
Search framework: selection of research questions and clinical themes on ACP and clinical practice

A multidisciplinary group of authors was assembled to develop the recommendations: a research coordinator, a geriatrician, two GPs, an expert in dementia care, a nurse, two psychologists and the director of the Flanders Federation for Palliative Care. Collectively, they have extensive experience in palliative, primary and dementia care in different settings in Flanders (Belgium). Based on their own experience and obstacles they have encountered in practice, this author group formulated clinical research questions related to ACP in people with dementia. Obstacles are defined as those areas in the ACP process that cause ACP not to be initiated at the appropriate time or not to be performed at all. The clarity, applicability and completeness of each clinical research question was evaluated in semi-structured interviews by SM and DN with 28 GPs, of whom 14 also act as coordinating advisory physicians or CAPs in a nursing home and of whom 14 are heads of residential care, all from different nursing homes in Flanders and all familiar with the concept and practice of ACP. Through discussion and consensus within the team of authors, these were categorized to six main clinical themes to guide the literature search (see Table 1).

Search for evidence

We undertook a stepwise approach to search the scientific literature for evidence about ACP in people with dementia related to the six selected clinical themes. Publications were included if (i) they were published in Dutch, French, English or German, (ii) their main theme was ACP in people with dementia, or, if a guideline,

Table 1 The six clinical themes and examples of research
questions used to search for evidence

Theme 1	Mental capacity
E.g.:	How can mental capacity be defined in the context of healthcare for people living with dementia?
	How can mental capacity be evaluated?
Theme 2	Advance care planning in people living with dementia
E.g.:	What are the specific points of interest in the involvement of people living with dementia in advance care planning? For early stages: How do we deal with persons who lack disease insight? What if people are resistant to talk about future care? For mild stages of dementia in whom verbal communication is still possible? For people with dementia in whom verbal communication about ACP is too difficult or not possible
	What if the wishes of the mentally competent person (the 'then self') does not correspond to the actual wishes of the person now lacking in mental capacity (the 'now self') or to the 'best interests' of the person?
Theme 3	Family and environment of people living with dementia
E.g.:	What is the role of family and the immediate social circle in advance care planning throughout the different stages of dementia?
	How can healthcare professionals support families and those in the person's immediate environment in taking on these roles?
Theme 4	Specifics for advance care planning in people living with early onset dementia
E.g.:	Are there specific points of interest concerning people living with early onset dementia and advance care planning?
Theme 5	Documentation and registration of ACP
E.g.:	What aspects of ACP need to be registered? How do we transfer information to different settings?
Theme 6	Organizational issues
E.g.:	What is the role in the ACP process of different professionals? What are the optimal preconditions for ACP in different settings?

ACP was included in the goals, or was one of the outcome recommendations. Publications were excluded if ACP in people with dementia was not the focus of the article. Meta-analyses and systematic reviews were excluded if they were published before 2004, to avoid including publications that approach ACP too narrowly. The authors believe that the majority of publications only started defining ACP from 2004 onward as a more comprehensive process that is not limited to advance directives [27].

The search consisted of three steps to identify relevant 1) international guidelines, 2) systematic reviews and meta-analysis and 3) primary studies (randomised controlled trials and observational research). Search terms and a PRISMA flowchart are provided in Fig. 1. The quality assessment procedure is described below.

1) We searched for existing guidelines concerning ACP and dementia in guideline databases G-I-N (Guidelines International Network), NHS (National Health Service), NGC (National Guideline Clearinghouse), and a databank of the NZGG (New Zealand Guideline Group), making use of two EBM-search engines (TRIP and SUMSEARCH).

2) Systematic reviews and meta-analyses were searched for by two authors (SM and DN) using five major bibliographic databases (Cochrane Database of Systematic Reviews, Medline, Embase, CINAHL and PsycINFO).

3) Two authors independently performed a *focused* literature search in Medline and Embase for primary studies (randomised controlled trials or observational studies) to answer clinical questions which could not be answered through guidelines, systematic reviews and/or meta-analysis. In addition, by using the snowballing method and based on expert advice, additional articles that may have been missed were added if perceived relevant by the authors.

Quality assessment
The quality of the guidelines and systematic reviews and/or meta-analyses was independently checked by pairs of authors against the Appraisal of Guidelines Research and Evaluation (AGREE II) instrument [28] for guidelines and a checklist to assess the methodological quality of systematic reviews [29], as recommended by CEBAM and Cochrane Netherlands [30–35]. The AGREE II instrument is an international 23-item tool to assess the quality and reporting of practice guidelines that is organised into six domains. All items are rated on a 7-point scale (1 'strongly disagree' – 7 'strongly agree'). The checklist used for assessment of systematic reviews was developed by Cochrane Netherlands (http://netherlands.cochrane.org; only available in Dutch). It has been shortened by the authors. It now consists of 12 'yes – no – cannot answer/too little information in the paper' questions, organised into three categories: validity, importance and applicability. Questions for assessment include: 1) Was the search request adequately formulated? 2) Was the search performed adequately? 3) Was the selection procedure for the articles performed adequately? 4) Was the quality assessment performed adequately? 5) Is the description of how the data extraction was organised adequate? 6) Were the most important characteristics of the included research reported? 7) Was the meta-analysis carried out appropriately? 8) Is there statistical pooling? 9) Is the research valid? 10) Are the results adequately described? 11) Are the findings applicable in the region? 12) Is this applicable in daily practice? (translation by authors). The quality score is

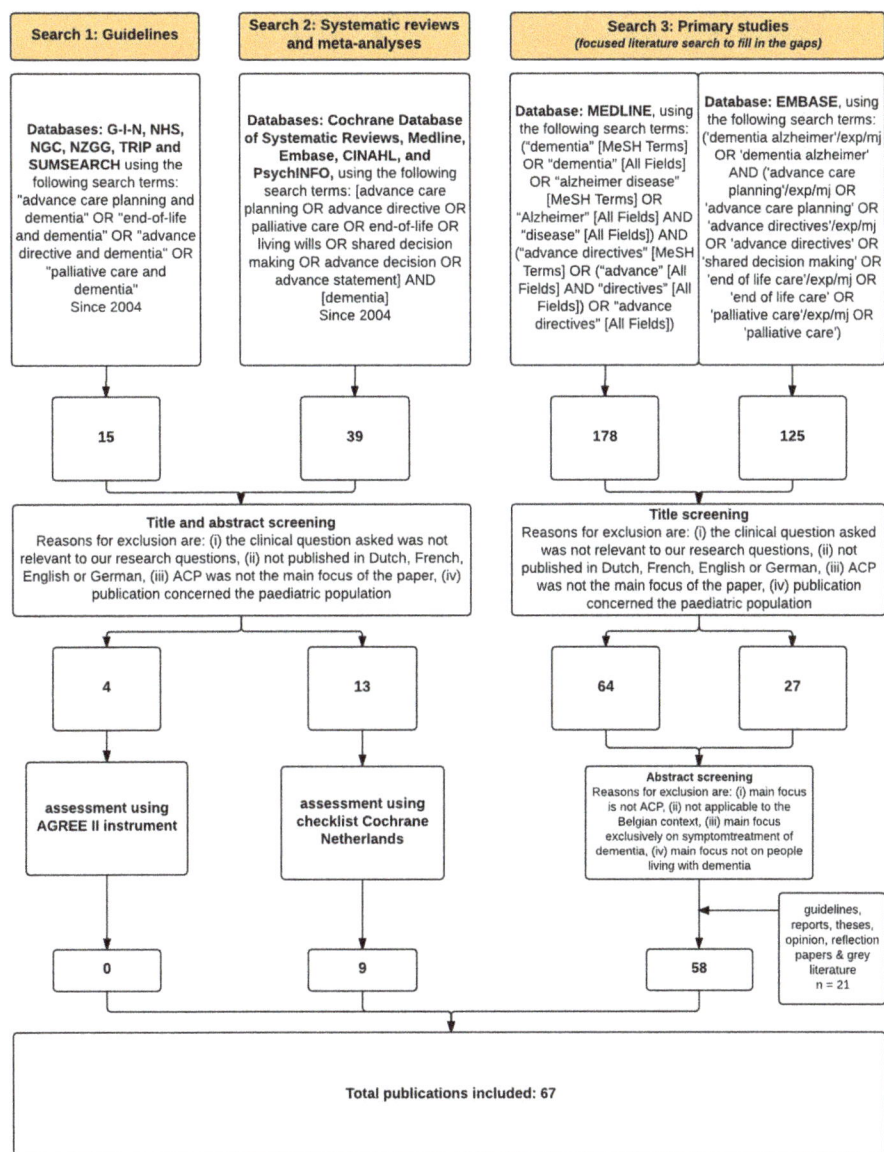

Fig. 1 PRISMA flow diagram of the study screening, eligibility, selection and inclusion process ACP advance care planning; G-I-N Guidelines International Network; NHS National Health Service; NGC National Guideline Clearinghouse; NZGG New Zealand Guidelines Group; TRIP Trip medical database; MeSH Medical Subject Headings; AGREE Appraisal of Guidelines for Research and Evaluation

the number of times 'yes' was applied to the questions (1 'low quality' - 12 'high quality'). As specified by the CEBAM procedure, we would have followed the scientific process of the ADAPTE procedure when the AGREE assessment was performed, to adapt useful guidelines to the local context through a process that can be found elsewhere [31–35]. However, none of the guidelines met these criteria and because of the limited number of systematic reviews on ACP and dementia the authors decided to include other primary studies (randomised controlled trials and observational research), opinion pieces and grey literature as well. An overview of all included publications is provided in Table 2.

2) Development of recommendations

Data extraction followed a structured process in which the research questions were divided by theme and given to a pair of authors for each of the six clinical themes. Each pair reviewed a selection of the included literature and extracted data ('key messages') that was applicable to their clinical research question. Extracted data was stored and structured in a Microsoft Excel™ matrix. These data were then used to inform the development of a first draft of possible recommendations drawn up by two authors (GA and LVdB). Two authors (GA and JS) additionally assessed the strength of each recommendation through critical appraisal of the evidence, against

Table 2 Overview and characteristics of publications included ($n = 67$)

Systematic reviews and meta-analysis ($n = 9$)

First author (year of publication)	Study type	Number of publications included (n)	Quality score ranging from 1 to 12* (number of items that could not be answered due to too little information in the paper)
1 Dening (2011)	Review	17	8 (4)
2 Robinson (2012)	Systematic review	4	7 (5)
3 Seeber (2012)	Review	43	6 (5)
4 Van der Steen (2010)	Systematic review	45	4 (8)
5 Sampson (2010)	Review (editorial)		2 (2)
6 Goodman (2010)	Integrative review	68	8 (3)
7 De Boer (2010)	Literature review	*Information not available*	3 (7)
8 Raymond (2014)	Critical synthesis	8	6 (3)
9 Van der Steen (2014)	Systematic review	33	7 (4)

Other ($n = 58$)

First author (year of publication)	Methods	Setting (sample, n)
Quantitative and experimental research		
1 Detering (2010)	Randomised controlled trial	Medical inpatients aged 80 or more ($n = 309$)
2 Vandervoort (2012)	Cross-sectional retrospective survey	Deceased residents with dementia in 345 nursing homes ($n = 764$)
3 De Gendt (2010)	Cross-sectional retrospective survey	Nursing home administrators ($n = 345$)
4 Benkendorf (1997)	Prospective cohort study	Patients > or = 19 years old with arrest of presumed cardiac cause, with locations at home or at a nursing home ($n = 2348$)
5 De Gendt (2013)	Cross-sectional retrospective survey	Deceased nursing home residents ($n = 1240$)
6 Sampson (2011)	Exploratory randomised controlled trial	Family caregivers of patients with severe dementia ($n = 33$; IG: $n = 22$; CG: $n = 11$)
7 Brazil (2015)	Cross-sectional survey	General practitioners ($n = 133$)
8 Grisso (1997)	Quasi-experimental trial	Acutely ill inpatients with a diagnosis of schizophrenia or schizoaffective disorder (IG: $n = 40$)
9 Givens (2009)	Prospective cohort study	Nursing home residents with advanced dementia and their healthcare proxies ($n = 223$)
10 Vandervoort (2013)	Cross-sectional retrospective survey	Deceased residents with dementia in 69 nursing homes ($n = 198$)
11 Baile (2002)	Questionnaires	Oncologists ($n = 167$)
12 Szafara (2012)	Prospective cohort study	Residents ($n = 1044$ US, $n = 513$ Netherlands)
13 van der Steen (2012)	Prospective cohort study	Residents with advanced dementia ($n = 94$)

Table 2 Overview and characteristics of publications included (n = 67) *(Continued)*

Qualitative research

14	Garand (2011)	Semi-structured interviews	Persons (n = 127) with a diagnosis of MCI or early AD (n = 72) or moderate to severe AD (n = 55)
15	de Boer (2012)	Semi-structured interviews	Individuals diagnosed with early-stage AD (n = 24)
16	Poppe (2013)	In-depth interviews	Patients with memory problems or mild dementia (n = 2) and eight carers (n = 8) and staff members from a memory clinic and a community mental health team (n = 11)
17	Chan (2011)	Semi-structured interviews	Nursing home residents (n = 42)
18	Piers (2013)	Semi-structured interviews	Elderly patients with limited prognosis (n = 38)
19	Ashton (2014)	Interviews	Family caregivers within a specialist dementia unit (n = 12)
20	Levi (2010)	Focus groups	Older individuals (n = 23)
21	Kim Suh (2011)	Interviews	Persons with AD (n = 188)
22	Shanley (2009)	Interviews	Managers from residential aged care facilities (n = 41)
23	Dening (2012)	Nominal group study	People with dementia (n = 6), carers (n = 5) and dyads of people with dementia and carers (n = 6) attending memory assessment services
24	Dening (2012)	Whole-systems qualitative study based on interviews and focus groups	Nine carers of people with dementia (n = 9) and focus groups (n = 6) with health care professionals with mixed professions (n = 26) and individual interviews with health care professionals with mixed professions (n = 15)
25	Hirschman (2006)	Semi-structured interviews	Family members of patients with advanced dementia (n = 30)
26	Hirschman (2008)	Semi-structured interviews	Family members of patients with advanced dementia (n = 30)
27	Dickinson (2013)	Semi-structured interviews	People with mild to moderate dementia (n = 17) and family carers (n = 29)
28	Hoe (2007)	Semi-structured interviews	Care recipient and caregiver dyads (n = 191)
29	Steeman (2007)	Interview study	Elderly people with probable mild dementia and their family members (n = 20)
30	Zimmerman (2015)	Interview study	Family members of decedents from 118 nursing home and residential settings (n = 264)
31	McMahan (2013)	Semi-structured focus groups	Focus groups with participants from a Veterans Affairs and county hospital and the community (n = 13)
32	Steeman (2013)	Longitudinal interview study	Elderly persons with early-stage dementia (n = 17)

Table 2 Overview and characteristics of publications included ($n = 67$) *(Continued)*

Mixed methods research			
33	Silvester (2012)	Survey (1) and review of existing ACP-related documentation (2)	(1) staff of aged care facilities ($n = 45$); (2) aged care facilities ($n = 12$)
34	Froggatt (2009)	Survey (1) and semi-structured interviews (2)	(1) care home managers ($n = 213$); (2) care home managers ($n = 15$)
35	de Boer (2011)	Survey (1) and semi-structured interviews (2)	(1) elderly care physicians ($n = 434$); (2) physicians ($n = 11$) and relatives ($n = 8$)
36	Van der steen (2014)	Five-round Delphi study	experts from 23 countries ($n = 64$)
Guidelines, reports, theses			
37	Van Mechelen (2014)	Guideline	NA
38	Clayton (2007)	Guideline	NA
39	WHO (2012)	Report	NA
40	Harle (2008)	Report	NA
41	Titler (2008)	Guideline	NA
42	Vellinga (2006)	Thesis	NA
43	Church (2007)	Guideline	NA
44	Conroy (2009)	Guideline	NA
45	American Medical Association (1999)	Guideline	NA
Opinion and reflection papers			
46	Harvey (2006)	NA	NA
47	Lemmens (2012)	NA	NA
48	Gillick (2012)	NA	NA
49	Scott (2012)	NA	NA
50	Berghmans (2001)	NA	NA
51	Burlà (2014)	NA	NA
52	Kim Suh (2006)	NA	NA
53	Gillick (2004)	NA	NA
54	Juthani-Mehta (2015)	NA	NA
55	Mold (1991)	NA	NA
56	Smith (2013)	hypothetical case report ($n = 2$)	2
Grey literature			
57	Van der steen (2011)	Leaflet *(Dutch)*	NA
58	Keirse (2009)	Leaflet *(Dutch)*	NA

NA Not Applicable, *GP* General Practitioner, *IG* Intervention Group, *CG* Control Group, *AD* Alzheimer's Disease
*Using the checklist that was developed by Cochrane Netherlands (http://netherlands.cochrane.org; only available in Dutch). It has been slightly adapted by the authors. It consists of 12 'yes – no - cannot answer/too little information in the paper' questions, organised into three domains (validity, importance and applicability): 1) Was the search request adequately formulated? 2) Was the search performed adequately? 3) Was the selection procedure for the articles performed adequately? 4) Was the quality assessment performed adequately? 5) Is the description of how the data extraction was organised adequate? 6) Were the most important characteristics of the included research reported? 7) Was the meta-analysis carried out appropriately? 8) Was there statistical pooling? 9) Is the research valid? 10) Are the results adequately described? 11) Are the findings applicable in the region? 12) Is this applicable in daily practice? (translation by authors). The quality score is the number of times 'yes' was applied to the questions (1 'low quality' - 12 'high quality')

the criteria of the Grading of Recommendations Assessment, Development and Evaluation (GRADE) working group [30–35]. The quality of the included literature and each recommendation can be found in Table 2 and Table 3.

When there was not enough evidence on a clinical research question, the author group formulated an expert opinion. Each step in the decision process was discussed and approved within the author group. The recommendations were finally re-organized into eight domains.

3) Validation process

Because high-quality evidence was lacking for many of the clinical research questions, we conducted additional validation of the recommendations. The results of this validation round were discussed within the author group and recommendations were revised if necessary and applicable.

1) To assess the clarity, acceptability and importance of each formulated recommendation, an online survey was set up. This survey was then e-mailed or sent with the newsletter of the Flemish Expertise Centre on Dementia Care and the Flemish Council for the Elderly to potential end users (healthcare professionals working with people living with dementia) across settings (primary care, home care, residential care and hospitals) in Flanders. The respondents were asked to score each recommendation on a scale of 1 to 7 for (i) clarity, (ii) acceptability and (iii) importance. As a result of this validation survey the authors provided more information for some of the terms used in the recommendation. For example: 'care goals' were defined more clearly by providing several examples such as "prolonging life, preserving function or control, optimal comfort, improving quality of life, a 'good death' or support from those close to them".

2) To evaluate possible barriers to the implementation of each recommendation, we organised two meetings of established peer review groups of GPs and geriatricians on March 8 and April 28, 2016 to provide feedback. Nearly 97% of all physicians in Belgium are affiliated with peer review groups like these and are obliged to attend two out of four meetings per year for accreditation [36].

3) Finally, we provided several experts (other than the authors) with the first draft of the recommendations (informed by 1 and 2) for them to formulate comments to improve them. Experts are healthcare professionals specifically selected by the authors from different disciplines, all with an extensive knowledge of the daily practice of dementia care and ACP.

Results

Selection of research questions and clinical themes

The research questions and clinical themes that needed to be addressed according to the multidisciplinary author group are provided in Table 1.

Search for evidence and expert and user validation

Figure 1 summarises the flow of selected publications through the review of all literature. A total of 67 publications constituted the evidence and validation base upon which the recommendations were developed (Table 2). In total, 51 end users, 10 experts, 12 GPs and 12 geriatricians confirmed the importance, relevance and clarity of the recommendations and helped to further define them. Characteristics of the participants in the validation process are described in Table 4.

Recommendations

We formulated 32 recommendations covering eight domains: 1) initiation of ACP, 2) evaluation of mental capacity, 3) holding ACP conversations, 4) the role and importance of those close to the person with dementia, 5) ACP when it is difficult or no longer possible to communicate verbally, 6) documentation of wishes and preferences, including information transfer, 7) end-of-life decision-making and 8) preconditions for optimal implementation. The main recommendations within each of the eight main domains are stated in bold and described below. The recommendations are presented in Table 3, with accompanying scores indicating their strength and supporting references.

Initiation of ACP

Start ACP as early as possible and integrate ACP into the daily care of people living with dementia, ideally before diagnosis or any cognitive decline [9, 25, 37–42]. Preferably, ACP should be performed on several occasions. These conversations can vary from short to lengthy discussions depending on how the person with dementia feels and how much time there is. They can be planned or occur spontaneously when the opportunity arises [23, 37–41, 43]. There are several key triggers for ACP conversations identified in the literature: admission to a nursing home, initiation of palliative care, deterioration of the condition or upon request. Specifically for dementia, **key moments might be the period around diagnosis** [38, 44], **while discussing the overall general care plan and/or when changes occur in health status, place of residence or financial situation** [45]. **Be alert for triggers and opportunities to start ACP and make use of any opportunity to talk about ACP** [46, 47]. Given the fluctuating cognitive capacities of people with

Table 3 Recommendations

	Recommendations[a]	Quality of the recommendation, according to GRADE[b]
Domain 1	Initiation of ACP	
1	Start ACP as early as possible and integrate ACP into the daily care of people living with dementia [10, 37, 106] [11, 38–43] Specific key moments might be: - the period around the diagnosis of dementia [39, 44] - when discussing the general care plan - when changes occur in the health status, place of residence or financial situation [45]	1C
2	Be alert for triggers and opportunities to start ACP and make use of any opportunity to talk about ACP [46, 47]	1C
3	The healthcare professional should initiate ACP conversations if the person living with dementia and/or those close to them do not do this themselves [37, 44–47] [38, 45–48]	1C
4	Consider the person as an individual and consider their specific situation when starting ACP conversations [43, 49]	1C
Domain 2	Evaluation of mental capacity	
5	Always assume maximal mental capacity [50, 51]	1C
6	Consider mental capacity as a fluctuating rather than static condition [52], and stay alert for signs of loss of capacity	1C
7	Judge mental capacity task-specifically i.e. for a certain decision at a particular moment in time [11, 50, 51]	1C
8	Always stay in contact with the person him/herself and ensure their maximum participation [1]	1C
9	Assess mental capacity through formal clinical assessment: - where there is doubt or disagreement between healthcare professionals and/or family - when the decisions can have far-reaching consequences - preferably by a multidisciplinary or interdisciplinary team with experience in dementia	NA*
Domain 3	Performing ACP conversations	
10	Adjust conversation style and content to the person's level and rhythm [59]	1C
11	Explore who the significant people in their life are and who can be involved in the ACP conversations, and explore who can become their legal representative [47, 52, 61]	1C
12	Lead the conversation but do not force it to become too formulaic or phased [59]	1C
13	Explore the person's disease awareness and their expectations, ideas and possible misconceptions concerning the disease trajectory [5]	1C
14	Where someone lacks disease awareness or is reluctant to talk about ACP, do not insist [106, 63]	1C
15	ACP conversations can best be held on several occasions and over a longer period of time [38, 106, 45] and cover several different topics such as the broader values of the person, their experience of the present and their fears about the future and the end of life, their future care goals, specific advance decisions about the end of life, advance directives	1C
16	Try to understand the whole person living with dementia; explore their life story, important values, norms, beliefs and preferences [17, 26]	1C
17	Explore the person's current experiences; ask what is the perception of the person living with dementia of their quality of life? What are their fears and concerns? [25, 106, 52, 65]	1C
18	Explore the person's fears and concerns for the future and for the end of life [106]	1C
19	If possible and desirable, guide the person in formulating their care goals [49, 66]	1C
20	If possible and desirable, guide the persons with formulating specific wishes concerning specific end-of-life decisions [45]	1C
21	Explore whether the person would like to have a written advance directive or if they have made one in the past [45]	1C

Table 3 Recommendations *(Continued)*

	Recommendations[a]	Quality of the recommendation, according to GRADE[b]
Domain 4	The role and importance of those close to them	
22	Involve family or significant others as early as possible in the ACP process and inform them about the role of a surrogate decision-maker [11, 26, 41]	1C
23	Evaluate their disease awareness and inform them about the expected disease trajectory and possible end-of-life decisions [17, 25, 43, 82, 83]	1C
24	Pay attention to their perceptions during the ACP process [11, 26, 52, 65, 85]	1B
Domain 5	ACP when it is difficult or no longer possible to communicate verbally	
25	Keep connected with the person living with dementia and ensure their maximum participation [1]: respond to their emotions, attend to non-verbal communication and observe their behaviour to know more about their current quality of life, fears and desires	1C
26	Actively involve family and others close to them in the ACP process and the expression of care goals and wishes concerning end-of-life decisions [11, 26, 82]	1C
Domain 6	Documentation of wishes and preferences, including information transfer	
27	Write down in the medical/care files of the person with dementia the outcomes of the ACP process, their values, preferences and care goals, and if applicable, the advance directive and legal representative [26, 87, 88]	1B
28	Regularly re-evaluate as part of the ACP process; decisions can be revised at all times [17, 26, 47]	1C
29	Communicate the outcomes of the ACP process within the care team, i.e. values, preferences and care goals, and if applicable advance directives or legal representatives, especially in the case of transfer to another care setting.	NA*
Domain 7	End-of-life decision-making	
30	Carefully weigh the wishes (expressed and/or written down earlier) against the current best interest of the person living with dementia, in consultation with those close to them and the healthcare professionals involved [83, 89, 90]	1C
Domain 8	Preconditions for optimal implementation of ACP	
31	Provide enough training opportunities for healthcare professionals to learn how to conduct ACP conversations. Adequate support is essential in making healthcare professionals confident about engaging in ACP [11, 17, 26, 94, 114]	1C
32	Integrate ACP into the mission and policy of the organization and embed it in the organizational culture [62, 91, 95–97] [61, 96–98] [62, 96–98]	1C

NA Not applicable, *ACP* Advance care planning

[a]Recommendations without references were added only by the experts and end users during the consensus procedure

[b]Grading scores go from 1A to 2B, 1A representing a strong recommendation, based on a high level of evidence and 2C representing a weak recommendation and low to very low level of evidence. A grading score of 1C represents 'strong recommendation but low to very low level of evidence' meaning that this recommendation can be applied to patients and to care but may still change once higher-quality evidence is available. A grading score of 1B represents 'strong recommendation and moderate level of evidence' meaning that this recommendation has enough support for it to be applied in practice. More information on GRADE scores can be found on the website of the GRADE working group

dementia it is important to make use of spontaneous opportunities.

Because research has shown that ACP conversations are not often initiated by the person living with dementia him/herself, **healthcare professionals should initiate them** unless the person and/or those close to them do this [37, 45–47]. Although GPs play an important role, all healthcare professionals can be involved in discussing elements of ACP [46, 47] according to their own skills [37, 45–47]. It is important to have a trusting relationship with the person and those close to them, to have some knowledge of the disease trajectory [37, 48] and to communicate with the GP.

Each individual patient and situation is different. Hence, when starting ACP conversations, one needs to **consider the person as an individual and consider their specific situation** [43, 49].

Evaluation of mental capacity

When performing ACP with people living with dementia, their mental capacity should be considered. However, a diagnosis of dementia should not automatically be equated with loss of mental capacity. Healthcare professionals should consider the following principles:

Always assume full mental capacity [50, 51] and regard it **as a fluctuating, not static, condition** situated on a continuum [52]. **Stay alert for signals of loss of**

Table 4 Professional background of the participants involved during the validation process

Professional background	N
Survey participants (end users)	51
Nurse	17
Dementia reference person	8
Social worker	5
Occupational therapist	4
Physician	3
Other healthcare professionals in various settings	14
Experts	10
Geriatric psychiatrist	1
Neurologist	1
Social worker	2
Nurse	2
General practitioner	1
Occupational therapist	1
Psychologist	2
Peer-review groups	2
Family physicians	12
Geriatrician	12

mental capacity. **Judge mental capacity task-specifically** as the capacity for making a certain decision at a particular moment [9, 50, 51]. **Always stay in contact with the person him–/herself to ensure maximal participation** [1]. **A formal clinical assessment (including substantive clinical and neuropsychological examinations [53]) is only necessary in case of doubt or disagreement between healthcare professionals and/or those close to the person, or when decisions can have far-reaching consequences, and should then preferably be performed by a multidisciplinary team with expertise in dementia.** To be able to hold ACP conversations with people with dementia, a general clinical judgment of mental capacity as part of the conversation usually suffices. Available tools for making general clinical judgments of mental capacity are the MacArthur Competence Assessment Tool [54], the Vignette method [55] or the flow chart guide from Church et al. [56].

ACP conversations

In people with dementia, cognitive activity and abstract thinking – abilities which are needed to think about the future – can become difficult, even in mild cases [42]. Moreover, people with dementia are likely to live in the present and thinking about the future may cause fear or anxiety. This does not preclude ACP but does make ACP conversations more difficult [21, 57, 58]. To facilitate ACP conversations with people with dementia, the following recommendations apply:

When engaging in a conversation with a person who has mild/moderate dementia, **adjust the communication style and content to their own level and rhythm** [59], taking into account the principles of person-centred care [60].

Find out who are the significant people in their life, people who may be able to be involved in the ACP conversations, and who may be able to become their surrogate decision-makers (if not yet appointed), while explaining that these are people who can legally be appointed to act on behalf of a patient when s/he is no longer capable [47, 52, 61].

Lead the conversation but do not make it too phased, despite the fact that ACP is often described in such a way [59]. Because of a lack of disease awareness, decreasing decision-making ability and imaginative capacity and decreasing ability to process new information, it will often not be possible to follow a prescribed structure [25, 43, 62]. Supporting materials, if necessary and available, can be helpful (e.g. applications, books, etc.).

Explore the person's disease awareness and his/her expectations, ideas and possible misconceptions concerning the disease trajectory [5]. It is important to provide a balanced view of what living with dementia may entail.

If someone lacks disease awareness or is reluctant to talk about ACP, do not insist [42, 63]. It is important for people to decide their own information preferences. However, even if disease awareness is lacking, it remains important to explore someone's general values and concerns as part of the ACP process [9, 64].

ACP conversations are best held on several occasions over a period of time [37, 42, 45]. They can cover several different topics: the person's more general values, their experience of the present and fears about the future and the end of life, their future care goals, their specific advance decisions about the end of life and advance directives.

Learn to know who the person living with dementia is 'as a whole person': explore their life story and most important values, norms, ideas and preferences in order to understand who the person is, what the significant events in their life have been and what gives their life meaning [15, 25, 37, 45].

Explore people's current experiences in terms of quality of life, fears and concerns. ACP is not only about exploring the future, but includes a focus on the past and the present [4, 22, 63, 65]. **Explore the person's fears and concerns for the future and for the end of life** [42, 63].

If possible and desirable, guide the person in formulating his/her care goals [8, 49, 66, 67] i.e. prolonging life, preserving function or control, optimal comfort, improving quality of life, a 'good death' or support from those close to them [67, 68]. Be aware that such care goals can change throughout the disease trajectory [58, 69, 70].

If possible and desirable, guide the person in formulating specific wishes concerning specific end-of-life decisions [45]. Most people with dementia do not die suddenly. Often medical decisions with regard to the provision of antibiotics, hospital admission in case of urgent health problems, resuscitation and artificial fluids are relevant [2, 71, 72]. Provide the necessary information about different possible end-of-life decisions in dementia (e.g. non-treatment decisions), and prevent misconceptions with regard to the use of resuscitation [73–76], artificial food and fluids [77] and antibiotics near the end of life [78–80].

Explore whether the person would like to complete an advance directive or whether s/he has done so in the past [45]. It is important to stipulate that documenting wishes formally can be relevant for people living with dementia, especially those who don't have any close family or those who value being in control. However, professionals should be aware that in some situations, advance directives might not be specific enough to fully inform the decision-making process. Documented wishes will help guide end-of-life decision-making for physicians, other care professionals and those close to the person, and they will be most helpful if they are the result of a continuous and in-depth communication process.

These recommendations are mainly applicable to people who have mild or moderate dementia, with whom verbal communication is still possible. Part 5 focuses more on people with dementia who find it difficult or impossible to communicate verbally.

The role and importance of those close to the person with dementia

Because of the gradual loss of mental capacity in people living with dementia - more than in other diseases - they are often dependent on other people [81]. **Family or significant others should preferably be involved as early as possible in the ACP process and be informed about the role of a surrogate decision-maker** [9, 25, 40]. As part of the ACP process, it will be important to determine who can be involved in ACP conversations, but it can be difficult to determine when to involve them and how many people to involve. If a legal representative is appointed, they should be involved in ACP conversations [82]. If there is no legal representative, it will be useful to consider who will be the first point of contact for professionals, and how information is transferred among other family members. Every family is unique, so the involvement of family and those close to the person with dementia should be evaluated on a case-by-case basis, along with the person with dementia themselves.

Evaluate the disease awareness of those close to the person and inform them of the expected disease trajectory and possible end-of-life decisions [15, 23, 43, 83, 84]. The information preferences of those close to the person with dementia should also be explored. Make sure the information about the disease trajectory is correct and make sure it is balanced and qualified. In many cases the person with dementia does not experience his/her disease as something 'negative' in the way that the family does [82, 85].

Pay attention to the needs of those close to the person during the ACP process [9, 25, 63, 65, 86]. Sufficient support, education and information are important, as is addressing the concerns, experiences, expectations and fears of the family. Family can be unprepared or feel guilty [87]. Pay attention to the emotional process of family members and consider that family dynamics might change over time. It is not always easy to harmonise the views of those close to the person with dementia.

ACP when it is difficult or no longer possible to communicate verbally

In moderate/severe dementia, where verbal communication is difficult or no longer possible, formulating care goals or specific care preferences is difficult. **Keep a connection with the person with dementia and ensure their maximum participation** [1, 42]. **Respond to their emotions, attend to non-verbal communication and observe behaviour to understand more about their current quality of life, fears and desires** [63]. People's emotions can give direction to the decision-making process [42]. Subsequently, **actively involve family or other close people in the ACP process and the expression of care goals and wishes concerning end-of-life decisions** [9, 25, 83] to get an understanding of the life story of the person with dementia and to interpret certain aspects of their behaviour or emotions.

Documentation of wishes and preferences, including information transfer

After every planned or unplanned ACP discussion, healthcare professionals should **write down the outcome in the patient's medical/care files, e.g. the values, wishes or care goals of the person and, where relevant, details of an advance directive or legal representative** [25, 88, 89]. If the person wishes, support them in formulating specific wishes and advance decisions concerning the end of their life, explore whether they have made a formal written advance directive in the past or if they want to make one now [45] and provide information about the advantages and disadvantages of advance directives [2, 71]. It is recommended that **ACP documentation is evaluated regularly as part of the ACP process**, for example in anticipation of a 'response shift' [15, 25, 40, 47, 70]. **Decisions can be revised at all times**.

The outcomes of the ACP process should be communicated within the care team, i.e. values, preferences and care goals and any advance directives or legal representatives, particularly upon transfer to another care setting. This can be done verbally or in writing. Make sure relevant information is available to other care providers in the shared sections of the care file or is easily accessible when needed, especially upon transfer to another care setting. Information sharing should always take professional confidentiality into account [66].

End-of-life decision-making

Despite all good intentions, ACP cannot anticipate all possible scenarios. The disease trajectory is not always predictable and the emotional burden on those close to the person with dementia can often lead to a certain amount of confusion and lack of clarity about providing care. When end-of-life decisions need to be made, it is important to **weigh carefully the wishes expressed and/or written down earlier against the current best interest of the person living with dementia, in consultation with the person's close circle and the healthcare professionals involved** [84, 90, 91]. End-of-life decision-making entails shared decision-making and as much consensus amongst healthcare providers and those close to the person as possible [84, 90, 91]. Materials such as the Framework for Weighing Previously Expressed Preferences v. Best Interest can support professionals and family in making these decisions, by asking questions such as: 'is the clinical situation an emergency that allows no time for deliberation?', 'in view of the person's values and goals, how likely is it that the benefits of the intervention outweigh the burdens?', 'to what degree does the advance directive fit the situation at hand?', 'how much leeway did the patient allow the surrogate in overriding the advance directive?' or 'how well does the surrogate represent the patient's best interests?' [87].

Preconditions for optimal implementation of ACP

The optimal implementation of ACP requires improved public understanding of end-of-life care issues [92] and patients who are more informed or educated about ACP [92]. Additionally, **the provision of sufficient training opportunities for healthcare professionals to learn how to conduct ACP conversations is important. Adequate support in practice is essential in making healthcare professionals confident about engaging in ACP** [9, 20, 25, 93, 94]. Training should at least entail the basic principles of ACP, the legal, deontological and ethical framework, the importance and effectiveness of ACP, a discussion of the professionals' own barriers to

ACP, general communication techniques and active listening skills, documentation of advance directives, communication with other professionals and how to make decisions at certain times [9, 20, 25, 93, 94]. Interactive sessions with role-plays, regular come-back sessions and a specific focus on attitudes towards talking about death and dying are also important [5, 25, 62, 95, 96]. These training programmes should be organised for GPs, nurses and social care workers, as the skills they provide often function as an important facilitator between physician and patient [92, 97].

Integrate ACP into the mission and policy of the organization and embed ACP in the organizational culture [62, 97–99]. ACP should be part of daily practice and this requires a supportive culture within the community or facility and an open attitude to conversations about end-of-life care and dementia among healthcare professionals. Within the facility there should be a clear statement of intent and a formal policy concerning ACP and how to embed it in routine care [1, 62, 92, 97–99].

Discussion

There are few guidelines available for healthcare professionals concerning ACP in people living with dementia, especially those with early onset dementia. And those guidelines are often not developed using high-quality research, mainly because such research is lacking. Difficulties implementing ACP in this population and the evaluation of "active ingredients" necessary to successfully change outcomes are not fully addressed in research and high-quality evaluation research such as randomised design studies are still rare [6, 8]. By maintaining a systematic approach, we could define a unique set of recommendations to provide ACP to people living with dementia and those close to them. In doing, so we integrated the available expertise in dementia care in a wide range of settings in Flanders with the existing evidence on ACP as reported in the scientific literature.

Compared with ACP in other diseases where lack of mental capacity is a less pronounced problem, performing ACP in dementia entails several significant and specific attention points. The most important concerns the involvement of those close to the person with dementia. Family members, next-of-kin and other significant people are an important point of contact in communication and decision-making in end-of-life care for people with dementia, as their mental capacity gradually declines and verbal communication becomes more difficult or even impossible [1]. Involvement of these people from the initial stages of the condition is of the utmost importance in providing end-of-life care that corresponds to the wishes and preferences of the person with dementia.

A second element very specific to ACP in people with dementia is the trajectory of the decrease in mental capacity [81]. The clinical question of the evaluation of mental capacity as part of the ACP process was heavily debated by the author group and within the expert panel and proved to be something which is difficult to do in practice. Because of these discussions, we concluded that mental capacity should be considered as a continuum that fluctuates over time and is task-specific. In addition, we recommend that formal, in-depth, multidisciplinary assessments of capacity should not always be performed before or during ACP conversations. However, it is important that care professionals hold ACP conversations at different points over a period of time, making use of spontaneous remarks on ACP-related issues by patients or those close to them, as well as having planned conversations. Such conversations will not always follow a predefined or structured format and will vary in content, length and depth depending on the physical, cognitive and psychological state of the person. In some cases, e.g. when high-stake decisions need to be made, formal multidisciplinary assessment and referral will be necessary. However, further research is needed to substantiate this recommendation.

ACP is an important part of care, especially in older people and those living with dementia. Older people themselves indicate that they find ACP valuable [17, 63] and there is an important body of literature suggesting that it has a positive impact on outcomes, ranging from family satisfaction with care to concordance between end-of-life care and patient wishes, especially for older people and those living in nursing homes [100, 101]. There is additional evidence, albeit of variable quality, which shows that ACP has the potential to reduce inappropriate hospital admissions and healthcare costs in nursing homes where end-of-life care spending is already high [39, 102]. Further high-quality research, however, would strengthen the arguments for ACP becoming part of routine dementia care and provide information on how it can be carried out effectively and sustainably [103]. More specifically, we found insufficient research to support recommendations on issues such as a uniform definition of lack of mental capacity, contraindications for initiating ACP and what to do if a person living with dementia does not want to involve those close to them.

To the best of our knowledge, this is the first practical guideline developed to improve the performance of healthcare professionals in providing ACP to people living with dementia across settings. Until now, existing guidelines from guideline development groups (GDGs) such as the National Institute for Health and Clinical Excellence have only highlighted a few recommendations concerning advance care planning, and these are limited to 'discuss the use of advance directives and identify surrogates' and 'discuss cardiopulmonary resuscitation in advance and inform patients about poor outcomes in

advanced dementia' [26, 104]. Nonetheless, evidence shows that ACP may be more effective in meeting a patient's preferences when it entails more than just written documents and a conversation [39, 101]. Local initiatives have tried to provide guidance in ACP specifically for people living with dementia, but standardization and consistency are lacking [105]. By consulting both experts and end users with different professional backgrounds, we have been able to include broad multidisciplinary support at a regional level for these recommendations. In addition, rather than just requiring the experts to agree or disagree with predefined statements, they were actively involved in specifying the statements so that greater consensus could be achieved. We consider this an important feature of our work.

However, readers must be aware of several limitations of this study. The first limitation is the rather small number of experts ($n = 10$) and end users ($n = 51$) who replied to the survey, and the limited number of peer-review groups ($n = 2$). In addition, the main source from which the recommendations are derived is low-quality systematic reviews, studies in which the quality of evidence was not assessed formally, and from the opinions of professionals or experts. We also wish to make clear that professionals must be aware of the policies and legislation that govern the jurisdiction in which they work and that they must abide by existing policies and legislation when applying the recommendations. Additionally, healthcare professionals should of course apply these recommendations in their workplaces to serve as a general guide, but follow them subject to their own judgment and each individual case. The recommendations serve neither as an action programme nor as a strict guideline but provide a list of attention points for healthcare professionals involved in dementia care. We recommend that they should additionally be trained to perform ACP, because merely providing and disseminating a guideline like this will not be enough to improve their practice [106]. The results of this study can serve as a tool to educate healthcare professionals.

The final guideline requires further testing in clinical practice. However, initial feedback from experienced healthcare professionals and other experts has indicated that it can be helpful in terms of initiation, organisation and implementation of ACP and when holding discussions on end-of-life care. Such guidelines are shown to play an important role in enabling good care up to the end of life which is provided according to high ethical and quality standards [1].

Conclusion

Little high-quality evidence is available on ACP in dementia care. By combining the available evidence with expert and user opinions, we have defined a unique set of recommendations for ACP in people living with dementia. These recommendations will be used for the development of a Flemish guideline for ACP in people living with dementia and can serve as a valuable tool to educate healthcare professionals on how to perform ACP across settings.

Abbreviations
ACP: Advance care planning; CAP: Coordinating and advising physician; GP: General practitioner

Acknowledgements
We thank Sofie Masschelein (SM) and Dorien Nickmans (DN) and the experts who provided feedback and refinement throughout the development of the recommendations: Satya Buggenhout, Patrick Cras, Myriam De Schynkel, Aline De Vleminck, Manu Keirse, Jo Lisaerde, Gerda Okerman, Jurn Verschraegen and Sandra Vertongen. We would also like to thank all the people who replied to the survey, the people who participated in the peer-review groups and Sylvie Tack for reviewing the legal section of the Flemish guideline. Ruth Piers is supported by Fund Marie-Thérèse De Lava, King Baudouin Foundation, Belgium.

Authors' contributions
All authors carried out the concept and design of the study, the collection of data, the analysis and the interpretation of the data. The drafting of the manuscript was led by RP, GA, JG and LVdB. All authors read and approved the final manuscript.

Competing interest
The authors declare that they have no competing interests.

Author details
[1]Department of Geriatric Medicine, Ghent University Hospital, Ghent, Belgium. [2]End-of-life Care Research Group, Vrije Universiteit Brussel (VUB) and Ghent University, Laarbeeklaan 103, 1090 Brussels, Belgium. [3]Flanders Federation for Palliative Care, Vilvoorde, Belgium. [4]Department of Public Health and Primary Care, ACHG, KU Leuven, Leuven, Belgium. [5]Department of Sociology, University of Antwerp, Antwerp, Belgium. [6]Flemish Expertise Centre on Dementia Care, Antwerp, Belgium. [7]Academic Centre for Nursing and Midwifery, KULeuven, Leuven, Belgium. [8]Department of Geriatric Medicine, Ghent University Hospital, Ghent, Belgium. [9]Department of Family Medicine and Chronic Care, Vrije Universiteit Brussel (VUB), Laarbeeklaan 103, 1090 Brussels, Belgium.

References
1. World Health Organization, Alzheimer's Disease International. Dementia: a public health priority. Geneva: World Health Organization; 2012. http://apps. who.int/.../75263. ISBN: 9789241564458
2. Givens JL, Kiely DK, Carey K, Mitchell SL. Healthcare proxies of nursing home residents with advanced dementia: decisions they confront and their satisfaction with decision-making: Healthcare Proxy Decision-Making Satisfaction. J Am Geriatric Soc. 2009;57:1149–55.
3. Sampson EL, Burns A, Richards M. Improving end-of-life care for people with dementia. Br J Psychiatry. 2011;199:357–9.
4. Exley C, Bamford C, Hughes J, Robinson L. Advance care planning: an opportunity for person-centered care for people living with dementia. Dementia. 2009;8:419–24.
5. Van Mechelen W. Vroegtijdige Zorgplanning. Richtlijn, Versie: 1.0. In: Federatie Palliatieve Zorg Vlaanderen vzw; 2014.
6. Seymour J, Horne G. Advance Care Planning for the end of life: an overview. In: Adv Care Plan End Life Care. Oxford: Oxford University Press. p. 16–27. http://www.oxfordscholarship.com/view/10.1093/acprof:oso/9780199561636.001.0001/acprof-9780199561636.
7. Royal College of Physicians of London. Concise guidance to good practice: a series of evidence-based guidelines for clinical management. Number 12: advance care planning National Guidelines. In: Royal College of Physicians of London; 2009.
8. Dixon J, Karagiannidou M, Knapp M. The effectiveness of advance care planning in improving end-of-life outcomes for people with dementia and their Carers: a systematic review and critical discussion. J Pain Symptom Manag. 2018;55:132–150.e1.
9. Dening KH, Jones L, Sampson EL. Advance care planning for people with dementia: a review. Int Psychogeriatr. 2011;23:1535–51.
10. Vandervoort A, Houttekier D, Vander Stichele R, van der Steen JT, Van den Block L. Quality of dying in nursing home residents dying with dementia: does advanced care planning matter? A Nationwide postmortem study. Montazeri a. PLoS One. 2014;9:e91130.
11. Vandervoort A, Houttekier D, Van den Block L, van der Steen JT, Stichele RV, Deliens L. Advance care planning and physician orders in nursing home residents with dementia: a Nationwide retrospective study among professional caregivers and relatives. J Pain Symptom Manag. 2014;47:245–56.
12. De Gendt C, Bilsen J, Mortier F, Vander Stichele R, Medical DL. End-of-life decision-making and terminal sedation among very old patients. Gerontology. 2009:99–105.
13. Meeussen K, Van den Block L, Echteld M, Bossuyt N, Bilsen J, Van Casteren V, et al. Advance care planning in Belgium and the Netherlands: a Nationwide retrospective study via sentinel networks of general practitioners. J Pain Symptom Manag. 2011;42:565–77.
14. Wickson-Griffiths A, Kaasalainen S, Ploeg J, McAiney C. A review of advance care planning programs in long-term care homes: are they dementia friendly? Nurs Res Pract. 2014;2014:1–11.
15. Ashton SE, Roe B, Jack B, McClelland B. End of life care: The experiences of advance care planning amongst family caregivers of people with advanced dementia - A qualitative study. Dementia [Internet]. 2014 [cited 2015 Apr 10]; Available from: http://dem.sagepub.com/cgi/doi/10.1177/1471301214548521
16. Stewart F, Goddard C, Schiff R, Hall S. Advanced care planning in care homes for older people: a qualitative study of the views of care staff and families. Age Ageing. 2011;40:330–5.
17. Sharp T, Moran E, Kuhn I, Barclay S. Do the elderly have a voice? Advance care planning discussions with frail and older individuals: a systematic literature review and narrative synthesis. Br J Gen Pract. 2013;63:657–68.
18. Lovell A, Yates P. Advance care planning in palliative care: a systematic literature review of the contextual factors influencing its uptake 2008-2012. Palliat Med. 2014;28:1026–35.
19. Black BS, Fogarty LA, Phillips H, Finucane T, Loreck DJ, Baker A, et al. Surrogate decision makers' understanding of dementia patients' prior wishes for end-of-life care. J Aging Health. 2009;21:627–50.
20. Ke L-S, Huang X, O'Connor M, Lee S. Nurses' views regarding implementing advance care planning for older people: a systematic review and synthesis of qualitative studies. J Clin Nurs. 2015;24(15-16):2057–73. https://doi.org/10.1111/jocn.12853.
21. Dickinson C, Bamford C, Exley C, Emmett C, Hughes J, Robinson L. Planning for tomorrow whilst living for today: the views of people with dementia and their families on advance care planning. Int Psychogeriatr. 2013;25:2011–21.
22. Lorenz KA, Lynn J, Dy SM, Shugarman LR, Wilkinson A, Mularski RA, et al. Evidence for improving palliative care at the end of life: a systematic review. Ann Intern Med. 2008;148:147–59.

23. Dening KH, Jones L, Sampson EL. Preferences for end-of-life care: a nominal group study of people with dementia and their family carers. Palliat Med. 2013;27(5):409–17. https://doi.org/10.1177/0269216312464094.
24. Dempsey D. Advance care planning for people with dementia: benefits and challenges. Int J Palliat Nurs. 2013;19:227–34.
25. van der Steen JT. Dying with dementia: what we know after more than a decade of research. J Alzheimers Dis. 2010;22:37–55.
26. Ngo J, Holroyd-Leduc JM. Systematic review of recent dementia practice guidelines. Age Ageing. 2015;44:25–33.
27. Briggs L. Shifting the focus of advance care planning: using an in-depth interview to build and strengthen relationships. J Palliat Med. 2004;7:341–9.
28. Maymone MB de C, Gan SD, Bigby M. Evaluating the strength of clinical recommendations in the medical literature: GRADE, SORT, and AGREE. J Invest Dermatol. 2014;134:e25.
29. Shea BJ, Hamel C, Wells GA, Bouter LM, Kristjansson E, Grimshaw J, et al. AMSTAR is a reliable and valid measurement tool to assess the methodological quality of systematic reviews. J Clin Epidemiol. 2009;62:1013–20.
30. Tools & Checklists | Cochrane Netherlands [Internet]. [cited 2017 Jun 14]. Available from: http://www.belgium.cochrane.org/en/information-resources/tools-checklists.
31. The ADAPTE Collaboration. The ADAPTE process: Resource Toolkit for Guideline Adaptation. Version 2.0. [Internet]. 2009. Available from: http://www.g-i-n.net
32. Fervers B, Burgers JS, Voellinger R, Brouwers M, Browman GP, Graham ID, et al. Guideline adaptation: an approach to enhance efficiency in guideline development and improve utilisation. BMJ Qual Saf. 2011;20:228–36.
33. Attia A. Adaptation of international evidence based clinical practice guidelines: the ADAPTE process. Middle East Fertil Soc J. 2013;18:123–6.
34. Van Royen P. GRADE. Een systeem om niveau van bewijskracht en graad van aanbeveling aan te geven. Huisarts Nu. 2008;37:505–9.
35. Atkins D, Best D, Briss PA, Eccles M, Falck-Ytter Y, Flottorp S, Guyatt GH, Harbour RT, Haugh MC, Henry D, Hill S, Jaeschke R, Leng G, Liberati A, Magrini N, Mason J, Middleton P, Mrukowicz J, O'Connell D, Oxman AD, Phillips B, Schünemann HJ, Edejer T, Varonen H, Vist GE, Williams JW Jr, Zaza S. GRADE Working Group. Grading quality of evidence and strength of recommendations. BMJ. 2004;328(7454):1490.
36. Reyniers T, Houttekier D, Cohen J, Pasman HR, Deliens L. What justifies a hospital admission at the end of life? A focus group study on perspectives of family physicians and nurses. Palliat Med. 2014;28:941–8.
37. Burlá C, Rego G, Nunes R. Alzheimer, dementia and the living will: a proposal. Med Health Care Philos. 2014;17:389–95.
38. Garand L, Dew MA, Lingler JH, DeKosky ST. Incidence and predictors of advance care planning among persons with cognitive impairment. Am J Geriatr Psychiatry Off J Am Assoc Geriatr Psychiatry. 2011;19:712–20.
39. Robinson L, Dickinson C, Rousseau N, Beyer F, Clark A, Hughes J, et al. A systematic review of the effectiveness of advance care planning interventions for people with cognitive impairment and dementia. Age Ageing. 2012;41:263–9.
40. Sampson EL. Palliative care for people with dementia. Br Med Bull. 2010;96:159–74.
41. Vandervoort A, Van den Block L, van der Steen JT, Vander Stichele R, Bilsen J, Deliens L. Advance directives and physicians' orders in nursing home residents with dementia in Flanders, Belgium: prevalence and associated outcomes. Int Psychogeriatr. 2012;7:1133–43.
42. de Boer ME, Dröes R-M, Jonker C, Eefsting JA, Hertogh CMPM. Thoughts on the future: the perspectives of elderly people with early-stage Alzheimer's disease and the implications for advance care planning. AJOB Prim Res. 2012;3:14–22.
43. van der Steen JT, Van Soest-Poortvliet MC, Hallie-Heierman M, Onwuteaka-Philipsen BD, Deliens L, de Boer ME, et al. Factors associated with initiation of advance care planning in dementia: a systematic review. J Alzheimers Dis. 2014;40:743–57.
44. Poppe M, Burleigh S, Banerjee S. Qualitative evaluation of advanced care planning in early dementia (ACP-ED). Forloni G, editor. PLoS One. 2013;8:e60412.
45. Hirschman KB, Kapo JM, Karlawish JHT. Identifying the factors that facilitate or hinder advance planning by persons with dementia. Alzheimer Dis Assoc Disord. 2008;22:293–8.
46. Brazil K, Carter G, Galway K, Watson M, van der Steen JT. General practitioners' perceptions on advance care planning for patients living with dementia. BMC Palliat Care [Internet]. 2015 [cited 2015 May 4];14. Available from: http://www.biomedcentral.com/1472-684X/14/14
47. Scott IA, Mitchell GK, Reymond E J, Daly MP. Difficult but necessary conversations — the case for advance care planning. Med J Aust. 2013;199:662–6.
48. Seeber AA, Hijdra A, Vermeulen M, Willems DL. Discussions about treatment restrictions in chronic neurologic diseases: a structured review. Neurology. 2012;78:590–7.
49. Bélanger E, Rodríguez C, Groleau D. Shared decision-making in palliative care: a systematic mixed studies review using narrative synthesis. Palliat Med. 2011;25:242–61.
50. Kim SYH, Appelbaum PS. The capacity to appoint a proxy and the possibility of concurrent proxy directives. Behav Sci Law. 2006;24:469–78.
51. Capacity BRL. consent. Curr Opin Psychiatry. 2001;14:491–9.
52. Robinson L, Tang E, Taylor J-P. Dementia: Timely diagnosis and early intervention. BMJ. 2015;350:h3029–9.
53. Welie SPK, Dute J, Nys H, van Wijmen FCB. Patient incompetence and substitute decision-making: an analysis of the role of the health care professional in Dutch law. Health Policy Amst Neth 2005;73:21–40.
54. Grisso T, Appelbaum P, Hill-Fotouhi C. The MacCAT-T: a clinicial tool to assess patients' capacities to make treatment decisions. Psychiatr Serv. 1997; 48:1415.
55. Vellinga A. To know or not to be: development of an instrument to assess decision-making capacity of cognitively impaired elderly patients. [S.l.]: s.n.]; 2006.
56. Church M, Watts S. Assessment of mental capacity: a flow chart guide. Psychiatr Bull. 2007;31:304–7.
57. Dening KH, Greenish W, Jones L, Mandal U, Sampson EL. Barriers to providing end-of-life care for people with dementia: a whole-system qualitative study. BMJ Support Palliat Care. 2012;2:103–7.
58. de Boer ME, Dröes R-M, Jonker C, Eefsting JA, Hertogh CMPM. Advance directives for euthanasia in dementia: how do they affect resident care in Dutch nursing homes? Experiences of physicians and relatives. J Am Geriatr Soc. 2011;59:989–96.
59. Chan HY, Pang SM. Readiness of Chinese frail old age home residents towards end-of-life care decision making: readiness towards end-of-life decision making. J Clin Nurs. 2011;20:1454–61.
60. The American Geriatrics Society Expert Panel on Person-Centered Care. Person-centered care: a definition and essential elements. J Am Geriatr Soc. 2016;64:15–8.
61. Séchaud L, Goulet C, Morin D, Mazzocato C. Advance care planning for institutionalised older people: an integrative review of the literature. Int J Older People Nursing. 2014;9:159–68.
62. Raymond M, Warner A, Davies N, Nicholas N, Manthorpe J, Iliffe S. Palliative and end of life care for people with dementia: lessons for clinical commissioners. Prim Health Care Res Dev. 2014;15:406–17.
63. Piers RD, van Eechoud IJ, Van Camp S, Grypdonck M, Deveugele M, Verbeke NC, et al. Advance care planning in terminally ill and frail older persons. Patient Educ Couns. 2013;90:323–9.
64. Hirschman KB, Kapo JM, Karlawish JHT. Why doesn't a family member of a person with advanced dementia use a substituted judgment when making a decision for that person? Am J Geriatr Psychiatry Off J Am Assoc Geriatr Psychiatry. 2006;14:659–67.
65. Levi BH, Dellasega C, Whitehead M, Green MJ. What influences individuals to engage in advance care planning? Am J Hosp Palliat Med. 2010;27:306–12.
66. Clayton JM, Hancock KM, Butow PN, Tattersall MH, Currow DC, Adler J, et al. Clinical practice guidelines for communicating prognosis and end-of-life issues with adults in the advanced stages of a life-limiting illness, and their caregivers. Med J Aust. 2007;187:478.
67. van der Steen JT, Radbruch L, Hertogh CM, de Boer ME, Hughes JC, Larkin P, et al. White paper defining optimal palliative care in older people with dementia: a Delphi study and recommendations from the European Association for Palliative Care. Palliat Med. 2014;28:197–209.
68. Mold JW, Blake GH, Becker LA. Goal-oriented medical care. Fam Med. 1991; 23:46–51.
69. American Medical Association. Education for Physicians on End-of-life Care (EPEC) Project. Plenary 3 Elem Models End–Life Care [Internet]. 1999. Available from: https://scholarworks.iupui.edu/handle/1805/708
70. Steeman E, Tournoy J, Grypdonck M, Godderis J, De Casterlé BD. Managing identity in early-stage dementia: maintaining a sense of being valued. Ageing Soc. 2013;33:216–42.

71. McMahan RD, Knight SJ, Fried TR, Sudore RL. Advance care planning beyond advance directives: perspectives from patients and surrogates. J Pain Symptom Manag. 2013;46:355–65.

72. Vandervoort A, Van den Block L, van der Steen JT, Volicer L, Stichele RV, Houttekier D, et al. Nursing home residents dying with dementia in Flanders, Belgium: a Nationwide postmortem study on clinical characteristics and quality of dying. J Am Med Dir Assoc. 2013;14:485–92.

73. Benkendorf R, Swor RA, Jackson R, Rivera-Rivera EJ, Demrick A. Outcomes of cardiac arrest in the nursing home: destiny or futility? [see comment]. Prehospital Emerg Care Off J Natl Assoc EMS Physicians Natl Assoc State EMS Dir. 1997;1:68–72.

74. van Gijn MS, Frijns D, van de Glind EMM, C van Munster B, Hamaker ME. The chance of survival and the functional outcome after in-hospital cardiopulmonary resuscitation in older people: a systematic review. Age Ageing 2014;43:456–463.

75. Ebell MH, Afonso AM. Pre-arrest predictors of failure to survive after in-hospital cardiopulmonary resuscitation: a meta-analysis. Fam Pract. 2011;28:505–15.

76. Volicer L. End-of-Life care for people with dementia in residential care settings [Internet]. Alzheimer's Association Chicago, IL; 2005 [cited 2016 Jul 13]. Available from: https://www.alz.org/documents/national/endoflifelitreview.pdf.

77. Van der Steen, Jenny, de Graas, T. Zorg rond het levenseinde voor mensen met de ziekte van Alzheimer of een andere vorm van dementie. Een handreiking voor familie en naasten. (Leaflet). VU Medisch Centrum - EMGO Instituut voor onderzoek naar gezondheid en zorg.; 2011.

78. Szafara KL, Kruse RL, Mehr DR, Ribbe MW, van der Steen JT. Mortality following nursing home-acquired lower respiratory infection: LRI severity, antibiotic treatment, and water intake. J Am Med Dir Assoc. 2012;13:376–83.

79. van der Steen JT, Lane P, Kowall NW, Knol DL, Volicer L. Antibiotics and mortality in patients with lower respiratory infection and advanced dementia. J Am Med Dir Assoc. 2012;13:156–61.

80. Juthani-Mehta M, Malani PN, Mitchell SL. Antimicrobials at the end of life: an opportunity to improve palliative care and infection management. JAMA. 2015;314:2017–8.

81. Mitchell SL, Teno JM, Kiely DK, Shaffer ML, Jones RN, Prigerson HG, et al. The clinical course of advanced dementia. N Engl J Med. 2009;361:1529–38.

82. Hoe J, Katona C, Orrell M, Livingston G. Quality of life in dementia: care recipient and caregiver perceptions of quality of life in dementia: the LASER-AD study. Int J Geriatr Psychiatry. 2007;22:1031–6.

83. Sampson EL, Jones L, Thuné-Boyle ICV, Kukkastenvehmas R, King M, Leurent B, et al. Palliative assessment and advance care planning in severe dementia: an exploratory randomized controlled trial of a complex intervention. Palliat Med. 2011;25:197–209.

84. Gillick MR. Doing the right thing: a geriatrician's perspective on medical care for the person with advanced dementia. J law med ethics J am Soc law. Med Ethics. 2012;40:51–6.

85. Steeman E, Godderis J, Grypdonck M, De Bal N, Dierckx de Casterlé B. Living with dementia from the perspective of older people: is it a positive story? Aging Ment Health. 2007;11:119–30.

86. Detering KM, Hancock AD, Reade MC, Silvester W. The impact of advance care planning on end of life care in elderly patients: randomised controlled trial. BMJ. 2010;340:c1345–5.

87. Smith AK, Lo B, Sudore R. When previously expressed wishes conflict with best interests. JAMA Intern Med. 2013;173:1241–5.

88. Shanley C, Whitmore E, Khoo A, Cartwright C, Walker A, Cumming RG. Understanding how advance care planning is approached in the residential aged care setting: a continuum model of practice as an explanatory device. Australas J Ageing. 2009;28:211–5.

89. Bernacki RE, Block SD. Communication about serious illness care goals: a review and synthesis of best practices. JAMA Intern Med. 2014;174:1994.

90. Harvey M. Advance Directives and the severely demented. J Med Philos. 2006;31:47–64.

91. Lemmens C. End-of-life decisions and demented patients. What to do if the patient's current and past wishes are in conflict with each other? Eur J Health Law. 2012;19:177–86.

92. Conroy S, Fade P, Fraser A, Schiff R, Guideline Development Group. Advance care planning: concise evidence-based guidelines. Clin Med Lond Engl. 2009;9:76–9.

93. De Gendt C, Bilsen J, Stichele RV, Deliens L. Nursing home policies regarding advance care planning in Flanders, Belgium. Eur J Pub Health. 2010;20:189–94.

94. Zimmerman S, Cohen L, van der Steen JT, Reed D, van Soest-Poortvliet MC, Hanson LC, et al. Measuring end-of-life care and outcomes in residential care/assisted living and nursing homes. J Pain Symptom Manag. 2015;49:666–79.

95. Baile WF, Lenzi R, Parker PA, Buckman R, Cohen L. Oncologists' attitudes toward and practices in giving bad news: an exploratory study. J Clin Oncol Off J Am Soc Clin Oncol. 2002;20:2189–96.

96. Keirse M, Vlaanderen OFPZ. Het levenseinde teruggeven aan de mensen. Vroegtijdige Plan Van Zorg Fed Palliat Zorgen Wemmel Downloadbare Broch Op Www Palliatief Be [Internet]. 2009 [cited 2016 Jul 13]; Available from: http://waasland.palliatieve.org/upload/file/VZP/VZP_brochure_zorgverlener_2008.pdf

97. Froggatt K, Vaughan S, Bernard C, Wild D. Advance care planning in care homes for older people: an English perspective. Palliat Med. 2009;23:332–8.

98. Beck ER, McIlfatrick S, Hasson F, Leavey G. Health care professionals' perspectives of advance care planning for people with dementia living in long-term care settings: A narrative review of the literature. Dementia. 2017; 16(4):486–12. https://doi.org/10.1177/1471301215604997. Epub 2015 Sep 16.

99. Silvester W, Fullam RS, Parslow RA, Lewis VJ, Sjanta R, Jackson L, et al. Quality of advance care planning policy and practice in residential aged care facilities in Australia. BMJ Support Palliat Care. 2012;bmjspcare:2012.

100. Martin RS, Hayes B, Gregorevic K, Lim WK. The effects of advance care planning interventions on nursing home residents: A systematic review. J Am Med Dir Assoc. 2016;17(4):284–93. https://doi.org/10.1016/j.jamda.2015.12.017.

101. Houben CHM, Spruit MA, Groenen MTJ, Wouters EFM, Janssen DJA. Efficacy of advance care planning: a systematic review and meta-analysis. J Am Med Dir Assoc. 2014;15:477–89.

102. Dixon J, Matosevic T, Knapp M. Economic evidence for advance care planning: Systematic review of evidence. Palliat Med. 2015;29(10):869–84. https://doi.org/10.1177/0269216315586659.

103. Penders YW, Gilissen J, Moreels S, Deliens L, Van den Block L. Palliative care service use by older people: Time trends from a mortality follow-back study between 2005 and 2014. Palliat Med. 2018;32(2):466–75. https://doi.org/10.1177/0269216317720833.

104. National Collaborating Centre for Mental Health. UK. Dementia: A NICE-SCIE Guideline on Supporting People With Dementia and Their Carers in Health and Social Care [Internet] Leicester (UK): British Psychological Society; 2007 [cited 2016 Jul 14] Available from. http://www.ncbi.nih.gov/books/NBK55459/

105. Rondia K, Raeymaekers P. Vroeger nadenken ...over later: reflecties over de toepassing van vroegtijdige zorgplanning in België (met bijzondere aandacht voor dementie). Brussel: Koning Boudewijnstichting; 2011.

106. Titler MG. The Evidence for Evidence-Based Practice Implementation. In: Hughes RG, editor. Patient Saf Qual Evid-Based Handb Nurses [Internet]. Rockville (MD): Agency for Healthcare Research and Quality (US); 2008 [cited 22 Aug 2016]. Available from: http://www.ncbi.nlm.nih.gov/books/NBK2659/

5

Place of death in patients with dementia and the association with comorbidities

Burkhard Dasch[1*] ⓘ, Claudia Bausewein[2] and Berend Feddersen[2]

Abstract

Background: Due to increasing life expectancy, more and more older people are suffering from dementia and comorbidities. To date, little information is available on place of death for dementia patients in Germany. In addition, the association of place of death and comorbidities is unknown.

Methods: A population-based cross-sectional survey was conducted in Westphalia–Lippe (Germany), based on the analysis of death certificates from 2011. Individuals with dementia ≥ 65 years were identified using the documented cause of death. In this context, all mentioned causes of death were included. In addition, ten selected comorbidities were also analyzed. The results were presented descriptively. Using multivariate logistic regression, place of death was analyzed for any association with comorbidities.

Results: A total of 10,364 death certificates were analyzed. Dementia was recorded in 1646 cases (15.9%; mean age 86.3 ± 6.9 years; 67.3% women). On average, 1.5 ± 1.0 selected comorbidities were present. Places of death were distributed as follows: home (19.9%), hospital (28.7%), palliative care unit (0.4%), nursing home (49.5%), hospice (0.9%), no details (0.7%). The death certificates documented cardiac failure in 43.6% of cases, pneumonia in 25.2%, and malignant tumour in 13.4%. An increased likelihood of dying in hospital compared to home or nursing home, respectively, was found for the following comorbidities (OR [95%-CI]): pneumonia (2.96 [2.01–4.35], $p = 0.001$); (2.38 [1.75–3.25], $p = 0.001$); renal failure (1.93 [1.26–2.97], $p = 0.003$); (1.65 [1.18–2.32], $p = 0.003$); and sepsis (13.73 [4.88–38.63], $p = 0.001$); (7.34 [4.21–12.78], $p = 0.001$).

Conclusion: The most common place of death in patients with dementia is the retirement or nursing home, followed by hospital and home. Specific comorbidities, such as pneumonia or sepsis, correlated with an increased probability of dying in hospital.

Keywords: Dementia, Place of death, Comorbidities, Death certificate, Observational study, End-of-life care

* Correspondence: burkhard.dasch@bergmannsheil.de
[1]Department of Anesthesiology, Intensive Care Medicine, Palliative Care Medicine and Pain Management, Berufsgenossenschaftliches Universitätsklinikum Bergmannsheil gGmbH Bochum, Medical Faculty of Ruhr University Bochum, Bürkle-de-la-Camp-Platz 1, 44789 Bochum, Germany
Full list of author information is available at the end of the article

Background

The proportion of people developing a dementia-related disease increases with increasing age. Older people's state of health is also usually characterized by comorbidity — i.e., they suffer from several diseases simultaneously.

In Germany, it is estimated that about 1.6 million people are currently diagnosed with dementia [1]. The absolute numbers of affected people have been estimated as 8.7 million in Europe in 2013 [2] and 46.8 million worldwide in 2015 [3]. Due to the age-dependency of the disease process and continually rising life expectancy, particularly in Western industrialized countries, the prevalence of the disease will increase further in the future. On the basis of predicted population trends in Germany, the number of patients with the condition will increase by around 40,000 annually and will rise to about 3 million by 2050 [1].

There is currently no treatment for dementia and the condition usually progresses very slowly. The duration of the disease cannot be reliably predicted in the individual case. Overall, the age-specific mortality rate is at least double that for individuals without dementia [4, 5]. Sampson et al. demonstrated in a prospective cohort of people with advanced dementia in the UK that 37% of these people died during a 9-months observational period [6]. Similar mortality rates have been reported in other countries [7–9].

During the course of the disease, people with severe dementia lose almost all their learned skills and abilities. They consequently require extensive nursing and medical support in many life situations. This represents a major health-policy and social challenge. It also affects end-of-life care. The disease is increasingly regarded as life-limiting by physicians, and the need for palliative care in patients in the advanced staged of dementia has been noted [10, 11].

Place of death is regarded as a kind of quality indicator for evaluating end-of-life care. Surveys on place of death show that most people clearly prefer to die at home rather than in institutions [12–14].

The place of death is not listed in official statistics in Germany, since the information given on the death certificate is not further analyzed by the relevant authorities. Studies on place of death for the general population in Germany show that hospitals are by far the most frequent place of death, followed by the home environment, retirement or nursing homes, hospices, and palliative care units [15].

Hardly any data regarding place of death are available for individuals with dementia in Germany. Escobar Pinzon et al. showed that in the federal state of Rhineland–Palatinate in 2008 42.4% of those with dementia died at home, followed by nursing homes (26.9%), hospitals (26.2%) and palliative

institutions (hospices and/or palliative units; 3.2%) [16]. International studies show that individuals with dementia mainly die in institutions, with nursing homes and hospitals to some extent, being the most frequent place of death in most countries [16–22].

Older people with dementia often suffer from multiple additional diseases [23]. On average, two to eight other chronic diseases are present [24, 25]. In 3971 patients with dementia aged over 64 receiving care from family physicians in Spain, at least three other diagnoses were present in 70% with the most frequent being arterial hypertension, osteoarthrosis (in both women and men), as well as anxiety disorder/neurosis in women and benign prostate hypertrophy in men [26]. In the UK, arterial hypertension (53.4%), chronic pain (33.5%), depression (23.5%), presbyacusis (22.3%), coronary heart disease (21.6%), and chronic renal failure (20.8%) were the most frequent comorbidities in 4999 patients with dementia [27]. Overall, patients with dementia have a higher prevalence of complex situations that indicate functional limitations (including immobility, dysphagia, and impaired hearing), depression, and frailty syndrome (reduced physical activity, weakness, fatigue, weight loss) [28]. In addition, these patients have more often emergency hospital admissions compared to patients without dementia, and the number of hospital admissions increases with the severity of the disease [29, 30]. The reasons for hospital admission are often bronchial and urogenital infections, falls, or fractures, as well as delirium [31, 32]. Although it appears obvious from the clinical point of view that comorbidities contribute to the place of death for patients with dementia, hardly any scientific evidence is available on the topic.

The aim of the present study was to describe the place of death of patients with dementia in Germany on the basis of analyzed death certificates and to investigate the extent to which specific comorbidities are associated with the place of death.

Methods
Design
This was a population-based epidemiological cross-sectional study based on death certificates for the study region in 2011.

Study region
The study region included selected urban areas (the cities of Bochum and Münster) and rural areas (the districts of Borken and Coesfeld) in Westphalia–Lippe in the federal state of North Rhine–Westphalia (Germany). On December 31st 2010, the study region's population was 1,243,957,

representing 1.5% of the total population of Germany at that time.

Study data

The study used a complete dataset of death certificates for the study region. In all, 12,914 death certificates were available for 2011, which were archived in each local public health department and had to be analyzed on site due to data protection regulations. Information was collected about age, sex, time of death, place of death, manner of death, and cause of death. The main focus of the analysis was on the cause of death in patients with dementia. Ten other selected diseases documented by the physicians on the death certificate were also examined: pneumonia, aspiration, sepsis, cardiac failure, myocardial infarction, intracerebral bleeding (ICB) and/or cerebral stroke, malignant neoplasia, chronic obstructive pulmonary disease (COPD), renal failure, and Parkinson's disease.

As cases of dementia mainly become clinically manifest in the elderly, the analyses was restricted to deceased persons whose age at death was 65 or over and who had a natural cause of death ($n = 10,364$).

Documentation of cause of death

In accordance with German law, all deaths have to be certified by a physician. The form and structure of the death certificate are the responsibility of each federal state in Germany and are not standardized. In all 16 federal states, however, the question of the cause of death largely follows the scheme set out by the World Health Organization. Efforts have been made to develop a standard federal death certificate, but the project has so far been blocked by several states. It is also intended to introduce an electronic death certificate in Germany, as has been demanded at the European Union level, but this project has not yet been implemented [33].

The present study used death certificates from the state of North Rhine–Westphalia. Documentation of the cause of death is specified as follows here: "Section I," I.a) "immediate cause of death" — i.e., the disease that led directly to death; I.b) "this is a result of" — i.e., a disease that is derived from the underlying condition and causally contributed to the death; I.c) "the underlying cause" — i.e., the disease causally leading to death and giving rise to the diseases described in I.a and I.b. In addition, the physician is able to record other diseases that were not immediately part of the causal chain leading to the death in "Section II." The heading "Epicrisis" also provides an opportunity to document additional medical details on the sequence of the disease, accident occurrence, etc.

The analysis of death certificates is carried out in a standardized fashion in all federal states. The non-confidential section (time of death, manner of death, place of death) and the confidential section (cause of death) in the medical certificate are first sent to the local civil registry office where the patient was registered with his or her place of residence, and an official death statistic bulletin is drawn up. During this official procedure, the medical information about place of death is unfortunately not included. The death certificate is then sent on to the responsible public health office. There, the medical officer of health checks among other matters whether the stated diagnoses are compatible with the sex and age of the deceased and in general whether sufficient information about the cause of death is given. In a third step, the information is then transferred to the state statistical offices, where it is combined with the death statistic bulletin. Trained signatories once again check the medical details on the cause of death and finally determine the underlying disease in accordance with the regulations in the *International Statistical Classification of Diseases and Related Health Problems* (ICD), volume 2 [34]. This involves monocausal statistics on the cause of death — i.e., only one underlying disease is recorded and represented ("one cause per death"). The other diagnoses noted on the death certificate are ignored. Finally, this information is sent to the Federal Office of Statistics, which publishes annually cause-of-death statistics for the whole of Germany.

In contrast to the official cause-of-death statistics in Germany, the present study made use of all medical information available on the cause of death (Sections I.a, I.b, I.c, Section II, and epicrisis) in order to identify patients with dementia and other selected diseases. However, the medically documented diagnosis was not further differentiated according to Section I, Section II, or epicrisis. The reason for this was the highly time-consuming logistic effort involved in obtaining the documentation in each local public health office in the study region.

Persons with dementia-related disease

In accordance with ICD-10, patients with a dementia-related disease constituted the study population if the medical details on the cause of death were described as follows: Alzheimer's disease (F00, G30), vascular dementia (F01), dementia in other diseases classified elsewhere (F02), and unspecified dementia (F03).

Comorbidities

All death certificates were analyzed for ten additional comorbid conditions and classified in accordance with ICD-10: pneumonia (J12.0–J18.9), aspiration (J69.0, J60.1, J69.8; J95.4; T17.2–T17.9), sepsis (A39.2–39.4, A40, A41, B37.7, R52.7), cardiac failure (I09, I25.1, I25.3–I25.9, I50), myocardial infarction (I21, I22, I24, I25.2), intracerebral bleeding (ICB) or cerebral stroke

(I60, I61, I62, I63, I64, I69), malignant neoplasia (C00–C97), chronic obstructive pulmonary disease (COPD) (J41, J42, J44), renal failure (N17, N18, N19), and Parkinson's disease (G20).

Definition of place of death

The place of death was classified in the study as home environment, hospital, palliative care unit, retirement home or nursing home, hospice, and other locations. The category "home environment" combined the deceased person's private residence as well as other private homes that were not the home of the deceased individual. Hospitals, psychiatric clinics, and sanatoriums were included under "hospital" as place of death. Palliative care units were counted as a separate place of death. The category "retirement or nursing home" included all institutions involving old age homes, retirement homes, geriatric care homes, sheltered housing, and short-term care. "Other locations" represented other public areas, family physicians' practices, and leisure centers.

Statistical analyses

To assess the prevalence, the absolute number of individuals aged 65 or over with a dementia-related disease was counted and related to the overall number of deaths in that age group (relative frequency). An analysis stratified by sex and specific age groups (65–69, 70–74, 75–79, 80–84, 85–89, 90–94, ≥ 95 years) was also carried out. In addition, the data were subjected to direct age standardization. For this purpose, the age-specific mortality rate in the study population was calculated, weighted with the age-specific rate in a standard population, and added up. The "Old European Standard Population" was used as the standard population.

The characteristics of the study population were listed by sex, age, selected comorbidities and number of comorbidities (no.: 1, 2, 3, 4, ≥ 5), and a subdivision relative to place of death was also carried out. It was investigated whether individuals who died at home with dementia differed significantly from those with a different place of death (hospital, palliative care unit, retirement or nursing home, hospice, other location, no details). For this purpose, unpaired t-tests were used for continuous data and the chi-squared test for categorical data, or in the case of cell numbers fewer than five, Fisher's exact test was used.

Places of death were represented using absolute and relative frequencies, and sex-specific differences were tested using the chi-squared test. As no deaths at "other places" were observed, that category was not listed further in the results.

An association between "explanatory factors" and the dependent variable "place of death" was tested using a multivariate logic regression model. The target variable

"home" (0) was investigated relative to the place of death "hospital" (1) and the place of death "retirement or nursing home" (1); in a second step, the place of death "retirement or nursing home" (0) was investigated relative to the places of death "hospital" (1). Due to very low results, the places of death "palliative care unit" ($n = 6$) and "hospice" ($n = 14$) were not subjected to multivariate regression analysis.

"Independent factors" were sex (women (1) vs. men (0)) and the median age of the deceased persons (≥ 86.7 y (1) vs. < 86.7 y (0)). In addition, the multivariate regression model considered all ten comorbidities — pneumonia, aspiration, sepsis, cardiac failure, myocardial infarction, intracerebral bleeding (ICB) or cerebral stroke, malignant tumour, chronic obstructive pulmonary disease (COPD), renal failure, and Parkinson's disease. The process of modeling followed primarily clinical aspects. The aim was to analyze the statistical impact of each explanatory variable (sex, age, diseases) on the dependent variable "place of death". Accordingly, we used a block method and not a stepwise regression procedure (forward selection or backward elimination). Under these conditions, we accepted a possibly poorer adjustment of the statistical model. Odds ratios with 95% confidence intervals were generated from this model. The Wald test was used to examine whether the independent variable had any significant influence on the target variable. The quality of the statistical model was expressed using Nagelkerke pseudo-R^2 coefficients.

To minimize the global increase in the probability of alpha error due to multiple testing of the same sample, the significance level was set at $p < 0.01$ (two-sided). All analyses were carried out using the statistics program IBM SPSS Statistics, version 23.

Ethics approval and data protection

The study was submitted to the Ethics Committee of the Ruhr University of Bochum and approved after examination (registry no. 4522-12). Letters were sent to the public health offices requesting access to the death certificates archived there. Permission to collect data and carry out the scientific analysis, while observing legal data protection regulations, was officially granted. The data had to be recorded locally in the public health offices.

Results

A total of 10,364 death certificates of patients who had died at the age of 65 or over were analyzed. Dementia was described in 1646 cases, representing a relative frequency of 15.9%. A larger proportion of women (19.5%) than men (11.4%) were affected. The standardized prevalence of all individuals with a dementia-related disease was 8.0% (women 9.0%, men 6.9%; data not shown). One in ten deceased persons aged 75–79 suffered from dementia. In the 95 or older age group, one in four men and one in three women were affected by the disease (Fig. 1).

Overall, 67.3% of the deceased patients were women. Of deaths in retirement or nursing homes from dementia, two-thirds were women. Of deaths in hospital, just under half were men. The mean age was 86.3 ± 6.9 years. On average, 1.5 ± 1.0 other comorbidities were present. No comorbidity was present in 14.9% of cases, one additional condition was present in 40.6%, and three comorbidities were present in 10.6% of the cases. The most frequent accompanying disease was cardiac failure (43.6%). Pneumonia was documented in one-quarter of the cases, and cancer in just over one in ten. Patients with dementia who died in hospital suffered significantly more often from pneumonia, aspiration, sepsis, and renal failure compared to patients with dementia who died at home. Patients with dementia who died in hospices had malignant tumours more often compared to those who had received terminal care in the home environment (71.4% vs. 12.8%; $p < 0.01$) (Table 1).

Patients with dementia dying in hospital had a high proportion of infectious diseases (such as pneumonia or sepsis), aspiration, and renal failure in comparison with other places of death that were investigated. In contrast, septic conditions were only rarely noted in death certificates for those who died at home (1.2%), while cardiac failure was the most frequent in that location with 45.9%. In retirement or nursing homes, the frequency of documented pneumonia was similar to that for deaths in the home environment (19.9%) which was much lower

in comparison with hospitals (39.1%). In hospices, dementia patients mainly died of tumours (Fig. 2).

Retirement or nursing homes were by far the most frequent place of death. Approximately every second patient died there. Hospitals represented the second most frequent place of death (28.7%). Only one in five deaths occurred in the home environment. Palliative care units and hospices played a subordinate role, with a total of 1.3%. Stratified by sex, women died more often in retirement or nursing homes, while men by contrast died more often in hospital (Fig. 3).

In the multivariate regression analysis, very elderly patients with dementia (86 years, ≥ 0.5 quantile) and women had a higher odds of dying in retirement or nursing homes compared to the home setting (OR 1.59 [95%-CI 1.21–2.08], $p = 0.001$; OR 1.55 [95%-CI 1.16–2.08], $p = 0.003$) and a lower odds of dying in hospital compared to retirement or nursing homes (OR 0.50 [95%-CI 0.38–0.64], $p = 0.001$; OR 0.50 [95%-CI 0.38–0.66], $p = 0.001$). There was a statistical association between pneumonia, sepsis, and renal failure and hospitals as a place of death. In comparison with deaths at home, the odds of dying in hospital was three times higher when there was a medically documented pneumonia (OR 2.96 [95%-CI 2.01–4.35], $p = 0.001$), while in the presence of renal failure it was twice as high (OR 1.93 [95%-CI 1.26–2.97], $p = 0.003$) and with sepsis 14 times higher (OR 13.73 [95%-CI 4.88–38.63], $p = 0.001$). Similarly, in comparison with deaths in retirement or nursing homes, the odds of dying in hospital was also higher in the presence of pneumonia (OR 2.38 [95%-CI 1.75–3.25], $p = 0.001$), sepsis

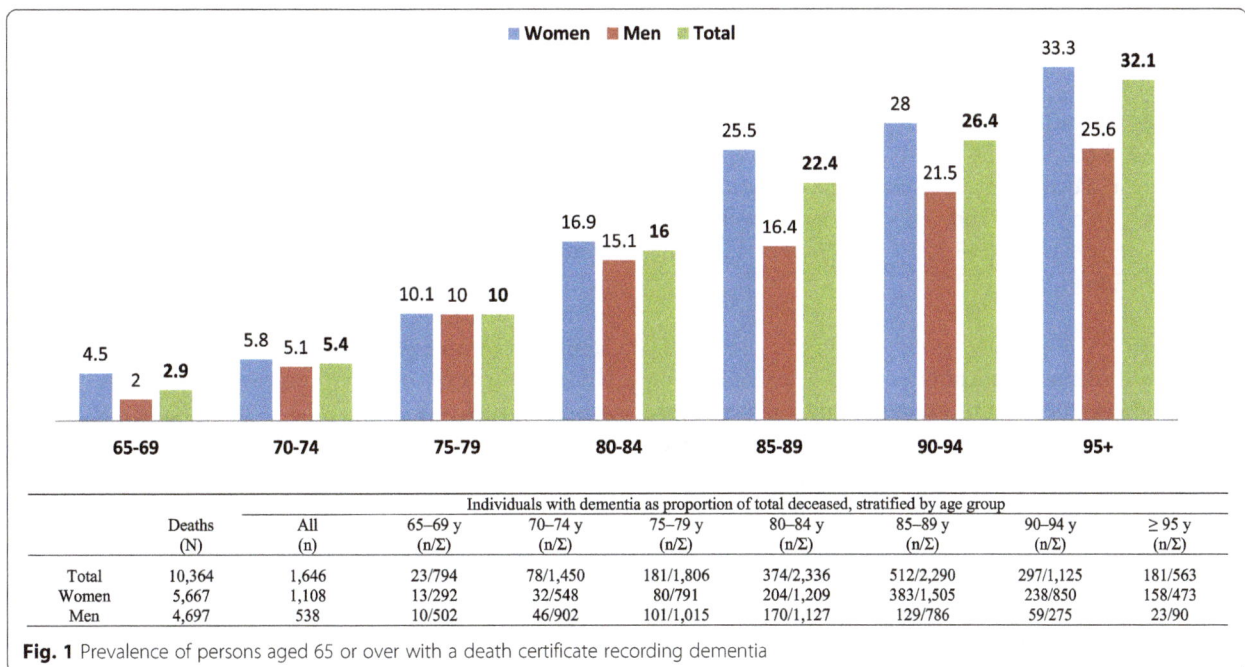

Fig. 1 Prevalence of persons aged 65 or over with a death certificate recording dementia

| | Deaths (N) | All (n) | Individuals with dementia as proportion of total deceased, stratified by age group | | | | | | |
			65–69 y (n/Σ)	70–74 y (n/Σ)	75–79 y (n/Σ)	80–84 y (n/Σ)	85–89 y (n/Σ)	90–94 y (n/Σ)	≥ 95 y (n/Σ)
Total	10,364	1,646	23/794	78/1,450	181/1,806	374/2,336	512/2,290	297/1,125	181/563
Women	5,667	1,108	13/292	32/548	80/791	204/1,209	383/1,505	238/850	158/473
Men	4,697	538	10/502	46/902	101/1,015	170/1,127	129/786	59/275	23/90

Table 1 Characteristics of deceased persons with dementia aged 65 or over, stratified by place of death

	Overall (n = 1646)		Home (n = 327)		Hospital (n = 473)		Palliative care unit (n = 6)		Retirement or nursing home (n = 815)		Hospice (n = 14)		No details (n = 11)	
	%	n	%	n	%	n	%	n	%	n	%	n	%	n
Women	67.3	1108	64.5	211	55.4*	262	83.3	5	75.6*	616	42.9	6	72.7	8
Men	32.7	538	35.5	116	44.6*	211	16.7	1	24.4*	199	57.1	8	27.3	3
Age (mean / SD)	86.3 ± 6.9		85.8 ± 6.8		84.2* ± 6.5		81.5 ± 7.4		87.8* ± 6.8		81.1 ± 6.7		84.5 ± 5.4	
Age (median, 0.5 quantile)	86.7		86.4		84.6		84.9		88.2		81.9		83.9	
Age (0.25 quantile)	82.0		81.7		80.1		74.5		83.6		79.3		80.7	
Age (0.75 quantile)	90.7		90.4		88.9		86.7		92.0		85.5		86.7	
Age, women (mean / SD)	87.7 ± 6.6		87.2 ± 6.6		85.8 ± 6.4		80.7 ± 7.9		88.8* ± 6.4		82.6* ± 2.4		84.7 ± 6.3	
Age, men (mean / SD)	83.3 ± 6.5		83.4 ± 6.4		82.1 ± 6.0		85.5 ± 0		84.7 ± 6.8		80.0 ± 8.7		84.1 ± 2.9	
Pneumonia	25.2	415	19.3	63	39.1*	185	0	0	19.9	162	28.6	4	9.1	1
Aspiration	10.0	164	9.5	31	15.6*	74	0	0	7.1	58	7.1	1	0	0
Sepsis	5.7	93	1.2	4	14.4*	68	0	0	2.3	19	7.1	1	9.1	1
Cardiac failure	43.6	718	45.9	150	44.2	209	50.0	3	42.8	349	14.3	2	45.5	5
Myocardial infarction	4.8	79	4.6	15	7.2	34	0	0	3.7	30	0	0	0	0
ICB and/or cerebral stroke	13.0	214	13.1	43	10.8	51	16.7	1	14.2	116	14.3	2	9.1	1
Malignant tumour	13.4	220	12.8	42	13.3	63	33.3	2	12.3	100	71.4*	10	27.3	3
COPD	6.1	100	5.8	19	7.6	36	16.7	1	5.2	42	7.1	1	9.1	1
Renal failure	15.4	253	12.5	41	19.7*	93	33.3	2	14.4	117	0	0	0	0
Parkinson's disease	9.4	154	8.0	26	11.4	54	16.7	1	9.0	73	0	0	0	0
Comorbidity (mean)	1.5 ± 1.0		1.3 ± 0.9		1.8 ± 1.0		1.7 ± 0.8		1.3 ± 0.9		1.5 ± 0.7		1.1 ± 0.8	
0 Comorbidity	14.9	245	16.8	55	5.9*	28	0.0	0	19.6	160	0.0	0	18.2	2
1 Comorbidity	40.6	669	45.3	148	33.4*	158	50.0	3	42.3	345	57.1	8	63.6	7
2 Comorbidities	31.1	512	27.8	91	39.1*	185	33.3	2	28.0	228	35.7	5	9.1	1
3 Comorbidities	10.6	175	8.6	28	15.9*	75	16.7	1	8.5	69	7.1	1	9.1	1
4 Comorbidities	2.2	36	1.5	5	4.9*	23	0.0	0	1.0	8	0.0	0	0.0	0
≥ 5 Comorbidities	0.5	9	0.0	0	0.8	4	0.0	0	0.6	5	0.0	0	0.0	0

COPD chronic obstructive pulmonary disease, ICB intracerebral bleeding, SD standard deviation
*Specific place of death vs. place of death "at home" (chi-squared test) $P < 0.01$

(OR 7.34 [95%-CI 4.21–12.78], $p = 0.001$) or renal failure (OR 1.65 [95%-CI 1.18–2.32], $p = 0.003$). There was also a correlation between the diagnosis of myocardial infarction and an increased probability of dying in hospital (OR 2.52 [95%-CI 1.45–4.36], $p = 0.001$) (Table 2).

Discussion

Patients with dementia most often died in retirement or nursing homes, followed by hospitals and the home environment. Palliative care units and hospices as places of death played only a minor role. An association was seen between selected comorbidities and an increased likelihood of dying in hospital.

In the present study, nearly one in two deaths among patients with dementia occurred in retirement or nursing homes in Westphalia-Lippe (Germany). This finding is not surprising, as it reflects the high level of nursing care required by dementia patients. Relatives who are caring for people with dementia usually have a strong wish to care for and look after the patient in the shared home environment. However, relatives dealing with dementia patients on a daily basis are exposed to a large number of problems and challenges. The time demands involved in caring often conflict with the carer's own family, and working life. Persons with dementia may also show depressive or even aggressive behavior in the course of their disease, as well as developing restlessness and/or a marked urge for movement. This can lead to a high level of physical and above all emotional burden on caring relatives, which may even cause social isolation [35, 36]. Caregivers usually belong to the patient's immediate family (first-degree relatives, children, spouses), or more rarely they may be friends or other people linked to the patient [37]. If relatives struggle to cope with the situation they can get potentially support from a home

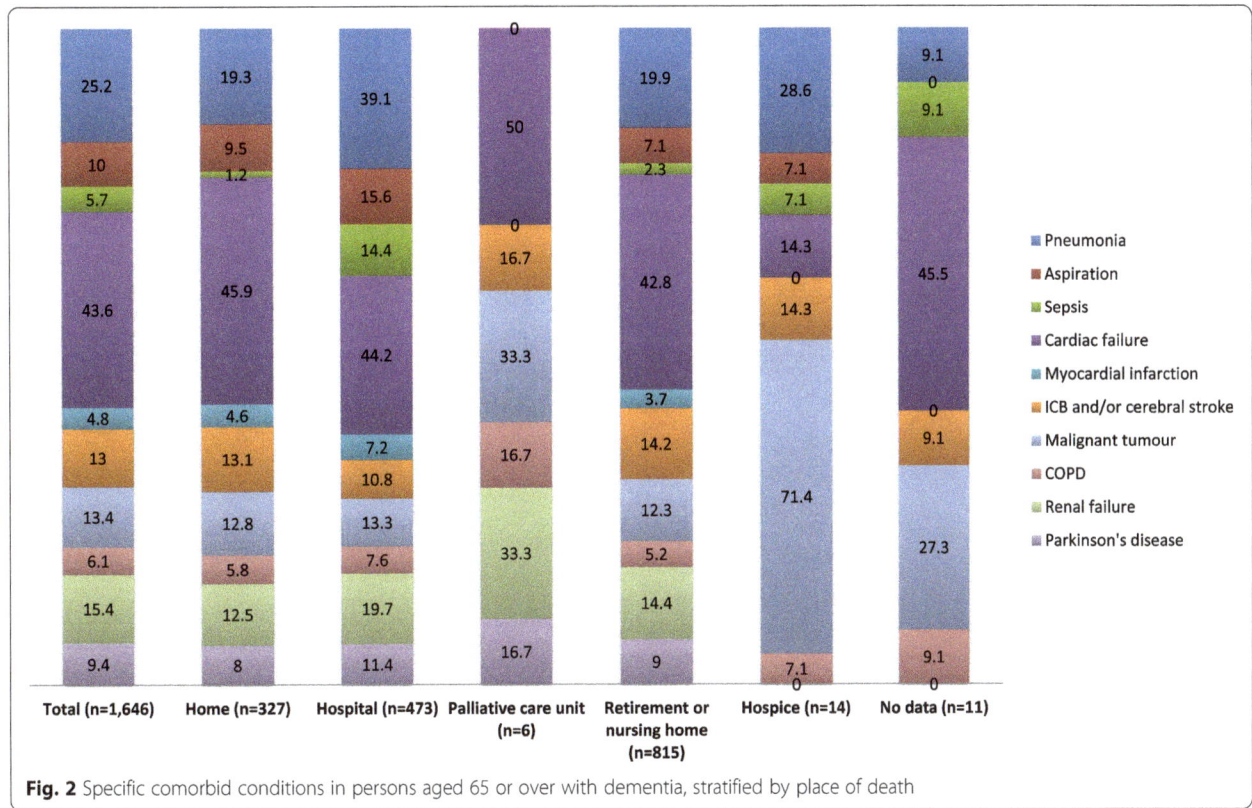

Fig. 2 Specific comorbid conditions in persons aged 65 or over with dementia, stratified by place of death

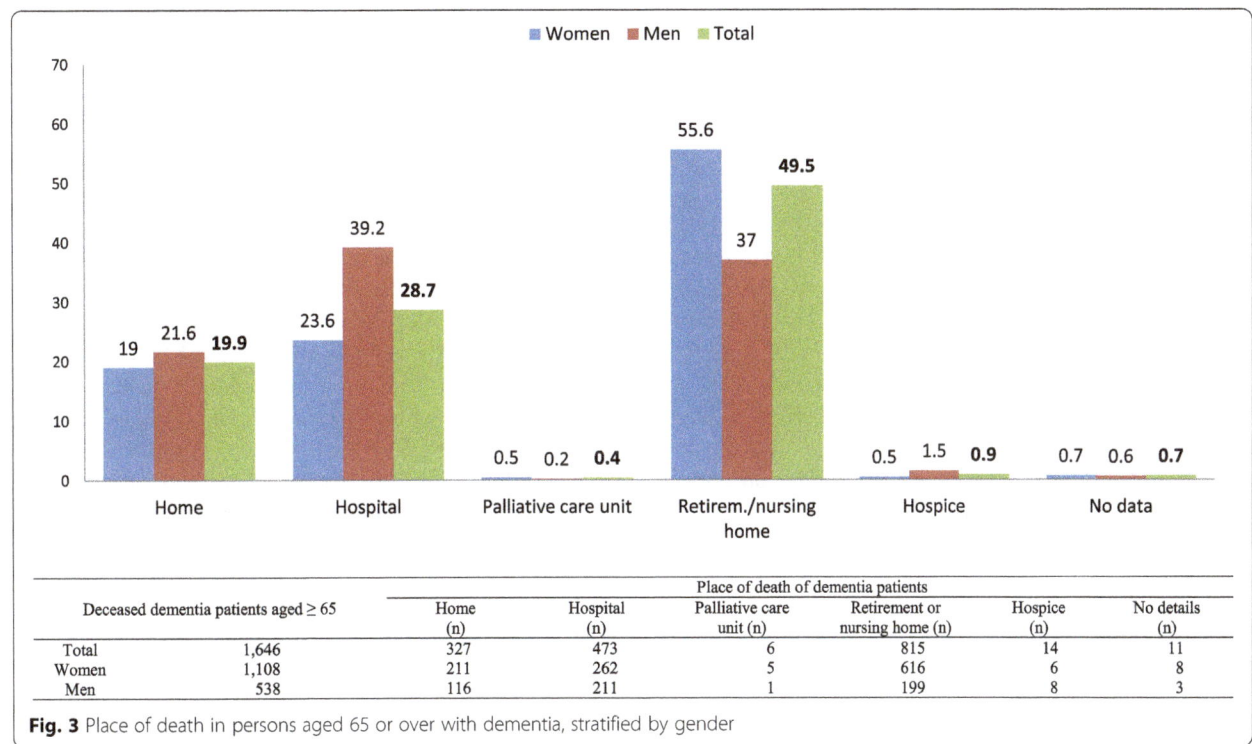

Deceased dementia patients aged ≥ 65		Place of death of dementia patients					
		Home (n)	Hospital (n)	Palliative care unit (n)	Retirement or nursing home (n)	Hospice (n)	No details (n)
Total	1,646	327	473	6	815	14	11
Women	1,108	211	262	5	616	6	8
Men	538	116	211	1	199	8	3

Fig. 3 Place of death in persons aged 65 or over with dementia, stratified by gender

Table 2 Association between place of death and specific comorbidities in persons aged 65 or over with dementia

	Hospital (1) vs. home (0)		Retirement or nursing home (1) vs. home (0)		Hospital (1) vs. retirement or nursing home (0)	
	OR (95% CI)	p value	OR (95% CI)	p value	OR (95% CI)	p value
Women (1) vs. men (0)	0.80 (0.58–1.11)	0.186	1.55 (1.16–2.08)*	0.003	0.50 (0.38–0.66)*	0.001
Age (median), ≥ 86.7 y (1) vs. < 86.7 y (0)	0.78 (0.57–1.08)	0.133	1.59 (1.21–2.08)*	0.001	0.50 (0.38–0.64)*	0.001
Pneumonia, yes (1) vs. no (0)	2.96 (2.01–4.35)*	0.001	1.25 (0.85–1.84)	0.249	2.38 (1.75–3.25)*	0.001
Aspiration, yes (1) vs. no (0)	1.26 (0.76–2.09)	0.380	0.66 (0.39–1.12)	0.126	1.68 (1.09–2.59)	0.018
Sepsis, yes (1) vs. no (0)	13.73 (4.88–38.63)*	0.001	1.71 (0.57–5.16)	0.338	7.34 (4.21–12.78)*	0.001
Cardiac failure, yes (1) vs. no (0)	1.29 (0.94–1.78)	0.113	0.82 (0.62–1.07)	0.145	1.51 (1.16–1.97)	0.012
Myocardial infarction, yes (1) vs. no (0)	2.19 (1.13–4.23)	0.019	0.86 (0.45–1.66)	0.661	2.52 (1.45–4.36)*	0.001
ICB /cerebral stroke, yes (1) vs. no (0)	1.01 (0.63–1.60)	0.984	1.10 (0.75–1.61)	0.642	0.87 (0.60–1.28)	0.471
Malignant tumour, yes (1) vs. no (0)	1.19 (0.75–1.87)	0.450	1.03 (0.69–1.53)	0.888	1.26 (0.87–1.83)	0.230
COPD, yes (1) vs. no (0)	1.28 (0.69–2.37)	0.439	0.98 (0.55–1.75)	0.957	1.42 (0.85–2.36)	0.182
Renal failure, yes (1) vs. no (0)	1.93 (1.26–2.97)*	0.003	1.15 (0.78–1.70)	0.483	1.65 (1.18–2.32)*	0.003
Parkinson's disease, yes (1) vs. no (0)	1.39 (0.82–2.35)	0.227	1.20 (0.75–1.94)	0.449	1.12 (0.74–1.70)	0.577
Nagelkerke R^2 (goodness of fit)	0.179		0.040		0.221	

OR odds ratio, CI confidence intervals, COPD chronic obstructive pulmonary disease, ICB intracerebral bleeding
*P < 0.01

help, a day or temporary nurse or a nursing service. However, these measures are often only effective in the shorter term. Alternative residential forms are available, such as "sheltered housing" or "dementia apartment-sharing," but a move to a nursing home is often the only practicable way of ensuring care.

This study has shown that (unsurprisingly) it is mainly very elderly people and women who die in retirement and nursing homes. This observation is explained by demographic change and changes in social life. Life expectancy has been increasing for decades in the Western industrialized countries, and this applies to Germany as well. In this country, the mean life expectancy is currently 83.1 years for women and 78.2 years for men [38]. Due to their lower life expectancy, men are more likely to be survived by their partners, and this also increases the probability that they will be cared for by relatives at home at the end of their lives. Also, due to the increasing age, there is a greater likelihood that women will be widowed or living alone when they are elderly and, with increasing physical problems will be dependent on assistance from strangers or institutions. The results of the 2011 population census in Germany also indicate that more and more people are living alone. The proportion of people living alone, for example, increased from 15.6% in 1996 to 19.6% in 2011 [39].

Surveys have shown that most people would prefer to die at home [12–14] and this also applies to people with dementia-related diseases [16]. The findings of the present study are in contrast to this wish of patients: only one in five persons with dementia died at home. The reasons for this remain speculative, but it may again

be linked to excessive stress on relatives caring for the patient and show that there is a need for relevant action to be taken in health care policy. This need has been recognized by the relevant German political decision-making body, and measures have been implemented [40]. The legal meaning of the term "status of requiring care" has been redefined and extended to mental and psychological illnesses. Patients with dementia have consequently had their previous benefit entitlement from the nursing insurance fund upgraded. In addition, relatives who have had to stop working in order to provide care are now receiving improved financial support from the state.

Advanced-stage dementia is increasingly being regarded as a terminal disease leading to death [10, 11, 41, 42]. Palliative care is appropriate in dementia, since it represents a "disease that does not respond to curative treatment" or a "life-threatening disease," as dementia itself is not curable. The treatment approach aims at achieving improvements in quality of life. The results of the present study show that in-patient palliative and hospice institutions were only playing a minor role in 2011 in comparison with all other places of death. Only 0.4% of all dementia patients who died received end-of-life care in a palliative care unit, and only 0.9% of them received care in a hospice. There might be several reasons for this observation. First, a health economic aspect. There were only 32,1 palliative care unit beds and 40,2 hospice beds in the study region relative to a population of 1 million — corresponding to two-thirds of the maximum number recommended by the European Association for Palliative Care (EAPC) [43]. Thus, there was a need for implementing further inpatient palliative care and hospice services in this region in 2011. Second, the life expectancy of patients with dementia. In many cases, the natural course of the disease often exceeds the official requirements that patients should only be admitted to hospices when the medical estimate of life expectancy is less than 3–6 months.

Several investigations indicate that patients with dementia are at increased risk of hospital admission compared to people without dementia [29, 30, 43–46]. The reasons for this are complex [6, 31, 32, 47–49]. The most frequent causes include respiratory and urogenital infections, fall-related injuries, neurological and psychiatric causes (syncope, confusion, delirium), pressure sores, and nutritional disturbances. There is a consensus in the research findings that many of these diseases could have been treatable in home care or in in-patient care institutions, so that hospital admission could have been avoided [50, 51]. Psychosocial factors also affect hospital admissions — for example, when the previous carer suddenly becomes unavailable.

Generally, a hospital stay is a severe burden for many people with dementia and it is also associated with a number of risks. These include prolongation of the hospitalization period, a decline in physical functional abilities, increased frequencies of nosocomial infections, and an increased likelihood of not being able to return to the home environment after the hospital treatment [52]. Sampson et al. concluded that an unplanned hospital stay significantly shortens the median survival time in patients with dementia [53].

In the present study group of deceased individuals in the general population aged 65 or older with dementia, in-patient deaths represented 28.7% of cases. A similar percentage was reported by Houttekier et al. in a European survey in 2003 [18]. The mean percentage of dementia patients aged 65 or over who died in hospital in that study was 27.4%, including all countries investigated (Belgium, Netherlands, England, Wales, and Scotland). The Netherlands showed a very low percentage, with only 2.8% of deaths occurring in in-patients. In this country, some general practitioners ("verpleeghuisarts") work exclusively in nursing homes enabling them to monitor the state of health of nursing-home patients tightly and offer medical treatment in a timely manner when physical changes occur. In most cases, hospital admissions can be avoided.

The medical information on cause of death that was analyzed in the present study showed that the deceased dementia patients had been suffering from a mean of 1.5 of the selected comorbidities. Cardiac failure was the most frequent comorbidity documented in the death certificates with almost one in two deaths, with the diagnoses of pneumonia, renal failure and malignant

tumours following in frequency. Cardiovascular diseases are the most common cause of death in Germany, followed by cancers. The diagnosis of dementia is already in third place [54]. The prevalence of cardiac failure, like that of dementia, increases with increasing age [55, 56], and this may have contributed to the high prevalence of cardiac failure in the present sample. Many patients with advanced dementia also suffer from dysphagia [57], which may make fluid intake much more difficult. This can lead to dehydration and prerenal kidney failure. In addition, there is a risk of aspiration of fluid and food particles potentially resulting in pneumonia leading to sepsis and multiple-organ failure causing death finally [58]. In several autopsy studies, pneumonia was the most frequent cause of death [59, 60]. These findings are supported by clinical data. Mitchell et al. [7], for example, noted in the CASCADE study that 41.1% of the patients developed at least one episode of pulmonary infection during the 18-month follow-up period. The infection was associated with a high mortality rate. In the Netherlands, the three most frequent causes of death in nursing-home residents with dementia were dehydration (38%), cardiovascular diseases (19%), and respiratory infections (18%) [61]. In the present study, the death certificates described pneumonia in 25.2% of cases and aspiration in 10.0%. Pneumonia and/or aspiration were particularly frequent on the death certificates of dementia patients who died in hospital (39.1 and 15.6%, respectively). Compared to home or nursing home deaths, the odds of dying in hospital with documented pneumonia was two to three times higher, and with aspiration by a factor of 1.3 or 1.7 higher. In addition, deceased hospital patients often had sepsis (14.4%), renal failure (19.7%), and myocardial infarction (7.2%). These results suggest that there is a high intensity of treatment in hospital at the end of life in dementia patients. Unfortunately, the study was not able to provide any further information on this.

Care for patients with dementia in the last phase of their lives represents a special challenge, since those affected are often unable to express their treatment preferences directly themselves, while established, evidence-based treatment pathways for this phase of disease are still largely lacking. Research results showing that physical symptoms are widespread in persons with dementia and that they even increase before death [6, 7, 16, 61].

In Germany, a new law was passed in 2015 to improve hospice and palliative care [62]. The law aims to strengthen comprehensive hospice and palliative care in Germany by implementing targeted measures in statutory health insurance and social care insurance. The measures are intended among other things to ensure networking among medical and nursing services, as well as attendant hospice services, and to guarantee cooperation among the health-care providers involved. The aim is to strengthen palliative care and hospice approaches in in-patient care institutions and hospitals and to offer information to health-insurance policy-holders in a targeted way about the hospice and palliative care services available, as well as enabling nursing-home residents to carry out individualized care planning for the last phase of life. The statutory framework conditions have been set out, but they require specific arrangements and a financial basis so that everyone in Germany — and particularly those with dementia — can be offered adequate palliative medical care adapted to their individual needs at the end of their lives.

Strengths and limitations

This study is based on the largest dataset ($n = 10,364$) analyzed to date on place of death in patients with dementia in Germany. No details were available regarding the place of death for only 0.7% of deceased persons with dementia aged 65 or over. As the study is related only to the selected study region of Westphalia–Lippe, the results are not representative of Germany as a whole.

The study design used a population-based cross-sectional survey. This methodological approach is very suitable for hypothesis generation, but it does not allow any causal conclusions to be drawn. The validity of such studies is also limited, since only a few variables are available for analysis. Important determining factors contributing to the place of death — such as the patient's and/or relatives' preference for place of death, marital status (single, married, divorced), residential situation (living alone or together with one or more other people), the amount of care required, information about treatments (chemotherapy, surgery, intensive-care procedures), links to a specialist team for palliative care, etc. — were not available for the analysis and could not be further explored for data protection reasons.

The medical details provided about the cause of death require critical reflection. For reasons of the logistics involved in obtaining the data, for example, this study did not differentiate among causes of death relative to the underlying disease, contributing factors and the final direct cause of death. On the other hand, for dementia and ten other diseases, it was possible to include all available information about the cause of death, which would otherwise not have been taken into account in the official statistics for cause of death. In consequence, the determined prevalence of dementia can be regarded as particularly reliable. The medical details about dementia given in the death certificates usually did not include either any information about the severity of the disease nor when it had started, so that in this respect no conclusions could be drawn. It should also be

critically noted that the duration of the diseases investigated was not taken into account in any way in the recording and analysis of the data, since this information could not be accurately traced from the medical details.

It is known that dementia-related diseases are not always perceived by physicians as representing an underlying disease leading to death, and are consequently often not stated on death certificates [63]. This affects dementia patients who are being cared for at home more often than those in nursing homes. Due to this documentation practice, the frequency of dementia observed in the present study, particularly in the home environment, may be lower than is really the case.

The quality of the data given in death certificates is generally viewed critically. The form of the medical documentation contributes to this [33]. Illegible handwriting and varying choices of words to describe diagnoses often make it difficult to classify the medical details in accordance with ICD-10. A lack of knowledge on the part of physicians involved about the purpose of the details given (establishing a causal chain) also contributes to this. In addition, physicians often do not have any precise medical information about the deceased person's clinical history. Without such knowledge, however, a precise cause of death can only be established with difficulty.

Conclusion

The most common place of death in people with dementia was the retirement and nursing home, followed by hospital. Only one-fifth died in the home environment.

End-of-life care for people with dementia represents a special challenge and requires a person-centered care approach with staff qualified in palliative care. In this context, existing nursing and medical care services and hospice services need to be further developed and extended to ensure that all individuals with dementia can receive adequate palliative care in accordance with their own individual needs at the end of their lives.

Abbreviations
CASCADE: Choices, Attitudes, and Strategies for Care of Advanced Dementia at the End-of-Life; COPD: Chronic obstructive pulmonary disease; EAPC: European Association for Palliative Care; ICB: Intracerebral bleeding; ICD: International Statistical Classification of Diseases and Related Health Problems

Acknowledgements
Data collection was ably supported by Laila Boutakmant, Hartmut Hofmeister, Marievonne Hofmeister, and Viola Willeke. Thanks are also due to the chief executives of the public health offices in Bochum, Borken, Coesfeld, and Münster (Germany).

Authors' contributions

BD conceived the study, developed the concept, acquired the data, carried out the analysis and wrote the initial drafts of the manuscript. CB provided statistical support, helped with interpretation of the data and results and draft the manuscript. BF helped with interpretation of the data and results. All authors contributed to the final draft of the manuscript. All authors read and approved the final manuscript.

Competing interests

The authors declare that they have no competing interests.

Author details

[1]Department of Anesthesiology, Intensive Care Medicine, Palliative Care Medicine and Pain Management, Berufsgenossenschaftliches Universitätsklinikum Bergmannsheil gGmbH Bochum, Medical Faculty of Ruhr University Bochum, Bürkle-de-la-Camp-Platz 1, 44789 Bochum, Germany. [2]Department of Palliative Medicine, Munich University Hospital, Ludwig-Maximilians- University Munich, Munich, Germany.

References

1. Deutsche Alzheimer Gesellschaft e.V. Die Häufigkeit von Demenzerkrankungen. Informationsblatt 1 [Internet]. Berlin: Deutsche Alzheimer Gesellschaft e.V; 2016. Available from: https://www.deutsche-alzheimer.de/fileadmin/alz/pdf/factsheets/infoblatt1_haeufigkeit_demenzerkrankungen_dalzg.pdf. Accessed 11 Sept 2017
2. Alzheimer Europe. Prevalence of dementia in Europe [internet]. Luxembourg: Alzheimer Europe Office; 2013. Available from: http://www.alzheimer-europe.org/Research/European-Collaboration-on-Dementia/Prevalence-of-dementia/Prevalence-of-dementia-in-Europe. Accessed 11 Sept 2017
3. Alzheimer's Disease International (ADI). World Alzheimer report 2016. Improving healthcare for people living with dementia. Summary sheet [internet]. London: Alzheimer's Disease International; 2016. Available from: https://www.alz.co.uk/research/worldalzheimerreport2016sheet.pdf. Accessed 11 Sept 2017
4. Lee M, Chodosh J. Dementia and life expectancy: what do we know? J Am Med Dir Assoc. 2009;10:466–71.
5. Dewey ME, Saz P. Dementia, cognitive impairment and mortality in persons aged 65 and over living in the community: a systematic review of the literature. Int J Geriatr Psychiatry. 2001;16:751–61.
6. Sampson EL, Candy B, Davis S, Gola AB, Harrington J, King M, et al. Living and dying with advanced dementia: a prospective cohort study of symptoms, service use and care at the end of life. Palliat Med. 2017;1: 269216317726443. https://doi.org/10.1177/0269216317726443.
7. Mitchell SL, Teno JM, Kiely DK, Shaffer ML, Jones RN, Prigerson HG, et al. The clinical course of advanced dementia. N Engl J Med. 2009;361:1529–38.
8. Van der Steen JT, Mitchell SL, Frijters DH, et al. Prediction of 6-month mortality in nursing home residents with advanced dementia: validity of a risk score. J Am Med Dir Assoc. 2007;8:464–8.
9. Toscani F, Van der Steen JT, Finetti S, et al. Critical decisions for older people with advanced dementia: a prospective study in long-term institutions and district home care. J Am Med Dir Assoc. 2015;16:535. e13–e20
10. Van der Steen JT, Radbruch L, Hertogh CMPM, de Boer ME, Hughes JC, Larkin P, et al. White paper defining optimal palliative care in older people with dementia: a Delphi study and recommendations from the European Association for Palliative Care. Palliat Med. 2014;28:197–209.
11. Alzheimer's Association. Dementia care practice recommendations for assisted living residences and nursing homes. Phase 3 end-of-life care [internet]. Chicago: Alzheimer's Association; 2007. Available from: https://www.alz.org/national/documents/brochure_dcprphase3.pdf Accessed 11 Sept 2017
12. Bell CL, Somogyi-Zalud E, Masaki KH. Factors associated with congruence between preferred and actual place of death. J Pain Symptom Manag. 2010; 39:591–604.
13. Escobar Pinzon LC, Claus M, Zepf KI, Letzel S, Fischbeck S, Weber M. Preference for place of death in Germany. J Palliat Med. 2011;14:1097–103.
14. Gomes B, Higginson IJ, Calanzani N, Cohen J, Deliens L, Daveson BA, et al. Preferences for place of death if faced with advanced cancer: a population survey in England, Flanders, Germany, Italy, the Netherlands, Portugal and Spain. Ann Oncol. 2012;23:2006–15.
15. Dasch B, Blum K, Gude P, Bausewein C. Place of death: trends over the course of a decade: a population-based study of death certificates from the years 2001 and 2011. Dtsch Arztebl Int. 2015;112:496–504.
16. Escobar Pinzon LCE, Claus M, Perrar KM, Zepf KI, Letzel S, Weber M. Dying with dementia: symptom burden, quality of care, and place of death. Dtsch Arztebl Int. 2013;110:195–202.
17. Mitchell SL, Teno JM, Miller SC, Mor V. A national study of the location of death for older persons with dementia. J Am Geriatr Soc. 2005;53:299–305.
18. Houttekier D, Cohen J, Bilsen J, Addington-Hall J, Onwuteaka-Philipsen BD, Deliens L. Place of death of older persons with dementia. A study in five European countries. J Am Geriatr Soc. 2010;58:751–6.
19. Sleeman KE, Ho YK, Verne J, Gao W, Higginson IJ, GUIDE Care project. Reversal of English trend towards hospital death in dementia: a population-based study of place of death and associated individual and regional factors, 2001-2010. BMC Neurol. 2014;14:59.
20. Reyniers T, Deliens L, Pasman HR, Morin L, Addington-Hall J, Frova L, et al. International variation in place of death of older people who died from dementia in 14 European and non-European countries. J Am Med Dir Assoc. 2015;16:165–71.
21. Black H, Waugh C, Munoz-Arroyo R, Carnon A, Allan A, Clark D, et al. Predictors of place of death in south West Scotland 2000-2010: retrospective cohort study. Palliat Med. 2016;30:764–71.
22. National End of Life Care Intelligence Network. Deaths from Alzheimer's disease, dementia and senility in England [internet]. London: National End of Life Care Intelligence Network; 2010. Available from: http://www.endoflifecare-intelligence.org.uk/resources/publications/deaths_from_alzheimers. Accessed 11 Sept 2017
23. Bunn F, Burn A-M, Goodman C, Rait G, Norton S, Robinson L, et al. Comorbidity and dementia: a scoping review of the literature. BMC Med. 2014;12:192.
24. Sanderson M, Wang J, Davis DR, Lane MJ, Cornman CB, Fadden MK. Co-morbidity associated with dementia. Am J Alzheimers Dis Other Demen. 2002;17:73–8.
25. Schubert CC, Boustani M, Callahan CM, Perkins AJ, Carney CP, Fox C, et al. Comorbidity profile of dementia patients in primary care: are they sicker? J Am Geriatr Soc. 2006;54:104–9.
26. Poblador-Plou B, Calderón-Larrañaga A, Marta-Moreno J, Hancco-Saavedra J, Sicras-Mainar A, Soljak M, et al. Comorbidity of dementia: a cross-sectional study of primary care older patients. BMC Psychiatry. 2014;14:84.
27. Browne J, Edwards DA, Rhodes KM, Brimicombe DJ, Payne RA. Association of comorbidity and health service usage among patients with dementia in the UK: a population-based study. BMJ Open. 2017;7:e012546.
28. Beekmann M, van den Bussche H, Glaeske G, Hoffmann F. Geriatric morbidity patterns and need for long-term care in patients with dementia. Psychiatr Prax. 2012;39:242–7.
29. Pinkert C, Holle B. People with dementia in acute hospitals. Literature review of prevalence and reasons for hospital admission. Z Gerontol Geriatr. 2012;45:728–34.
30. Phelan EA, Borson S, Grothaus L, Balch S, Larson EB. Association of incident dementia with hospitalizations. JAMA. 2012;307:165–72.
31. Toot S, Devine M, Akporobaro A, Orrell M. Causes of hospital admission for people with dementia: a systematic review and meta-analysis. J Am Med Dir Assoc. 2013;14:463–70.
32. Sampson EL, Blanchard MR, Jones L, Tookman A, King M. Dementia in the acute hospital: prospective cohort study of prevalence and mortality. Br J Psychiatry J Ment Sci. 2009;195:61–6.
33. Schelhase T, Weber S. Mortality statistics in Germany. Problems and perspectives. Bundesgesundheitsblatt Gesundheitsforschung Gesundheitsschutz. 2007;50:969–76.

34. World Health Organization. International statistical classification of diseases and related health problems. Geneva: World Health Organization; 2010.

35. Schulz R, O'Brien AT, Bookwala J, Fleissner K. Psychiatric and physical morbidity effects of dementia caregiving: prevalence, correlates, and causes. Gerontologist. 1995;35:771–91.

36. von Känel R, Mills PJ, Mausbach BT, Dimsdale JE, Patterson TL, Ziegler MG, et al. Effect of Alzheimer caregiving on circulating levels of C-reactive protein and other biomarkers relevant to cardiovascular disease risk: a longitudinal study. Gerontology. 2012;58:354–65.

37. Langa KM, Plassman BL, Wallace RB, Herzog AR, Heeringa SG, Ofstedal MB, et al. The aging, demographics, and memory study: study design and methods. Neuroepidemiology. 2005;25:181–91.

38. Statistisches Bundesamt. Regionale Unterschiede in der Lebenserwartung haben in den letzten 20 Jahren abgenommen. Pressemitteilung Nr. 378 vom 20.10.2016. [Internet]. Wiesbaden: Statisches Bundesamt; 2016. Available from: https://www.destatis.de/DE/PresseService/Presse/Pressemitteilungen/2016/10/PD16_378_12621.html. Accessed 11 Sept 2017

39. Statistisches Bundesamt. Alleinlebende in Deutschland. Ergebnisse des Mikrozensus 2011, Wiesbaden 2012 [Internet]. Wiesbaden: Statistisches Bundesamt; 2012. Available from: https://www.destatis.de/DE/PresseService/Presse/Pressekonferenzen/2012/Alleinlebende/begleitmaterial_PDF.pdf?__blob=publicationFile. Accessed 11th Sept 2017

40. Bundesministerium für Gesundheit. Pflegestärkungsgesetze [Internet]. Available from: http://www.pflegestaerkungsgesetz.de/. Accessed 11 Sept 2017.

41. Sampson EL. Palliative care for people with dementia. Br Med Bull. 2010;96:159–74.

42. van der Steen JT. Dying with dementia: what we know after more than a decade of research. J Alzheimers Dis. 2010;22:37–55.

43. European Association for Palliative Care (EAPC). White paper on standards and norms for hospice and palliative care in Europe [internet]. Vilvoorde: European Association for Palliative Care; 2009. Available from: http://www.eapcnet.eu/Themes/Resources/Organisation/EAPCStandardsNorms.aspx. Accessed 11 Sept 2017

44. Bynum JPW, Rabins PV, Weller W, Niefeld M, Anderson GF, Wu AW. The relationship between a dementia diagnosis, chronic illness, medicare expenditures, and hospital use. J Am Geriatr Soc. 2004;52:187–94.

45. Robert Bosch Stiftung. General Hospital Study (GHoSt). Zusammenfassung einer repräsentativen Studie zu kognitiven Störungen und Demenz in den Allgemeinkrankenhäusern von Baden-Württemberg und Bayern [Internet]. Stuttgart: Robert Bosch Stiftung; 2016. Available from: http://www.bosch-stiftung.de/de/publikation/general-hospital-study-ghost. Accessed 11 Sept 2017

46. Gozalo P, Teno JM, Mitchell SL, Skinner J, Bynum J, Tyler D, et al. End-of-life transitions among nursing home residents with cognitive issues. N Engl J Med. 2011;365:1212–21.

47. Andrieu S, Reynish E, Nourhashemi F, Shakespeare A, Moulias S, Ousset PJ, et al. Predictive factors of acute hospitalization in 134 patients with Alzheimer's disease: a one year prospective study. Int J Geriatr Psychiatry. 2002;17:422–6.

48. Natalwala A, Potluri R, Uppal H, Heun R. Reasons for hospital admissions in dementia patients in Birmingham, UK, during 2002–2007. Dement Geriatr Cogn Disord. 2008;26:499–505.

49. Givens JL, Selby K, Goldfeld KS, Mitchell SL. Hospital transfers of nursing home residents with advanced dementia. J Am Geriatr Soc. 2012;60:905–9

50. Feng Z, Coots LA, Kaganova Y, Wiener JM. Hospital and ED use among Medicare beneficiaries with dementia varies by setting and proximity to death. Health Aff (Millwood). 2014;33:683–90.

51. Porell FW, Carter M. Discretionary hospitalization of nursing home residents with and without Alzheimer's disease: a multilevel analysis. J Aging Health. 2005;17:207–38.

52. Andrews J. A guide to creating a dementia-friendly ward. Nurs Times. 2013;109:20–1.

53. Sampson EL, Leurent B, Blanchard MR, Jones L, King M. Survival of people with dementia after unplanned acute hospital admission: a prospective cohort study. Int J Geriatr Psychiatry. 2013;28:1015–22.

54. Statistisches Bundesamt. Zahl der Todesfälle im Jahr 2015 um 6,5% gestiegen. Pressemitteilung Nr. 022 vom 19.01.2017 [Internet]. Wiesbaden: Statisches Bundesamt; 2017. Available from: https://www.destatis.de/DE/PresseService/Presse/Pressemitteilungen/2017/01/PD17_022_232.html;jsessionid=1DD81EE7B10D3F2E4D527744B160DB56.cae1. Accessed 11 Sept 2017

55. McMurray JJ, Stewart S. Epidemiology, aetiology, and prognosis of heart failure. Heart Br Card Soc. 2000;83:596–602.

56. Neumann T, Biermann J, Erbel R, Neumann A, Wasem J, Ertl G, et al. Heart failure: the commonest reason for hospital admission in Germany: medical and economic perspectives. Dtsch Arztebl Int. 2009;106:269–75.

57. Mitchell SL. Advanced dementia. N Engl J Med. 2015;373:1276–7.

58. van der Steen JT, Ooms ME, Adèr HJ, Ribbe MW, van der Wal G. Withholding antibiotic treatment in pneumonia patients with dementia: a quantitative observational study. Arch Intern Med. 2002;162:1753–60.

59. Magaki S, Yong WH, Khanlou N, Tung S, Vinters HV. Comorbidity in dementia: update of an ongoing autopsy study. J Am Geriatr Soc. 2014;62:1722–8.

60. Burns A, Jacoby R, Luthert P, Levy R. Cause of death in Alzheimer's disease. Age Ageing. 1990;19:341–4.

61. Hendriks SA, Smalbrugge M, Hertogh CMPM, van der Steen JT. Dying with dementia: symptoms, treatment, and quality of life in the last week of life. J Pain Symptom Manag. 2014;47:710–20.

62. Hiddemann T. Das neue Hospiz- und Palliativgesetz, ein Beitrag zur würdevollen Versorgung am Ende des Lebens [Internet]. Berlin: Bundesministerium für Gesundheit; n.d. Available from: https://www.biva.de/wp-content/uploads/Hiddemann.pdf. Accessed 11 Sept 2017

63. Perera G, Stewart R, Higginson IJ, Sleeman KE. Reporting of clinically diagnosed dementia on death certificates: retrospective cohort study. Age Ageing. 2016;45:668–73.

6

Health service utilisation during the last year of life: a prospective, longitudinal study of the pathways of patients with chronic kidney disease stages 3-5

Shirley Chambers[1,2*] (iD), Helen Healy[3,4,5], Wendy E. Hoy[4,5], Adrian Kark[3], Sharad Ratanjee[3], Geoffrey Mitchell[2,4,5], Carol Douglas[6], Patsy Yates[1,2,7] and Ann Bonner[1,2,3,4]

Abstract

Background: Chronic kidney disease (CKD) is a growing global problem affecting around 10% of many countries' populations. Providing appropriate palliative care services (PCS) to those with advanced kidney disease is becoming paramount. Palliative/supportive care alongside usual CKD clinical treatment is gaining acceptance in nephrology services although the collaboration with and use of PCS is not consistent.

Methods: The goal of this study was to track and quantify the health service utilisation of people with CKD stages 3-5 over the last 12 months of life. Patients were recruited from a kidney health service (Queensland, Australia) for this prospective, longitudinal study. Data were collected for 12 months (or until death, whichever was sooner) during 2015-17 from administrative health sources. Emergency department presentations (EDP) and inpatient admissions (IPA) (collectively referred to as critical events) were reviewed by two Nephrologists to gauge if the events were avoidable.

Results: Participants (n = 19) with a median age of 78 years (range 42-90), were mostly male (63%), 79% had CKD stage 5, and were heavy users of health services during the study period. Fifteen patients (79%) collectively recorded 44 EDP; 61% occurred after-hours, 91% were triaged as imminently and potentially life-threatening and 73% were admitted. Seventy-four IPA were collectively recorded across 16 patients (84%); 14% occurred on weekends or public holidays. Median length of stay was 3 days (range 1-29). The median number of EDP and IPA per patient was 1 and 2 (range 0-12 and 0-20) respectively. The most common trigger to both EDP (30%) and IPA (15%) was respiratory distress. By study end 37% of patients died, 63% were known to PCS and 11% rejected a referral to a PCS. All critical events were deemed unavoidable.

Conclusions: Few patients avoided using acute health care services in a 12 month period, highlighting the high service needs of this cohort throughout the long, slow decline of CKD. Proactive end-of-life care earlier in the disease trajectory through integrating renal and palliative care teams may avoid acute presentations to hospital through better symptom management and planned care pathways.

Keywords: Chronic kidney disease, Palliative care, Supportive care, Conservative care, End of life, Patient tracking, Health service utilisation, Critical events

* Correspondence: se.connell@qut.edu.au
[1]Faculty of Health, Queensland University of Technology, Brisbane, Australia
[2]National Health and Medical Research Council, Centre for Research Excellence in End of Life Care, Brisbane, Australia
Full list of author information is available at the end of the article

Background

The prevalence and burden of chronic kidney disease (CKD) is increasing globally [1], and is a public health problem affecting more than 10% of people in advanced economies [2]. CKD is characterised by a sustained reduction in kidney function (estimated glomerular filtration rate [eGFR] ≤ 60 ml/min/1.73m^2 [3] with the leading causes being diabetes and hypertension [4]. In Australia, where the prevalence of CKD is around 10% [5], the greatest growth in incidence is in those aged over 65 years [6] who tend to have more comorbid conditions, and greater frailty [7], collectively translating to a greater need for health care services [8].

Health care utilisation patterns map a range of activities in the delivery of health care including service planning, resource allocation and analyses/research [9]. National health statistics, such as from admitted patient data [10–12], health expenditure data [13] and other major reports of activities [14], provide a glimpse of how some patient groups use health services. For example, Medicare expenses for CKD in the USA were around $50 billion USD in 2013, accounting for nearly 20% of all Medicare spending [14]. In the UK (2009-10) CKD stages 3-5 alone cost the National Health Service (NHS) around £1.45 billion annually, which equates to around 1.3% of all NHS spending [15]. In Australia CKD is associated with 17% of all hospitalisations [5]. Ngu et al. found that inpatient admissions (IPA) due to CKD in Australia significantly increased over a four-year period from 5.2% to 8.6% of all hospital admissions, and of intensive care admissions from 8.3% to 13.3% [11]. CKD is often related to, or is an underlying condition in, many other admitted disease groups, such as cardiovascular and diabetes [14]. It is a signal for heavy use of health services, reflecting the medical complexity of this group of patients [8].

There is compelling evidence that early integration of palliative care into usual cancer care provides benefits for patients and health systems [16]. While palliative care services (PCS) support patients in their terminal phases of cancer, the seamless integration of PCS into other clinical teams is less established [17]. It has been estimated that, globally, adults with non-malignant conditions make up around 65% of those needing palliative care [18] even though patients with a cancer diagnosis still dominate PCS utilisation [19]. The demand from people with terminal failure across a range of solid organs is also growing in Australia although access to PCS is low with only about 30% of the total PCS being provided to non-cancer patients [20]. In response palliative care is now broadening its scope to include these patient groups [21], notwithstanding the paucity of data about their specific palliative care needs [22]. Palliative care is an important care pathway in advanced CKD (eGFR < 30 ml/min/m^2) as well as end stage kidney disease (ESKD eGFR < 15 ml/min/m^2) to manage high symptom burden [23]

and the comorbid disease loads in a population characterised by increasing age and frailty. Moreover, ESKD differs from most other terminal organ failure, where, for patients across the lifespan, dialysis can artificially prolong life for decades unlike other devices [24]. For instance, ventricular assist devices are restricted to a far narrower range of patients and are less readily available in many countries. Alternatively, conservative care is another management pathway where patients decide to not commence, or have been medically advised against, dialysis. Patients may also move from the dialysis to the conservative care pathway to stop dialysis [25]. In patients who opt not to have dialysis and instead follow a conservative care pathway, 20% are still alive 3 years later [26]. Compared with terminal cancer, the patterns of health service use [21, 27] and functional decline [28] in advanced CKD are less predictable. These are all important points of differentiation likely to necessitate the re-design of cancer focused PCS to align with the needs of the CKD population. An approach that is gaining acceptance in nephrology teams is combining palliative care and nephrology expertise to create transdisciplinary skillsets particularly important in the domains of symptom control and medication management [24]. The patients' use and experiences of health services are likely key outcomes of this re-design. This study aimed to understand the health service utilisation patterns in a cohort with advanced CKD whose prognosis was less than a year of life. The results will be translated into the redesign of appropriate palliative care/kidney transdisciplinary teams.

Aims

This study aimed to quantify patients' health service use over the 12 month period prior to their (anticipated) death. Specifically, this study reports on emergency department presentations (EDP) and inpatient admissions (IPA) (collectively referred to as critical events) and PCS utilisation. A secondary aim was to report on patients' symptoms, physical functioning and quality of life over the same period and this has been previously published [29]. Due to the substantial symptom burden [29] and slow functional decline of patients with advanced and progressive CKD, programs that integrate palliative/supportive care into usual clinical kidney care could assist with easing symptom burden particularly in these patients' last 12 months of life.

Methods
Design

For this prospective, longitudinal, observational study, demographic, clinical and health administrative data were collected at regular intervals from patients' medical records and from hospital-based administrative health databases for a 12 month period, or until their death.

Setting and sample

Nephrologists (HH, SR and AK) identified potential patients for this study from a kidney health service within the Metro North Hospital and Health Service (Queensland, Australia) throughout 2015-16. The hospitals frequented by the patients are all situated within the same Queensland Health Hospital and Health Service, and are referred to as Hospitals 1 (which has a consultancy only PCS on site), 2 and 3 (which both have a PCS and a dedicated palliative care inpatient unit on site). Hospital 1 is a major referral tertiary hospital (1000-bed) for Hospitals 2 and 3. This hospital provides comprehensive renal care. Hospital 2 is a 250-bed regional hospital that has an onsite satellite dialysis unit and outpatient services but not the other components of a renal service. Hospital 3 is a major teaching hospital (624-bed) that does not have a dedicated renal unit. Hospitals 2 and 3 do not have the capacity to deal with complex renal emergencies so any presenting patients are transferred to the renal service at Hospital 1.

The convenience sample were eligible if they were English speaking adults (≥18 year of age), with CKD stages 3-5 with a prognosis of < 12 months (clinician identified by answering 'no' to the surprise question, "would you be surprised if the patient died in the following 12 months?"), and were cognitively sound and competent to give informed consent. Exclusion criteria were extreme psychological or social distress likely to bias the collection of interviewer administered surveys (determined by clinical and/or research staff), patients who died within 48 h of qualifying for the study, or who resided > 2 h' drive from the recruitment site (to enable in-person data collection). Patients included those who were receiving conservative care (CKD stages 4 and 5) and those receiving dialysis. Our target was to track 20 patients.

Data sources and tools

Clinical and administrative health data were collected from Queensland Health sources at the appropriate intervals throughout the study period to capture patients' medical history, emergency department presentations (EDP), inpatient admissions (IPA), and referrals to other health services. Comorbidities were collected from patients' medical records. See Tables 1 and 2 for details.

Expert consultant review of critical events

Critical events for the purpose of this study refer to: a) emergency department presentations (EDP); and b) inpatient admissions (IPA). Two nephrologists (AK and SR) reviewed patients' critical events retrospectively to determine if the events were avoidable or not. They were provided with a summary of each critical event alongside comprehensive chart notes of medical (diagnostic and

Table 1 Demographic, clinical and administrative health data collected and timing

Data Collected	Data Collection Time Points		
	Study Entry	3Mthly[a]	Study End
Demographic details	√		√
Medical history	√	√	√
Emergency department presentations		√	√
Inpatient admissions		√	√
Other health service use		√	√
Co-morbidities			√

[a]Cycle continues until patient's death

treatment), social and psychological details, and additional health service utilisation around each event. This was a subjective process using the experience and expertise of the reviewing medical practitioners.

Analysis

Unique study codes were assigned to the patients on study entry. Descriptive statistics and frequency distributions were generated from the patients' demographic and clinical characteristics and service usage. Data sourced from Queensland Health administrative databases were triangulated with medical chart notes to identify and resolve discrepancies. Triggers to EDP were identified by collating and categorising the 'Reason for Presentation' and other clinical notes as found in EDIS. Triggers to IPA were identified by collating and categorising the Australian Refined-Diagnostic Related Groups (AR-DRG) [30], as recorded in HBCIS, and associated

Table 2 Clinical and administrative health data sources (Queensland Health) and corresponding information retrieved

Data Source (Administering department)	Information Collected
Emergency Department Information System (EDIS)	*Emergency department presentations:* presentation date and timing, hospital location, demographic details, mode of arrival (e.g., ambulance), triage category[a], reason for presentation and departure status
Hospital Based Corporate Information System (HBCIS)	*Inpatient admissions:* admission date, hospital location, demographic details, care type, admission status, reason for admission (AR-DRG), length of stay, discharge date and destination
Medical records[b]	Health history (including comorbidities), diagnostic and treatment details, demographic details, health service referrals and use, and other relevant details

AR-DRG Australian Refined-Diagnostic Related Group [30]
[a]Triage categories: 1: immediately life-threatening; 2: imminently life-threatening; 3: potentially life-threatening; 4: potentially serious; 5: less urgent [31]
[b]Hard copy or electronic

medical notes extracted from patient charts of each admission. Authors AB (expert renal nurse) and SC (non-clinical researcher) collaborated to ensure clinical information was categorised appropriately. Comorbidity scores were calculated using the Charlson Comorbidity index [32].

Results

Of the 49 potentially eligible patients identified we recruited our target of 20 with two withdrawing within the first 2 months. They were replaced with two more patients from the potentially eligible group. One further patient withdrew at month 4, leaving a final sample of $n = 19$.

Demographic characteristics

Patients' median age at study entry was 78 years (range 42-90). Most patients were male (63%), married/defacto (53%) and co-residing with others (84%). Most were in CKD stage 5 (79%). Seven patients (37%) died during the study; of these, one died from a non-CKD related event (car accident). Nine patients (47%) were receiving conservative care throughout the study and the remaining 10 were on a haemodialysis pathway (53%). See Table 3 for full details.

Emergency department presentations (EDP)

Fifteen patients recorded 44 emergency department presentations (EDP) collectively at the participating hospitals. Patients receiving conservative care were more likely to present to Hospital 2 whereas those receiving haemodialysis presented to Hospital 1. Place of residence can dictate which hospital the patient is taken to in an emergency, which may explain the four hospital transfers where patients presented to one emergency department (ED) and then were transferred onto Hospital 1.

Patients in the dialysis group presented to the ED after-hours more often than those in the conservative group (43% versus 16% respectively). Most patients (89% of EDP) arrived at the ED by ambulance. These EDP were significant with 40 EDP (91%) triaged as categories 2 and 3 (Imminently and potentially life-threatening respectively) [32] and 73% admitted, i.e., transition to IPA. Patients spent considerable time in the ED (median 6.4 h [range 1.8 to 24.8 h]). Seven patients (42%) presented at EDs three or more times during the study period. Frequent attendance at ED was less common in the conservative group ($n = 2/9$; 22% of group) compared to the dialysis group ($n = 5/10$; 50% of group). See Table 4 for additional detail.

Triggers to EDP

The most common triggers for EDP were respiratory distress, pain (which was separated into chest pain and other pain), hypotension and falls. Respiratory distress

Table 3 Patients' demographic, diagnostic, comorbidity and death details

Characteristics	N = 19 All N (% All)	n = 9 Conservative n (% Group)	n = 10 Dialysis n (% Group)
Gender			
Male	12 (63)	5 (56)	7 (70)
Age (years)			
Median (range)	78 (42-90)	86 (72-90)	74 (42-90)
< 60 years	3 (16)	0 (0)	3 (30)
60-80	8 (42)	3 (33)	5 (50)
> 80	8 (42)	6 (67)	2 (20)
Marital status			
Married/Defacto	10 (53)	5 (56)	5 (50)
Living arrangements			
Lives with others	16 (84)[a]	7 (78)[b]	9 (90)[c]
Lives alone	3 (16)	2 (22)	1 (10)
CKD stage			
Stage 4	4 (21)	4 (44)	–
Stage 5	15 (79)	5 (56)	10 (100)
Comorbidity index			
Median (range)	8 (3-11)	9 (7-10)	6.5 (3-11)
Deaths during study period			
Number[d]	7 (37)	4 (44)	3 (30)
Median (range) days from study entry[d]	148 (92-330)	217 (92-330)	103 (101-228)

Note: Percentages may not equal 100% due to rounding,
[a]Three patients lived in nursing homes and one patient shared a house - not with a carer
[b]Two patients lived in nursing homes
[c]One patient lived in a nursing home and one patient shared a house - not with a carer
[d]Includes a patient who died as a result of an accident

was the most common trigger for EDP for the dialysis group (32% of EDP) whereas pain was the most common trigger in the conservative group (38% of EDP). See Table 5 for more details.

Inpatient admissions (IPA)

During the study period, 16 patients (84%) recorded 74 inpatient admissions (IPA) collectively, excluding routine dialysis admissions, across participating hospitals. Patients receiving dialysis were principally admitted to Hospital 1 (90% of group's IPA). The conservative group recorded a similar number of IPA on weekends or public holidays (13%), as the dialysis group (14%). Most of the IPA were sourced via an ED (49%) although some patients were sent to an outpatient renal clinic or the dialysis unit from an ED so the source of their admissions was classified in hospital databases from those areas. There were other patients who had routine dialysis and

Table 4 Emergency department Presentations (EDP) during study period[a]

Variables of Interest	N = 19 All 44 EDP # EDP (% All EDP)	n = 9 Conservative 13 EDP # EDP (% Group's EDP)	n = 10 Dialysis 31 EDP # EDP (% Group' EDP)
Hospital			
1	26 (59)	2 (15)	24 (77)
2	17 (39)	11 (85)	6 (19)
3	1 (2)	0 (0)	1 (3)
Main modes of arrival			
Ambulance	39 (89)	10 (77)	29 (94)
Walk in	4 (9)	3 (23)	1 (3)
After-hours presentations[b]	26 (61)	7 (16)	19 (43)
Triage category			
Category 1	0 (0)	0 (0)	0 (0)
Category 2	17 (39)	1 (8)	16 (52)
Category 3	23 (52)	10 (77)	13 (42)
Category 4	3 (7)	2 (15)	1 (3)
Category 5	1 (2)	0 (0)	1 (3)
Departure status			
Admitted	32 (73)	9 (69)	23 (74)
Transfer to other hospital	4 (9)	1 (8)	3 (10)
Home	4[c] (9)	3 (23)	1[2] (3)
Dialysis clinic	4 (9)	N/A	4 (13)
Length of stay in ED (hours)			
Median (range)	6.4 (1.8 - 24.8)	5 (3.1 - 13.1)	1.5 (1.8 - 24.8)
Number of EDP per patient			
Median (range)	1 (0-12)	1 (0-4)	2 (0-12)
	n (% All Patients)	n (% Group)	n (% Group)
0	4 (21)	2 (22)	2 (20)
1-2	8 (42)	5 (56)	3 (30)
3-5	6 (32)	2 (22)	4 (40)
6 +	1 (5)	0 (0)	1 (10)

Note: Totals may not add up to 100% due to rounding
EDP Emergency department presentation/s
[a]As per EDIS data
[b]After-hours defined as between the hours of 5 pm and 7 am on week days plus all weekend days and public holidays
[c]Includes one patient who declined admission

Table 5 Five most often recorded triggers to emergency department presentations (EDP)

Triggers[a]	N = 19 All # EDP (% All EDP)	n = 9 Conservative # EDP (% Group's EDP)	n = 10 Dialysis # EDP (% Group's EDP)
Respiratory distress	13 (30)	3 (23)	10 (32)
Pain (other than chest)	8 (18)	5 (38)	3 (10)
Chest pain	6 (14)	1 (8)	5 (16)
Hypotension	6 (14)	1 (8)	5 (16)
Falls	5 (11)	4 (31)	0 (0)

EDP Emergency Department Presentation/s
[a]These triggers are not mutually exclusive, i.e., the patient may have presented with more than one trigger

changes were the source of few IPA (8%). Some patient transfers were from hospitals not participating in the study hence the corresponding EDP were not captured. Most Care Types were recorded as *Acute* (92% of IPA), with very few recorded as *Palliative* (5% IPA).

Most IPA resulted in patients returning home (76%). Five of the six illness-related deaths of study patients were recorded at the participating hospitals. If a patient did not die in a recruitment hospital, and we were not informed of their place of death by relatives (carers), their place of death for the purpose of this study is unknown. The length of stay of IPA was similar for all patients combined (Median 3 days; range 1-29) and per group. Of particular interest, $n = 14$ patients recorded multiple IPA during the study period. See Table 6 for additional information relating to the patients' IPA during the study period.

Triggers to IPA
The most often recorded triggers for IPA were similar to those for EDP; this is not surprising as most EDP (73%) resulted in an IPA. These triggers were respiratory distress, chest pain, cardiac events, 'other' pain, and vascular access issues such as fistula repairs. See Table 7 for more details.

Consultant review of critical events
All critical events were deemed to be unavoidable taking into consideration the context of each patient's clinical presentation, treatment care pathway and social situation.

Palliative care service referral status
During this study, the kidney health service which spans the three study sites received funding to commence an integrated Kidney Supportive Care program (KSCp) (comprised of a renal and palliative care multidisciplinary team) which is provided earlier in the CKD trajectory to primarily focus on symptom management and decision-making. This program interfaces with the renal

then were admitted to an acute ward. Most admissions (58%) were classified as an 'emergency'. The code descriptor *Episode Change* (also known as a statistical admission) can be used to document a change in the patient's Care Type [30], for example from acute to palliative, rehabilitation or maintenance, and back to acute, while not being physically moved from the hospital ward, and to describe the IPA source, admission status or discharge destination. In this study episode

Table 6 Inpatient admissions (IPA) during study period[a]

Variables of Interest	N = 19 All 74 IPA[b] # IPA (% All IPA)	n = 9 Conservative 16 IPA # IPA (% Group's IPA)	n = 10 Dialysis 58 IPA[b] # IPA (% Group's IPA)
Hospital			
1	59 (80)	7 (44)	52 (90)
2	14 (19)	9 (56)	5 (9)
3	1 (1)	0 (0)	1 (2)
Weekend/public holidays	10 (14)	2 (13)	8 (14)
Source of IPA			
Emergency Department	36 (49)	10 (63)	26 (45)
Outpatient Department	15 (20)	4 (25)	11 (19)
Transfer	9 (12)	1 (6)	7 (12)
Routine IPA	8 (11)	0 (0)	9 (16)
Episode change	6 (8)	1 (6)	5 (9)
Admission status			
Emergency	43 (58)	10 (63)	33 (57)
Elective	15 (20)	5 (31)	10 (17)
Not assigned	15 (20)	1 (6)	14 (24)
Episode change	1 (1)	0 (0)	1 (2)
Care type			
Acute	68 (92)	15 (94)	53 (91)
Palliative	4 (5)	1 (6)	3 (5)
Maintenance	1 (1)	0 (0)	1 (2)
Rehabilitation	1 (1)	0 (0)	1 (2)
Discharge destination			
Home	56 (76)	11 (69)	45 (78)
Transfer	6 (8)	1 (6)	5 (9)
Episode change	6 (8)	1 (6)	5 (9)
Died	5 (7)	2 (13)	3 (5)
Aged care facility (initial)	1 (1)	1 (6)	0 (0)
Length of stay (days)			
Median (range)	3 (1-29)	3.5 (1-29)	3 (1-26)
Number of IPA per patient			
Median (range)	2 (0-20)	2 (0-3)	5 (0-20)
	N (% All Patients)	n (% Group)	n (% Group)
0	3 (16)	1 (11)	2 (20)
1-2	8 (42)	6 (67)	2 (20)
3-5	3 (16)	2 (22)	1 (10)
6+	5 (26)	0 (0)	5 (50)

Note: Totals may not add up to 100% due to rounding
IPA Inpatient admission/s
[a]As per HBCIS data [30]
[b]Excluding routine dialysis admissions

treating team, the patient's general practitioner, and when required, refers seamlessly to PCS. Table 8 provides details of referrals to PCS or to the new KSCp. Two patients undergoing conservative treatment were engaged with a PCS at study entry. Six of the seven patients who died during their study participation were referred to a PCS either prior to or during the study. Only one patient was referred to both services. Twelve patients were referred to and/or were receiving care from either of these services by the time of their death or by study end. Two patients

Table 7 Five most often recorded triggers for inpatient admissions (IPA)

Trigger[a]	All N = 19 # IPA (% All IPA)	Conservative n = 9 # IPA (% Group's IPA)	Dialysis n = 10 # IPA (% Group's IPA)
Respiratory distress	11 (15)	0 (0)	11 (19)
Chest pain	8 (11)	1 (25)	7 (14)
Cardiac event	6 (8)	0 (0)	6 (10)
Other pain	6 (8)	2 (13)	4 (7)
Vascular access issues	6 (8)	0 (0)	6 (10)

IPA Inpatient Admission/s
[a]These triggers are not mutually exclusive, i.e., the patient may present with more than one trigger

(both receiving dialysis), who were still living at study end, were offered a referral to the KSCp but rejected the suggestion reporting they were not ready for supportive care discussions. Referrals to PCS were received very close to three patients' deaths (3, 11 and 16 days prior to death).

Discussion

We prospectively followed each patient, anticipated to be in their last year of life, for a maximum of 12 months to describe critical health service events and the use of PCS, and while the sample was small, it does reflect the heterogeneity of the advanced CKD population at this site. The study cohort were heavy users of health services as a whole, however the dialysis subgroup in particular were responsible for most of the health service use during the study period. Almost all study patients had at least one EDP with most arriving at the ED by ambulance followed by admission to an acute ward. All critical events were unavoidable, and many critical events occurred after-hours. The most frequent trigger for EDP and IPA was respiratory distress. Most patients

Table 8 Palliative care referral status of patients across study period

Palliative care status	All N = 19 n (% All Patients)	Conservative n = 9 n (% Group)	Dialysis n = 10 n (% Group)
Known to PCS at study entry	4[a] (21)	4[a] (44)	0 (0)
Referred to KSCp during study	5[b] (26)	1[b] (11)	4 (40)
Referred to PCS during study	5[c] (26)	3[c] (33)	2 (20)
Total known to PCS/KSCp by study end	12 (63)	6 (67)	6 (60)
Refused referral to KSCp	2 (11)	0 (0)	2 (20)

PCS Palliative Care Service, KSCp Kidney Supportive Care Program
[a]Two of these patients were not actively engaged with a PCS at study entry
[b]One of these patients was already known to a PCS at study entry
[c]Two of these patients were known to, but were not actively engaged with, a PCS at study entry

who died during the study were engaged with a PCS prior to death although overall there were fewer deaths than anticipated.

Previous studies identifying patterns in health service utilisation in those with CKD are limited by their retrospective design, reliance on various forms of administrative health and insurance data [8, 11, 33] and/or incomplete capture of individual patient-level data. These limitations are shared by previous Australian studies of service use near the end of life [34–37]. Unlike reports from the Australian Hospital Statistics [10, 12, 38] which report collated service utilisation data (with the unit of measure being the occasion of service), this study reports the type as well as the number of critical events experienced by individual patients during their study participation.

Several other studies report people with advanced CKD are high users of health services [8, 11, 39]. The later stages of CKD is characterised by multiple comorbidities, [40], high symptom burden [23, 41–44] and a highly variable premature life expectancy [45–48]. Our findings of multiple critical events recorded for individual patients during the study period align with the literature. Patients receiving dialysis recorded more critical events per patient than the conservative group, excluding routine dialysis admissions, even though they were younger than the conservative group. Typically the group of patients who opt for conservative care tend to be on average older with more comorbidities [26, 49] than those who opt for dialysis. While Quinn et al. found fewer IPA per patient in a haemodialysis cohort than our study, they did find that patient groups who are known to be heavy users of inpatient services, such as cardiology, had fewer IPA than patients with ESKD [39]. However Quinn and colleagues did not select patients on the basis of a prognosis of less than 12 months [39]. Nevertheless, both our study and Quinn's report relatively high consumption of health resources by patients with advanced CKD. Our study is not representative of the Australian population which showed EDP by ambulance was lower at 24% in 2015-16 Australia wide compared to 89% in our study [50]. Furthermore, around 29% of all EDP in Australia during this time resulted in an IPA [50] compared with 73% of our cohort, highlighting the high service needs of the advanced CKD cohort.

The duration of IPA in CKD cohorts varies widely across studies [21, 39, 51]. These studies are heterogeneous, with differences including study patient selection. We did, however, find that the median length of stay of IPA in our study group was shorter than the Australian average of 5.5 days [12] notwithstanding the study selection criterion of the last 12 months of life. These differences in duration of IPA may reflect whole of hospital systems and practices at the study sites. Of interest, in those who died during the study, four had a palliative care related IPA. Given that all patients were expected to die within 12 months and had substantial symptom burden [29], these findings confirm the literature in that this patient group are not being referred early enough for palliative care/community services [52] even though in Australia, withdrawal from haemodialysis is the leading cause of death in these patients [53].

The after-hours initiated critical events captured during the study period are high. This may be because patients lack access to and/or knowledge of appropriate support, such as 24 h community services (e.g., general practitioners and domiciliary nursing services) and advice. In the area where this study took place, 24 h palliative care nursing care is available, however it is limited to those who are in the terminal phase of their disease. Another explanation is the complexity of the study patient cohort, with all critical events recorded during this study deemed to be unavoidable. We found that respiratory distress was the most common trigger to both EDP and IPA compared to findings in other studies of patients with CKD [8] or cancer [54] where pain was more likely to trigger an EDP. Patients with advanced CKD will benefit from palliative care input to initiate end-of-life discussions and to help determine future goals of care [55] such as their preferred place of care and withdrawal from dialysis. Furthermore, in collaboration with renal services, PCS can provide support with symptom management, and psychological support and education for both the patient and carer to manage expected exacerbation of symptoms such as breathlessness and pain [24]. Access to PCS earlier in the illness trajectory, rather than in the terminal phase, will ensure end-of-life decisions are made without urgency [56]. Proactive planning by PCS to address known triggers that could lead to acute health service use, particularly for events that occur after hours, are likely to reduce patients' use of these services or at the least reduce the length of IPA [57].

There are limitations inherent when using administrative health data to inform research as these data are primarily gathered for financial, administrative management and departmental reporting purposes [58]. We found that patient transitions through acute services were often not transparent. For example, the percentage of EDP that resulted in an IPA did not equate to the percentage of IPA sourced from an ED which is probably due to sourcing two different databases (EDIS and HBCIS) and how the processes of transfers between hospitals, and episode changes, are recorded. We were able to quality assure dataset integrity in our study by validation against chart reviews. However this was only possible because of our small sample size. For example, one patient who presented to the ED of Hospital 2 was admitted to the ED Short Stay Unit while waiting for a transfer to Hospital 1 for specialist renal care. Hence, the admission source of the IPA at Hospital 1 was classified in the inpatient database (HBCIS) as a 'Transfer' rather than an admission from the 'Emergency Department'. Furthermore, the Admission Status code of *Not Assigned* does not provide any information of the nature of the IPA, such as emergency or elective. Research using large datasets is critically dependent on data integrity and the methodological approach used may lead to underestimating ED use and other health service use in the CKD patient population.

Major strengths of this study include its prospective, longitudinal design and our recruitment method. We recruited patients directly from a kidney service. Hence the patients were already known to have underlying CKD on study entry. Relying on administrative health data alone to identify cases by International Classification of Diseases (ICD-10) codes [59] or *Palliative Care* occasions of service (by classifications and categories) includes patients who develop renal failure secondary to other health conditions rather than having a pre-existing CKD diagnosis. Furthermore, we report on patients' multiple critical events during the study period and capture the triggers to, and geographical location of, these events. Nevertheless, there are also limitations to our study. Due to the small convenience sample, findings cannot be generalised. Bias may have been introduced into the study as: i) the patients were recruited from one kidney service, ii) recruitment was limited to patients who resided < 2 h drive from the recruitment site, iii) three investigators (HH, AK, and SR) were treating clinicians, and iv) two of these nephrologists (AK and SR) also reviewed the critical events. This has the potential to be both a limitation and strength of the study due to the nephrologists' extensive knowledge of the treatment used at the recruitment sites and/or of patients' specific conditions. Even though the patients in this study were chosen due to their limited prognosis, less died than would have been anticipated with a 12-month prognosis. A recent study found prognostication using the 'surprise question' in those in stages 4-5 CKD had moderate sensitivity and specificity (55% and 76% respectively) [60] which may explain why fewer participants died during our study. Therefore, comparison to previous studies (of patients nearing the end of life) should be treated with caution as previous studies may have selected their study population differently, for example, persons in the last 3 or 6 months of life. Despite these limitations, the findings provide insight into the critical events contributing to health service use. Undertaking this study proved the feasibility of i) recruiting a vulnerable CKD cohort, and ii) collecting health administrative data prospectively, that is, in almost 'real time' from a variety of health administrative sources. Furthermore, the triangulation of these data with comprehensive chart notes provided precision at the level of data elements of patients' complex health service utilisation.

Conclusion

The purpose of this study was to follow and quantify the use of health services by patients with CKD in their last 12 months of life. Most study patients were heavy users of acute health services which highlights their complex needs. Usage is validated by the distressing and potentially life threatening character of the triggers to the critical events. Therefore this cohort needs matching high quality care to manage their complex conditions and to avoid or reduce after-hours critical events. Nephrology experts worldwide note that the quality of care, particularly conservative and palliative care, is currently suboptimal for persons with advanced CKD [56]. It is therefore imperative to assemble timely, effective and sustainable high quality care pathways that meet patient need. Our findings will inform the design of, and methods used in, future multisite studies to provide evidence to inform the development of timely palliative care models that improve patient outcomes for those with advanced stages of CKD.

Implication for practice

The CKD population is heterogeneous in end-of-life trajectories with those in the conservative care group typically experiencing a long and slow decline of many months to several years to death whereas those who withdraw from haemodialysis die within 7-10 days. Traditional siloed models of renal and palliative care teams are the dominant model; re-design of clinical services is required to better match the needs of these vulnerable patients. For instance in the UK, one of the leaders in delivering kidney supportive care, only about 23% of renal units have an integrated renal/palliative care team [61], although most restrict this service to the conservative care group of patients. Renal nurses are also strategically placed to assess for symptom burden, increasing frailty, and to coordinate the care of at-risk patients receiving kidney replacement therapies. Referral of patients to integrated renal/palliative care teams earlier in the CKD trajectory may reduce triggers to critical events which contribute to EDP and IPA as well as providing a seamless conduit to specialist PCS when the terminal phase approaches.

Abbreviations

AR-DRG: Australian Refined-Diagnostic Related Group; CKD: Chronic Kidney Disease; ED: Emergency Department; EDIS: Emergency Department Information System; EDP: Emergency Department Presentation/s; eGFR: Estimated Glomerular Filtration Rate; ESKD: End Stage Kidney Disease; HBCIS: Hospital Based Corporate Information System; ICD-10 codes: International Classification of Diseases-10th Revision; IPA: Inpatient Admission/s; KSCp: Kidney Supportive Care Program; NHS: National Health Service; PCS: Palliative Care Service/s

Acknowledgements
Not applicable

Funding
This study was funded by the National Health and Medical Research Council Centre for Research Excellence in End of Life Care (NHMRC CRE ELC). The funding body had no role in determining the study design, nor in the collection, analysis and interpretation of the data, nor in the writing of this or any other manuscript developed from this study.

Authors' contributions
PY, SC, AB: Conceived the study. HH, AK, SR: Assisted recruitment. SC: Collected and analysed the data. SC, AB: drafted the manuscript. All authors reviewed the manuscript and approved the final submitted version.

Competing interests
The authors declare that they have no competing interests.

Author details
[1]Faculty of Health, Queensland University of Technology, Brisbane, Australia. [2]National Health and Medical Research Council, Centre for Research Excellence in End of Life Care, Brisbane, Australia. [3]Kidney Health Service, Metro North Hospital and Health Service, Queensland Health, Brisbane, Australia. [4]National Health and Medical Research Council, Chronic Kidney Disease Centre for Research Excellence, Brisbane, Australia. [5]Faculty of Medicine, University of Queensland, Brisbane, Australia. [6]Palliative Care Service, Royal Brisbane and Women's Hospital, Queensland Health, Brisbane, Australia. [7]Centre for Palliative Care Research and Education, Queensland Health, Brisbane, Australia.

References
1. GBD 2015 Disease and Injury Incidence and Prevalence Collaborators. Global, regional, and national incidence, prevalence, and years lived with disability for 310 diseases and injuries, 1990-2015: a systematic analysis for the global burden of disease study 2015. Lancet. 2016;388:1545–602.
2. Eckardt K-U, Coresh J, Devuyst O, Johnson RJ, Köttgen A, Levey AS, et al. Evolving importance of kidney disease: from subspecialty to global health burden. Lancet. 2013;382(9887):158–69.
3. Kidney Disease Improving Global Outcomes. Definition and classification of CKD. Kidney Int Suppl. 2013;3(1):19–62.
4. Webster AC, Nagler EV, Morton RL, Masson P. Chronic kidney disease. Lancet. 2017;389(10075):1238–52.
5. Australian Institute of Health and Welfare. Chronic kidney disease compendium. Web Report 2016. https://www.aihw.gov.au/reports/chronic-kidney-disease/chronic-kidney-disease-compendium/contents/how-many-australians-have-chronic-kidney-disease. Accessed 20 Oct 2016.
6. Australian Institute of Health and Welfare. Incidence of end-stage kidney disease in Australia 1997-2013, Cat. no. PHE 211. Canberra: AIHW; 2016.

7.   Kittiskulnam P, Sheshadri A, Johansen KL. Consequences of CKD on functioning. Semin Nephrol. 2016;36(4):305–18.

8.   Welch JL, Meek J, Bartlett Ellis RJ, Ambuehl R, Decker BS. Patterns of healthcare encounters experienced by patients with chronic kidney disease. J Renal Care. 2017;43(4):209–18.

9.   Katz L, Fink RV, Bozeman SR, McNeil BJ. Using health care utilization and publication patterns to characterize the research portfolio and to plan future reserach investments. PLoS One. 2014;9(12):e114873.

10. Australian Institute of Health and Welfare. Admitted patient care 2014-15: Australian hospital statistics, Health services series no. 68. Cat. No. HSE 172. Canberra: AIHW; 2016.

11. Ngu K, Reid D, Tobin A. Trends and outcomes of chronic kidney disease in intensive care: a 5-year study. Intern Med J. 2017;47(1):62–7.

12. Australian Institute of Health and Welfare. Admitted patient care 2015-16: Australian hospital statistics, Health services series no. 75. Cat. no. HSE 185. Canberra: AIHW; 2017.

13. Australian Institute of Health and Welfare. Australian health expenditure - demographics and diseases: hospital admitted patient expenditure 2004-05 to 2012-13, Health and welfare expenditure series no. 59. Cat. no. HWE 69. Canberra: AIHW; 2017.

14. United States Renal Data System (USRDS). United States renal data system annual data report: epidemiology of kidney disease in the United States. 2015. https://www.usrds.org/2015/view/Default.aspx. Accessed 20 Oct 2017.

15. Kerr M, Bray B, Medcalf J, O'Donoghue DJ, Matthews B. Estimating the financial cost of chronic kidney disease to the NHS in England. Nephrol Dial Transplant. 2012;27(Suppl 3):iii73–80.

16. Bakitas MA, El-Jawahri A, Farquhar M, Ferrell B, Grudzen C, Higginson I, et al. The TEAM approach to improving oncology outcomes by incorporating palliative care in practice. J Oncol Pract. 2017;13(9):557–66.

17. Hui D, Elsayem A, De La Cruz M, Berger A, Zhukovsky DS, Palla S, et al. Availability and integration of palliative care at US cancer centres. JAMA. 2010;303(11):1054–61.

18. Connor SR, Bermedo MCSB, Worldwide Palliative Care Alliance (WPCA). Global atlas of palliative care at the end of life. Geneva: WHO; 2014.

19. National Council for Palliative Care. National survey of patient activity data for specialist palliative care services: minimum data set (MDS) inpatient services trend report for 2014-15. 2015. http://www.ncpc.org.uk/sites/default/files/user/documents/MDS%20Inpatients%20final%20report%202014_2015_1.pdf. Accessed 30 Nov 2017.

20. Rosenwax L, Spilsbury K, McNamara BA, Semmens JB. A retrospective population based cohort study of access to specialist palliative care in the last year of life: who is still missing out a decade on? BMC Palliat Care. 2016;15:46.

21. Brady B, Redahan L, Donohoe CL, Mellotte GJ, Wall C, Higgins S. Renal patients at end of life: a 5-year retrospective review. Prog Palliat Care. 2017; 25(5):224–9.

22. Murtagh FE, Higginson IJ. Death from renal failure eighty years on: how far have we come? J Palliat Med. 2007;10(6):1286–8.

23. Murtagh FE, Addington-Hall JM, Edmonds PM, Donohoe P, Carey I, Jenkins K, et al. Symptoms in advanced renal disease: a cross-sectional survey of symptom prevalence in stage 5 chronic kidney disease managed without dialysis. J Palliat Med. 2007;10(6):1266–76.

24. Kane PM, Vinen K, Murtagh FE. Palliative care for advanced renal disease: a summary of the evidence and future direction. Palliat Med. 2013;27(9):817–21.

25. Murtagh FE, Burns A, Moranne O, Morton RL, Naicker S. Supportive care: comprehensive conservative care in end-stage kidney disease. Clin J Am Soc Nephrol. 2016;11(10):1909–14.

26. Morton RL, Webster AC, McGeechan K. Conservative management and end of life care in an Australian cohort with ESRD. Clin J Am Soc Nephrol. 2016; 11(12):2195–203.

27. Addington-Hall J, Fakhoury W, McCarthy M. Specialist palliative care in nonmalignant disease. Palliat Med. 1998;12(6):417–27.

28. Walker SR, Brar R, Eng F, Komenda P, Rigatto C, Prasad B, et al. Frailty and physical function in chronic kidney disease: the CanFIT study. Can J Kidney Health Dis. 2015;2:32.

29. Bonner A, Chambers S, Healy H, Hoy WE, Mitchell G, Kark A, et al. Tracking patients with advanced kidney disease in last 12 months of life. J Renal Care. 2018; https://doi.org/10.1111/jorc.12239.

30. Queensland Health. Queensland hospital admitted patient data collection (QHAPDC) manual 2017-2018. Brisbane: Queensland Health; 2017.

31. Queensland Government Queensland Health. Emergency Department Categories. Emergency Departments 2016. http://www.performance.health. qld.gov.au/hospitalperformance/ed-categories.aspx?hospital=1. Accessed 10 May 2017.

32. Charlson M, Szatrowski TP, Peterson J, Gold J. Validation of a combined comorbidity index. J Clin Epidemiol. 1994;47(11):1245–51.

33. Mix TCH, Peter WL, Ebben J, Xue J, Pereira BJG, Kausz AT, et al. Hospitalization during advancing chronic kidney disease. Am J Kidney Dis. 2003;42(5):972–81.

34. O'Connell DL, Goldsbury ED, Davidson P, Girgis A, Phillips JL, Piza M, et al. Acute hospital-based services utilisation during the last year of life in New South Wales, Australia: methods for a population-based study. BMJ Open. 2014;4:e004455.

35. Langton JM, Srasuebkul P, Reeve R, Parkinson B, Gu Y, Buckley NA, et al. Resource use, costs and quality of end-of-life care: observations in a cohort of elderly Australian cancer decedents. Implement Sci. 2015;10:25.

36. Rosenwax LK, McNamara BA, Murray K, McCabe RJ, Aoun SM, Currow DC. Hospital and emergency department use in the last year of life: a baseline for future modifications to end-of-life care. MJA. 2011;194(11):570–3.

37. Rosenwax LK, McNamara BA. Who receives specialist palliative care in Western Australia – and who misses out? Palliat Med. 2006;20(4):439–45.

38. Australian Institute of Health and Welfare. Emergency department care 2016-17 Australian hospital statistics, Health services series no. 80. HSE 184. Canberra: AIHW; 2017.

39. Quinn MP, Cardwell CR, Rainey A, McNamee PT, Kee F, Maxwell AP, et al. Patterns of hospitalisation before and following initiation of haemodialysis: a 5 year single Centre study. Postgrad Med J. 2011;87(1028):389–93.

40. Fraser SD, Roderick PJ, May CR, McIntyre N, McIntyre C, Fluck RJ, et al. The burden of comorbidity in people with chronic kidney disease stage 3: a cohort study. BMC Nephrol. 2015;16:193.

41. Murtagh FE, Addington-Hall J, Edmonds P, Donohoe P, Carey I, Jenkins K, et al. Symptoms in the month before death for stage 5 chronic kidney disease patients managed without dialysis. J Pain Symptom Manag. 2010;40(3):342–52.

42. Noble H, Meyer J, Bridges J, Bridges J, Kelly D, Johnson B. Patient experience of dialysis refusal or withdrawal - a review of the literature. J Renal Care. 2008;34(2):94–100.

43. Axelsson L, Alvariza A, Lindberg J, Ohlen J, Hakanson C, Reimertz H, et al. Unmet palliative care needs among patients with end-stage kidney disease: a national registry study about the last week of life. J Pain Symptom Manag. 2018;55(2):236–44.

44. Almutary H, Bonner A, Douglas C. Symptom burden in chronic kidney disease: a review of recent literature. J Renal Care. 2013;39(3):140–50.

45. O'Hare AM, Song MK, Kurella Tamura M, Moss AH. Research priorities for palliative care for older adults with advanced chronic kidney disease. J Palliat Med. 2017;20(5):453–60.

46. Davison SN, Moss AH. Supportive care: meeting the needs of patients with advanced chronic kidney disease. Clin J Am Soc Nephrol. 2016;11(10):1879–80.

47. Makar MS, Pun PH. Sudden cardiac death among hemodialysis patients. Am J Kidney Dis. 2017;69(5):684–95.

48. Ramesh S, Zalucky A, Hemmelgarn BR, Roberts DJ, Ahmed SB, Wilton SB, et al. Incidence of sudden cardiac death in adults with end-stage renal disease: a systematic review and meta-analysis. BMC Nephrol. 2016;17:78.

49. Tonkin-Crine S, Okamoto I, Leydon GM, Murtagh FE, Farrington K, Caskey F, et al. Understanding by older patients of dialysis and conservative management for chronic kidney failure. Am J Kidney Dis. 2015;65(3):443–50.

50. Australian Institute of Health and Welfare. Emergency department care 2015-16: Australian hospital statistics, Health services series, no. 72. Cat. no. HSE 182. Canberra: AIHW; 2016.

51. Spilsbury K, Rosenwax L, Arendts G, Semmens JB. The impact of community-based palliative care on acute hospital use in the last year of life is modified by time to death, age and underlying cause of death. A population-based retrospective cohort study. PLoS One. 2017;12(9): e0185275.

52. Redahan L, Brady B, Smyth A, Higgins S, Wall C. The use of palliative care services amongst end-stage kidney disease patients in an Irish tertiary referral Centre. Clin Kidney J. 2013;6(6):604–8.

53. ANZDATA Registry. 39th report, chapter 3: mortality in end stage kidney disease. Adelaide: Australia and New Zealand Dialysis and Transplant Registry; 2017. Available at: http://www.anzdata.org.au

54. van der Meer DM, Weiland TJ, Philip J, Jelinek GA, Boughey M, Knott J, et al. Presentation patterns and outcomes of patients with cancer accessing care

Health service utilisation during the last year of life: a prospective, longitudinal study of the pathways...

79

in emergency departments in Victoria, Australia. Support Care Cancer. 2016; 24(3):1251–60.

55. Bansal AD, Schell JO. A practical guide for the care of patients with end-stage renal disease near the end of life. Semin Dial. 2018;31(2):170–6.

56. Davison SN, Levin A, Moss AH, Jha V, Brown EA, Brennan F, et al. Executive summary of the KDIGO controversies conference on supportive care in chronic kidney disease: developing a roadmap to improving quality care. Kidney Int. 2015;88(3):447–59.

57. Smith S, Brick A, O'Hara S, Normand C. Evidence on the cost and cost effectiveness of palliative care: a literature review. Palliat Med. 2014;28:130–50.

58. Hashimoto RE, Brodt ED, Skelly AC, Dettori JR. Administrative database studies: goldmine or goose chase? Evid Based Spine Care J. 2014;5(2):74–6.

59. World Health Organisation. ICD-10: international statistical classification of diseases and related health problems. Volume 2 Instruction Manual. 2010. http://apps.who.int/classifications/icd10/browse/Content/statichtml/ICD10Volume2_en_2010.pdf. Accessed 16 Nov 2017.

60. Javier AD, Figueroa R, Siew ED, Salat H, Morse J, Stewart TG, et al. Reliability and utility of the surprise question in CKD stages 4 to 5. Am J Kidney Dis. 2017;70(1):93–101.

61. Okamoto I, Tonkin-Crine S, Rayner H, Murtagh FE, Farrington K, Caskey F, et al. Conservative care for ESRD in the United Kingdom: a national survey. Clin J Am Soc Nephrol. 2015;10(1):120–6.

7

The 'lived experience' of palliative care patients in one acute hospital setting

Anne Black[1][*] [iD], Tamsin McGlinchey[1], Maureen Gambles[1], John Ellershaw[2] and Catriona Rachel Mayland[1]

Abstract

Background: There is limited understanding of the 'lived experience' of palliative care patient within the acute care setting. Failing to engage with and understand the views of patients and those close to them, has fundamental consequences for future health delivery. Understanding 'patient experience' can enable care providers to ensure services are responsive and adaptive to individual patient need.

Methods: The aim of this study was to explore the 'lived experience' of a group of patients with palliative care needs who had recently been in-patients in one acute hospital trust in the north-west of England.
Qualitative research using narrative interviews was undertaken, and data was analysed using thematic analysis. A sample of 20 consecutive patients complying with the inclusion/exclusion criteria were recruited and interviewed.

Results: Patient Sample:
Of the 20 patients recruited, there was a fairly equal gender split; all had a cancer diagnosis and the majority were white British, with an age range of 43–87 years.
Findings from Interviews:
Overall inpatient experience was viewed positively. Individual narratives illustrated compassionate and responsive care, with the patient at the centre. Acts of compassion appeared to be expressed through the 'little things' staff could do for patients, i.e., time to talk, time to care, humanity and comfort measures. AHSPCT involvement resulted in perceived improvements in pain control and holistic wellbeing. However, challenges were evident, particularly regarding over-stretched staff and resources, and modes of communication, which seemed to impact on patient experience.

Conclusions: Listening to patients' experiences of care across the organisation provided a unique opportunity to impact upon delivery of care. Further research should focus on exploring issues such as: why some patients within the same organisation have a positive experience of care, while others may not; how do staff attitudes and behaviours impact on the experience of care; transitions of care from hospital to home, and the role of social networks.

Keywords: Patient experience, Narrative research, Palliative care, Hospital, Qualitative

* Correspondence: anne.black@rlbuht.nhs.uk
[1]Palliative Care Institute Liverpool, Cancer Research Centre, University of Liverpool, 200 London Road, Liverpool L3 9TA, UK
Full list of author information is available at the end of the article

Background

'Person centred' approaches to care delivery have been promoted as a core part of service design within the National Health Service (NHS) [1]. Crucially, person centred care promotes a care environment that is respectful, compassionate and responsive to the needs of individuals [2]. This is not a novel idea as the person centred ethos can be seen echoed in the core principles and values of the NHS; "[the NHS] touches our lives at times of most basic human need, when care and compassion are what matter most" [3]. Whilst this may be an attractive concept to underpin health care delivery policy, the term has been criticised for being applied without clarity of definition, causing subsequent discourse around the subject to be 'woolly', particularly with regard to informing actual care delivery [4].

A recent high profile review of care delivery in hospitals has shown that a lack of openness and compassion led, at times, to care that was "totally unacceptable and a fundamental breach of the values of the NHS" [5]. Furthermore, the Neuberger review highlighted a lack of 'patient centred' care and openness around decision making as barriers to good care [6]. A failure to engage meaningfully with patients may result in an approach to care delivery that 'does to' rather than 'works with' patients; privileging the perspective of healthcare professionals and clinically focused outcomes [7]. Indeed, a lack of compassion from health care providers has been cited as a major reason for dissatisfaction with the care that patients receive [8].

Failing to engage with and understand the views of patients and those close to them, has fundamental consequences for future health care delivery. Both government policy/guidance and the research literature continues to emphasise the importance of exploring the 'patient experience' in order to support service providers to provide care that is responsive and adaptive to individual patient need – ie person centred [2, 9–12]. By actively seeking the views of patients and families, the potential to ensure that these views are placed at the centre of service provision is enhanced. This perspective sits in accordance with the overarching values of the NHS Constitution [3] as well as National Guidance for End of Life Care [10, 12, 13]; therefore engaging service users should form part of ongoing service improvement strategies.

Predominantly however, assessing the 'user experience' has centred on measuring 'satisfaction', with a focus on comparison and monitoring. Some commentators suggest that current widely used approaches for measuring 'satisfaction' may not be sufficiently grounded in the values or experiences of patients, thus raising serious questions about the validity of the concept as a way of eliciting what is important to patients and the care they receive [14, 15]. In recent years assessment of the performance of healthcare organisations has begun to move beyond examining clinical care alone, to considering and embracing 'patient experience' as an important indicator of quality [9].

So how can we best uncover the views of patients who receive care in our NHS organisations, to better understand how well it meets their needs? Patient experience is complex and multifaceted, and requires more in depth methods to explore how patients and families experience the care they receive [9]. Taking time to actively engage patients to find out what is really important to them has the potential to unlock a richness of information not possible solely through 'satisfaction' questionnaires alone [16].

Much of the recent focus of both the media and the academic literature has been on the perceived deficits in care delivery for hospital in-patients nearing the end of life and their relatives and carers [6, 17]. We therefore chose to focus this study on a group of hospital in-patients who had life limiting illness and who were potentially nearing the end of life. In order to identify a suitable group of patients, we focused on inpatients who had received input during their stay from members of the Academic Hospital Specialist Palliative Care Team (AHSPCT) in one acute hospital trust in the North-West of England. The AHSPCT is an advisory service which takes referrals from across the hospital for patients with identified specialist palliative care needs. The role of the service is to assess patients' holistic needs in order to optimise comfort, well-being and quality of life, in the presence of incurable, advancing illness. The AHSPCT is a multi-professional team, and includes doctors, specialist nurses and allied health professionals.

Methods

The aim of this study was to explore the 'lived experience' of a group of patients with palliative care needs who had recently been in-patients in one acute hospital trust in the north-west of England.

Exploring the lived experience required a phenomenological approach whereby participants were encouraged to recount their experience, allowing issues that held most personal importance to them unfold. This approach allows the researcher 'enter the patients world', promoting understanding of their experience from the patients' perspective [18]. In-depth narrative interviews were undertaken using a conversational approach where patients were encouraged to direct and shape the discussion in accordance with their own experiences, views and particular concerns [19, 20], rather than responding to a pre-determined agenda.

Procedure

Identification and recruitment of patients

In order to promote the potential to sample a range of experience, a consecutive sample of 20 patients who had been referred to the AHSPCT were recruited to take part. Recruitment was coordinated by the main researcher (AB). AB, female, is a Clinical Nurse Specialist with the AHSPCT, who was seconded for 1 year to undertake this research project.

During the recruitment phase, AB attended the morning 'run through' meeting within the AHSPCT attended by the multi-disciplinary team, to prompt identification of patients who may be 'eligible' for this study. Patients were considered 'eligible' if they met the following inclusion criteria:

- Hospital inpatient > = 18 years of age
- Referred to the AHSPCT and seen on at least two occasions;
- Due to be discharged from hospital.

Patients were not approached for this study if the following exclusion criteria applied:

- Hospital inpatient < 18 years of age;
- Recognised to be in the last few days or hours of life;
- Unable to provide fully informed consent to participate;
- Died prior to discharge;
- Unable to communicate in English.

Information and consent

Potential participants were initially approached by a member of the clinical team, who informed them that this study was being conducted. If the patient expressed interest, they then met with the researcher (AB), who gave them a Patient Information Sheet (PIS) along with verbal information and offered the opportunity for questions. If the patient was agreeable, a mutually agreed date/time and place was arranged to conduct the interview following discharge from hospital. AB then checked their agreement to participate prior to undertaking the interview, and a consent form was signed by the participant.

Interviews

The interviews were conducted by the researcher (AB) in the patients' home following discharge. The researcher began the interviews with an open question:

'Thinking back to x number of days ago when you came into hospital, can you tell me everything that has happened'.

A topic guide of 'prompts' was also created to support this process. For example, prompts such as 'tell me more about', 'can you remember specific examples?' and 'how did you feel about that?' were used in order to elicit more detailed responses where this did not occur more naturally from the conversation. The interviews were conducted between October 2015 and September 2016.

It was important to consider issues of potential bias within the research process, for example the balance of power in the relationship between patients and the researcher [21, 22]. Considering this, the interviews were conducted in a place where the patient felt comfortable, and the researcher kept a field note diary to document thoughts and feelings in order to aid ongoing reflection. In addition a distress protocol was available should the patient become distressed during the interview.

Analysis

Each interview was transcribed verbatim, and transcripts were analysed using Thematic Analysis, facilitating exploration of how people ascribe meaning to their experiences in their interactions with the environment [23]. The analysis process began at the interview stage, with the researcher keeping a field note diary of thoughts, feelings and emotional responses to the interview process and content. The process of analysis was cyclical and iterative in nature. Transcription further promoted familiarisation with the data and generation of initial emerging themes. The transcripts were also analysed in conjunction with the original recordings, so that the researcher became fully immersed in the data [23]. Against each transcript, the main researcher (AB) made initial notes documenting any observations, questions and interpretations that arose from the reading and re-reading of the data. AB then coded each transcript and made an initial narrative summary of the key themes for in-depth discussion with the wider team (TM and CM). TM and CM also independently analysed 5 transcripts (20%) to gain first-hand experience of the words of participants, giving the potential for a richer interpretation. Where appropriate, consideration of relevant published literature further enhanced the evolving interpretation.

Results

Final sample

A total of 20 interviews were undertaken (see Fig. 1 for recruitment flow diagram) lasting between 15 min and 90 min, with a median time of 41 min.

As a result of the complex and palliative nature of the patient cohort, over half (53% $n = 296/560$) initially referred to the AHSPCT were either 'too ill' or 'dying' at the point of referral, meaning they were not eligible for inclusion. However, many patients who were approached for inclusion expressed interest in taking part in the study;

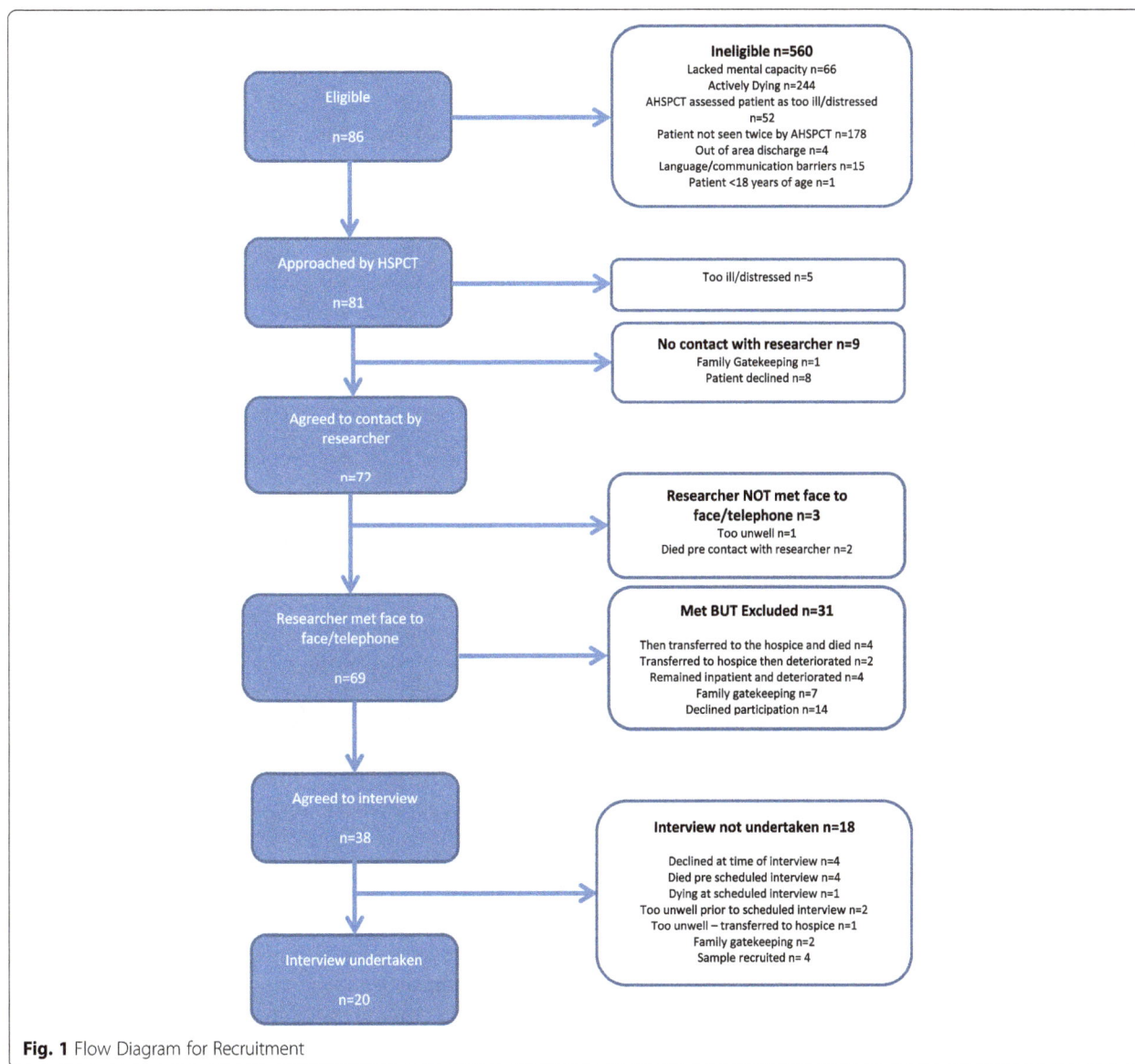

Fig. 1 Flow Diagram for Recruitment

of the 81 patients initially approached only 26 (32%) expressly declined. Thirty five patients (43%) initially showed interest but were unable to be recruited for the following reasons: deteriorating condition (n = 11); subsequent death (n = 10); family 'gate keeping' (n = 10); and the required sample had been reached (n = 4). The interviews took place no longer than 10 days following discharge home; 14/20 interviews took place within 6 days of discharge. Table 1 provides a summary of the demographic details of participating patients.

Findings from interviews
Four overarching themes were generated from the interview data and these are presented below.

Table 1 Demographic Details

Total No: Participants	20
Male	11 (55%)
Female	9 (45%)
Age Range	43–87 years
Diagnosis	20 cancer (100%)
Ethnicity	19 White British (95%) 1 Any other ethnic group (5%)
Median days - recruitment to Interview	6 days (IQR 5–7 days)
Median days - Interview to Date of Death (n = 17[a])	63 (IQR 35–218 days)

[a] 3 patients still alive at close of data collection period

Making Time – Taking Time

It was clear from the narratives that participants in this study were acutely aware of the pressures on the staff that were looking after them, including the busyness of the wards, and staff shortages:

"...sometimes they were run off their feet. They can't always come so you don't get bad tempered or anything, you just have to wait and know that they will come." (Betty).

"they're very, very busy and they're trying to fit you in and decide what's the best thing to do for you and they haven't got time to do, I wouldn't even call it value added, but to just communicate to you to say, 'right Mr P, this is what we plan to do and this is why we're doing it. There was none of that...because they are so busy and they haven't got time and resource in place to provide that information to you" (Bill).

Against this backdrop, the views of the participants highlighted how the mode and manner of communication and information giving, including the number of HCPs involved and the level of engagement, could further negatively impact their experience:

"...I saw four different teams, you know what I mean, so you do lose track that is; who and names (sic)... that was one of the problems I had anyway." (Gerry).

"That [lack of information] leaves you feeling as though...do they know any more, that they don't want to tell me? ...or is [it] a matter that they just don't know what's going on?" (Bill).

For some, it was perceived that it was not just busyness that meant that staff were less attentive than they would have liked, but individual differences in the way different staff approached their roles:

"Well it was sort of nurses, I mean, erm there was some of them were, it's hard to say, some of them were a lot better than others .. but there was others not so good; they would sit round chatting and things like that when there was, you know, basically, work to be done .. I mean you waited every night till nine o'clock to see which nurse .. was gonna come on and .. you know if they were good nurses .. you would have no problems" (Harry).

Understandably then, staff that went the extra mile to make time in their busy schedules and to take time to treat these patients as individuals, were highly valued:

"...it's just little things...that make a difference...they wanted to be there, they wanted to care. You could tell that they wanted to care...and they made time for me...they just seemed to care...to want to be there and help...they wanted to listen to what I have to say and understand how I feel ...one particular nurse, she just said to me one night, you're not you're normal self...do you need a hug? And I said, "Yeah, I do actually". So she gave me a hug and you know, she hugged me for a while until I was ready to stop having a hug..." (Tilly).

"nurses used to sit with me, not only about the medication, but they used to sit with me and listen to problems, about my health and what was going on and they used to sit with me for quite a while" (P7).

Experiencing and relieving pain

For some patients their in-patient stay was characterised by their experience of pain, and it was often what they remembered most about being in hospital.

"Erm, it's like you know if someone, they had like, erm, wood and paper and everything and they put a match to it and it went aflame, that's the way I feel, ya know when it hits my right leg...that's how the pain was, and I felt like a fire had gone off inside me." (Betty).

Where physical pain was not dealt with in an appropriate and timely manner, this was highlighted as having the potential to negatively impact the patient experience:

"...they [nurses] gave me paracetamol thinking it would help and I just sat up in the chair, I'd say for about three nights... they couldn't give me anything stronger because I wasn't written up for it so I was sat in the chair...trying to stop the pain and just ended up sitting up all night watching TV... just watching the clock until nine o'clock, until they came round with the medication" (Sadie).

"Sometimes we ask for medication and they'll say I'll get it for you, and you'd end up getting it eventually when they'd come round with the trolley two hours later..." (Bob).

When this was attended to however, the therapeutic value of this for patients made all the difference. The act of attending to patients' pain relief appeared to embody compassion, care, dignity, and being valued as a human being:

"That was great, and somebody's on your side, I can remember her coming up to me, whispers "I got you some more" [medication], oh thank God, yeah..." (Ritchie).

Interestingly, although initial anxiety was reported by some around whether the involvement of the Academic Hospital Specialist Palliative Care Team (AHSPCT) meant imminent death, it was their involvement, particularly with regards to pain management, that was highlighted as having had a positive impact:

"Oh the pain relief, they [AHSPCT] were absolutely marvellous...it was like someone waving a magic wand because after I'd seen them for a few occasions, about three times, er, I just, the next time they came to see me, I said it was the first time that I'd slept properly in about six weeks." (Sadie).

Loss of control and loss of self
Central to many patient stories, was the sense of 'struggle'; seeking to find sense and meaning in their lives in the face of an uncertain and changing future with a life limiting illness:

"I didn't know I was dying seven weeks ago...eight weeks ago I just had a bad back. I was actually working and doing stuff and planning my life and wanting to get better, expecting to get better, but now I'm dying and I'm not expecting to live, so I don't...I wanna understand what's happening to me and I wanna understand what's the likely scenario but there's a part of me that's terrified. I'm terrified of like being in agonising pain. I'm terrified of like losing meself (sic) to the pain; the pain steals your personality." (Tim).

Patients also described feeling 'labelled' by their illness, which in turn poses a challenge to their sense of 'self' and 'identity':

"Terminal, you know what I mean. Er, you do seem to feel a bit, a little bit different." (Terry).

Linked to this, some patients described the 'contagiousness' of cancer, and almost a sense of isolation, from having the 'label' of a cancer diagnosis:

"I suppose in the back of your mind...cancer is contagious...don't you, sounds silly doesn't it? ...I

suppose that's were you, er you think it's, it's a horrible word cancer, but it means a lot of things doesn't it?" (Charlie).

For some the hospital environment provided a 'secure' and 'supportive' environment during this time of flux, however once discharged home, patients described feeling 'alone' and less supported:

"...when you come home you're very much left to your own devices...now I'm in need of a bit of help and support...I feel as though I'm being provided with a poor...well not a poor service, but a limited service" (Bill).

Burden versus benefit of treatment interventions
From these patient stories, a picture emerged of wrestling with choices and decisions regarding treatment options. This illustrates the subjective values placed on 'life'; quality of life or the battle to survive at any cost.

"I know I'm not gonna get better, and I thought, why do it, you know? Why put me through anything that's intrusive at all? I really don't see the point; I really don't." (Wendy).

"...when you have a days like the last couple of days I've just felt ill...it's difficult to wanna like, battle on... fighting the sickness is horrible...I'm not sure if I wanna go back, to go back to radiotherapy though. I'm not sure I'd like it or trust it. I don't know how making me feel this ill; can be doing me any favours." (Tim).

The following patient quote illustrates the tensions that can arise when HCP and patients' perceptions of the focus of care are not aligned, impacting on patient choice, autonomy and dignity and shared decision making:

"...it changes when you become terminal. I could understand [considering all treatment interventions] before because then there is a real good case for it... once you go into the terminal thing then it's a case of not so much...it's a case of what can...make it better for now? And if the blood thinners was making me a lot worse so to me, my personal opinion, in that situation was let's just stop them. It might not have been somebody else's [wish] but nobody was actually saying...they were saying "This is what's going on" but [not asking] "what do you want to do?"" (Terry).

The following patient account highlights that when HCP 'take on board' what the patient wants, and work in partnership, this can alleviate the 'tension' and provide therapeutic benefits. This in turn impacts on patient autonomy, dignity and comfort, reinforcing the importance of active listening and shared decision making:

"[I felt] Jubilant...because like I say over a year and somebody's listened, and they've gone away, they've sorted it all out, done what they promised they'd do you know like oh we'll get it sorted, and we've heard that so many times, and no they did exactly what they said they'd do...that's all I could ask that somebody would listen, and take on board what the patient wants, as well as what the doctor's experiences are, obviously a two-way street, but when it comes to pain the patient knows what pain they're in, not the doctor." (Ritchie).

Discussion

This study has generated important information on the way in which patients' experience care currently, providing an opportunity for the acute hospital to generate recommendations, to consider how results from this study may inform future service design, education, training and resource utilisations. The results of this study illustrate that overall the in-patient experience was viewed positively for most patients, with accounts illustrating compassionate and responsive care. Challenges were highlighted, however, with regard to over stretched staff and resources, along with individual differences in the attitudes of staff, which was reported to have negatively impacted the experience of care for some patients. Whilst this study was undertaken in one acute hospital, these findings are likely to be of interest to all providers of in-patient care, as many of the themes and issues highlighted here may also resonate with those care services.

Where care delivery was timely, responsive, well led and compassionate, however, this appeared to contribute to patients feeling safe and valued as individuals rather than being 'processed' as commodities; a view reinforced in the literature and recent policy documents [10, 24, 25]. In this study, acts of compassion were experienced through the 'little things' that staff could do for patients such as; making and taking the time to talk, to care and to display characteristics of humanity. Indeed, one of the main components of 'good care' has been highlighted as feeling that 'you matter' [26]. This perspective supports the view that the smallest details of the patient experience can be the most meaningful [27]. The NHS is under relentless pressure to improve efficiency and throughput; however it is an imperative that the patient remains at the forefront of any improvement strategy [2].

For patients' in this study, modes of communication could have both positive and negative impacts on the patient experience. In particular, what information was given and how it was delivered appeared to impact on patients' understanding of services involved, their condition and the overall plan of care. Evidence suggests "effective communication is the core of every helping relationship, and listening is the foundation of every medical and social service interaction" [28], p57. Accounts from this study reinforce that when HCP's were able to 'connect' with patients beyond the 'physical' contact, this fostered a powerful sense of genuine human presence and care; effective communication, engagement and active listening, should be reflected within the culture of care in the organisation [29]. In recognition that 'dignity enhancing' or 'dignity preserving' care for palliative care patients is vitally important, the use of interventions such as the 'dignity model' has been highlighted as one way to ensure a person-centred approach in the acute hospital setting; promoting patient autonomy and recognition of the person as an individual [30].

For many patients in this study, pain appeared to be a major concern throughout their in-patient episode; a finding supported by previous studies [31–33]. Stories from this study reinforce the 'threat', highlighted by Pringle et al. [30], that untimely and unresponsive symptom assessment and control can be to patient dignity. For example patients described the seemingly all-encompassing nature of pain and the very real distress this caused when it was unremitting and unresolved. Specifically, some patients described 'a significant period of waiting for assessment and administration' of pain medication, impacting on their sense of dignity and wellbeing. Poignantly, patients described their relief when they felt that their pain was finally being attended to, underlining the significance of pain control to a patient's sense of being cared for and valued as a human being. The role of the AHSPCT was specifically highlighted in this regard, where despite initial uncertainty and anxiety from some patients associated with their understanding of the role of the AHSPCT [31, 34, 35] as noted in previous studies [30, 31, 36, 37], their involvement resulted in improvements in pain control and holistic wellbeing.

Throughout this study, patients' described the 'struggle' of living with a terminal illness, and the effect this had on their sense of self and life as they knew it before their diagnosis. This was a very important issue for patients, as their sense of 'self' had been ultimately changed, forcing them to renegotiate this in the face of uncertainty: "Death forces us to give an ultimate meaning to life and thereby transcend the apparent absurdity and meaninglessness of life in the face of death" [38].

Patients described feeling 'different' following their diagnosis, which echoes previous studies where the 'stigma' of cancer can have a negative impact on a patients sense of self, resulting in a 'renegotiation' of identity within the new context of their diagnosis [39]. It has also been suggested that over time the 'label' of a terminal illness can preclude 'sustaining self-images' resulting in 'diminished self-concept', as well as a fear of becoming a 'burden' to relatives as they readjust to the 'real world' [40]. This echoes with findings from this study, where for example despite the 'hustle and bustle' the hospital provided a 'safe haven' during this uncertain time [41], where patients could navigate and readjust within their 'renegotiation' of identity, self-worth, dignity and self-respect.

For some patients in this particular study, the distress prompted by this time of uncertainty extended beyond their inpatient admission. Some patients reported feeling 'alone' following discharge, indicating the potential for ongoing distress and need for additional support at this time. This resonates with the idea that 'structures' that underpin everyday life (such as social networks and relationships) can be 'disrupted' in light of serious chronic illness [42]. The 'chaos narrative' [43, 44] offers us another perspective that resonates with this study, for example the challenge of loss and adjustment faced by study participants when leaving the safe confines of hospital to return to the' real world'. Reinforcing the importance that care services should not 'end' at the point of discharge, ensuring that patients can be sufficiently supported.

Johnson suggests 'living with dignity' is bound up in the individual's sense of identity; through having one's human value acknowledged, irrespective of circumstances, 'personhood' and 'self-worth' [45]. Johnson also highlights the risk to dignity at the end of life (EOL) as health deteriorates being particularly concerning [45]. Therefore, as health professionals, it is crucial that we consider how we respect these views in our conduct with others, ensuring that our interactions are dignity enriching [45], seeing the 'person' in the patient, rather than merely their illness. This perspective is also highlighted by Chochinov [46] and Johnson [47], who describe the Patient Dignity Question (PDQ) as a means by which HPCs may enhance person-centred care, for people with palliative care needs in an acute hospital.

Strengths and limitations

This study provided a unique opportunity for one NHS organisation to explore what matters to patients with a life limiting illness, in the context on their in-patient stay. The approach that was taken, through listening to 'patient stories', reflects the traditions of hospice and palliative care, by giving time and space to listen and gain a greater understanding from the patients perspective [48].

However it has been recognised that involving patients with a palliative illness in research studies poses its own ethical and moral challenges. In this study for example

due to the vulnerability of the patient population, some were unable to be involved as they deteriorated or died prior to or after discharge from hospital. Despite ethical and methodological debates regarding the 'morality' and 'appropriateness' of involving this cohort of patients in this type of research [49], it was evident throughout recruitment, that patients had a desire to take part. Indeed there is growing evidence to suggest that in fact, palliative care patients do have a desire to take part in research [50, 51]. This adds to growing literature, critiquing the potentially constraining ethical guidelines, prompting the question of whether it is ethical to prohibit patients the chance to contribute to research [52, 53].

Also of note was that the majority of interviews took place within the last two months of the patient's life (17/20 had died by the end of the data collection period: October 2015 – September 2016). This is interesting given the reticence to involve patients in research as they are approaching the end of life, due to the assumption that it is an unwelcome burden for them at this time [46]. The inclusion criteria of this study however excluded patients that remained in hospital. It could be argued that this approach limited participation, possibly denying the opportunity for other palliative care patients to share their experiences and potentially silencing their voices. In addition, the sample was homogenous in terms of ethnicity and all had cancer, therefore future studies may seek to explore the views of a wider patient population, including patients that do not have a life-limiting illness. Interestingly, the referral criteria for the AHSPT are not limited to patients with a cancer diagnosis, yet these patients made up the total sample population for this study.

The issue of 'gatekeeping' was also important to consider, as for ten patients in this study family members specifically requested that the patient not be approached. Reasons for this included perceptions that the patient was too unwell, too tired, or it was 'not the right time' to be approached, despite some patients agreeing to meet or have contact with the researcher. However, there were examples where family 'gatekeepers' became part of the process [54], by facilitating access to the patient and by their presence in the interview itself, potentially shaping the stories that were being told. It is important to be mindful of these influences when undertaking this kind of research.

Conclusions

Despite the acknowledged organisational pressures, these patient narratives highlight the importance of concepts such as kindness, compassion and dignity; taking the time to 'care for patients' rather than time to 'do to patients', taking the time to listen to what is most important and taking the time to respond to the patient as an individual. When the patients' voice is heard and healthcare professionals 'see the person behind the name' rather than the illness, this provides opportunities for relationships to be built based on trust, confidence and mutual respect. This ultimately impacts on the patients' experience of care, and their perception of self-worth and identity and sense of dignity [46, 47]. The palliative nature of illness reinforced the 'preciousness' of time, underlining there is 'one chance to get it right' [55]. Having listened to our patients it is time to learn and change; this study has provided an opportunity for the 'patient voice' to be heard and the individual patient experience to be explored. Further research should focus on exploring issues such as: why some patients within the same organisation have a positive experience of care, while others may not; how do staff attitudes and behaviours impact on the experience of care; transitions of care from hospital to home; the role of social networks.

Abbreviations
AHSPCT: Academic Hospital Specialist Palliative Care Team; EOL: End of Life; NHS: National Health Service; PIS: Patient Information Sheet

Acknowledgements
The authors would like to thank, the AHSPCT, the Senior Management Team and the Patient and carer representatives on the project steering group and the Patient and Public Engagement Network, for all their help during the course of the study.

Funding
Academic Palliative and End of Life Care Centre.

Authors' contributions
AB,TM,MG,JE were involved in the process of designing the study. AB conducted the interviews. AB,TM,CRM participated in the data analysis process. AB, TM and CRM wrote the manuscript and MG and JE contributed to the drafting of the manuscript. All authors read and approved the final manuscript.

Ethics approval and consent to participate
When designing, and performing the study, the researchers were guided by ethical standard principles. The research project was reviewed and endorsed by the North West Wales Research Ethics Committee (15/WA/0237). All data collected was stored in line with the University of Liverpool data storage policy (http://www.liv.ac.uk/csd/regulations/informationsecuritypolicy.pdf), and handled in confidence in line with the Caldicott principles. Patients received verbal and written information about the study, and they provided their signed informed consent to participate before the interviews took place. Patients were also informed about the voluntary nature of their participation, and that they had the option to withdraw from the study without specifying a reason for doing so, at any time.

Competing interests
The authors declare that they have no competing interests.

Author details
[1]Palliative Care Institute Liverpool, Cancer Research Centre, University of Liverpool, 200 London Road, Liverpool L3 9TA, UK. [2]Royal Liverpool and Broadgreen University Hospitals NHS Trust, Prescot Street, Liverpool L7 8XP, UK.

References
1. Department of Health. The National Health Service (Revision of NHS Constitution Guiding Principles) Regulation. 2015. http://www.legislation.gov.uk/uksi/2015/1426/pdfs/uksi_20151426_en.pdf. Accessed 21 Nov 2017.
2. Goodrich J, Cornwell J. Seeing the person in the patient: the King's fund point of care Programme. J Holistic Healthcare. 2011;8:10–2.
3. Department of Health. The NHS Constitution – the NHS belongs to us all. 2013. https://www.gov.uk/government/uploads/system/uploads/attachment_data/file/480482/NHS_Constitution_WEB.pdf. Accessed 21 Nov 2017.
4. Brooker D. What is person-centred care in dementia? Rev Clin Gerontol. 2004;3:215–22.
5. The Mid Staffordshire NHS Foundation Trust: Public inquiry. 2013 http://webarchive.nationalarchives.gov.uk/20150407084231/http://www.midstaffspublicinquiry.com/report. Accessed 21 Nov 2017.
6. More care less pathway; a review of the Liverpool Care Pathway. 2014. https://assets.publishing.service.gov.uk/government/uploads/system/uploads/attachment_data/file/212450/Liverpool_Care_Pathway.pdf. Accessed 21 Nov 2017.
7. The Health Foundation. Person-centred care made simple: What everyone should know about person-centred care.2014. http://www.health.org.uk/publication/person-centred-care-made-simple. Accessed 21 Nov 2017.
8. Reader TW, Gillespie A, Roberts J. Patient complaints in healthcare systems: a systematic review and coding taxonomy. BMJ Qual Saf. 2014; https://doi.org/10.1136/bmjqs-2013-002437. Accessed 29th May 2018
9. Wolf JA, Niederhauser V, Marshburn D, LaVela SL. Defining patient experience. Patient Experience J. 2014;1:7–19.
10. Care Quality Commission. The five key questions we ask. 2016. http://www.cqc.org.uk/content/five-key-questions-we-ask. Accessed 21 Nov 2017.
11. Department of Health. End of life care strategy: promoting high quality care for adults at the end of their life. 2008 https://www.gov.uk/government/publications/end-of-life-care-strategy-promoting-high-quality-care-for-adults-at-the-end-of-their-life. Accessed 21 Nov 2017.
12. National Palliative and End of Life Care Partnership (NPELCP). Ambitions for Palliative and End of Life Care: a national framework for local action. 2015. http://endoflifecareambitions.org.uk. Accessed 21 Nov 2017.
13. National Institute for Clinical Excellence Care of dying adults in the last days of life. 2016. https://www.nice.org.uk/guidance/ng31. Accessed 21 Nov 2017.
14. Avis M, Bond M, Arthur A. Satisfying solutions? A review of some unresolved issues in the measurement of patient satisfaction. J Adv Nurs. 1995;22:316–22.
15. Wilcock PM, Brown GCS, Bateson J, Carver J, Machin S. Using patient stories to inspire quality improvement within the NHS modernization agency collaborative programmes. J Clin Nurs. 2003;12:422–30.
16. Aspinall F, Addington-Hall J, Hughes R, Higginson I. Using satisfaction to measure the quality of palliative care: a review of the literature. J Adv Nurs. 2003;42:324–39.
17. The Daily Telegraph. 2nd September 2009. Sentenced to Death on the NHS http://www.telegraph.co.uk/health/healthnews/6127514/Sentenced-to-death-on-the-NHS.html Accessed 22nd May 2018.
18. Charon R. Narrative Medicine: Honoring the stories of illness. Oxford: Oxford University Press; 2006.
19. Kvale S. InterViews: an introduction to qualitative research interviewing. 1st ed. London: Sage; 1996.
20. Polkinghorne DE. Narrative knowing and the human sciences. 1st ed. Albany: University of New York Press; 1988.
21. Sivell S, Prout H, Hopewell-Kelly N, Baillie J, Byrne A, Edwards M, Harrop E, Noble S, Sampson C, Nelson A, et al. Considerations and recommendations for conducting qualitative research interviews with palliative and end-of-life care patients in the home setting: a consensus paper. BMJ Support Palliat Care. 2015;0:1–7. https://doi.org/10.1111/1753-6405.12250.

22. Kendall S, Halliday LE. Undertaking ethical qualitative research in public health: are current ethical processes sufficient? Aust NZ J Publ Heal. 2014;(4):306–9.

23. Smith J, Jarman A, Osborne M. Doing interpretative phenomenological analysis. In: Murray M, Chamberlain K, editors. Qualitative Health Psychology: theories and methods. 1st ed. London: Sage; 1999. p. 218–40.

24. Institue of Medicine Crossing the Quality Chasm. Anew health system for the 21st century. Washington: National Academy Press; 2001.

25. Berghout M, Job v E, Leensvaart L, Cramm JM. Healthcare professionals' view on patient -centred care in hospitals. BMC Health Serv Res. 2015; 15:1–13.

26. Nolan MR, Davies S, Brown JM, Keady J, Nolan J, et al. Beyond 'person-centred' care: a new vision for gerontological nursing. J Clin Nurs. 2004; 13(3a):45–5333.

27. Frampton, SB, Charmel PA, Planetree, editors. Putting patients first: best practices in patient-centered care. 2nd ed. Wiley; 2009.

28. Langer N, Ribarich M. Using narratives in healthcare communication. Educ Gerontol. 2009;35:55–62.

29. Ciemens EL, Brant J, Kersten D, Mulete E, Dickerson DA. Qualitative analysis of patient and family perspectives of palliative care. J Palliat Med. 2015;18:282–5.

30. Pringle J, Johnston B, Buchanan D. Dignity and patient-centred care for people with palliative care needs in the acute hospital setting: a systematic review. Palliative Med. 2015;29:675–94.

31. Yang G, Ewing G, Booth S. What is the role of specialist palliative care in an acute hospital setting? A qualitative study exploring views of patients and carers. Palliative Med. 2011;26:1011–7.

32. Potter J, Hami F, Bryan T, Quigley C. Symptoms in 400 patients referred to palliative care services: prevalence and patterns. Palliative Med. 2003;17:310–4.

33. Rome RB, Luminais HH, Bourgeois DA, Blais CM. The role of palliative Care at the end of life. Oschsner Journal. 2011;11:348–52.

34. Seymour J, Ingleton C, Payne S, Beddow V. Specialist palliative care: patients' experiences. J Adv Nurs. 2003;44:24–33.

35. Connor A, Allport S, Dixon J, Somerville A-M. Patient perspective: what do palliative care patients think about their care? Int J Palliat Nurs. 2008:546–52.

36. Hanks GW, Robbins M, Sharp D, Forbes K, Done K, Peters TJ, Morgan H, Sykes J, Baxter K, Corfe F, Bidgood C. tHE imPaCT study: a randomised controlled trial to evaluate a hospital palliative care team. Brit J Cancer. 2002;87:733–9.

37. Higginson IJ, Finlay IG, Goodwin DM, Hood K, Edwards AGK, Douglas H-R, Normand CE. Is there evidence that palliative care teams Alter end-of-life experiences of patients and their caregivers? J Pain Symptom Manag. 2003;25:150–68.

38. Janssens R, Gordijin B. Clinical trials in palliative care: an ethical evaluation. Patient Edu Couns. 2000;41:55–62.

39. Matheison CM, Stam J. Renegotiating identity: cancer narratives. Sociol Health Ill. 1995;17:283–306.

40. Charmaz K. Loss of self; a fundamental form of suffering in the chronically ill. Sociol Health Ill. 1983;5:168–95.

41. Hockley J. Role of the hospital support team. Brit J Hosp Med. 1992;48:250–3.

42. Bury M. Chronic illness as biographical disruption. Sociol Health Ill. 1982;4:167–82.

43. Abma TA. Struggling with the fragility of life: a relational – narrative approach to ethics in palliative nursing. Nurs Ethics. 2005;(4):337–48.

44. Frank AW. The wounded storyteller .Body illness and ethics. 2nd ed: University of Chicago Press; 2013.

45. Johnson C. Living with dignity: a palliative approach to care at the end of life. ANMJ. 2017;25:30–3.

46. Chochinov HM. Dignity and the essence of medicine: the A, B, C, and D of dignity conserving care. Brit Med J. 2007;335:184–7.

47. Johnston B, Gaffney M, Pringle J, Buchanan D. The person behind the patient: a feasibility study using the patient dignity question for patients with palliative care needs in hospital. Int J Palliat Nurs. 2015; 21:71–7.

48. Bingley AF, Thomas C, Brown J, Reeve J, Payne S. Developing narrative research in supportive and palliative care: the focus on illness narratives. Palliative Med. 2008;22:653–8.

49. Duke S, Bennett H. A narrative review of the published ethical debates in palliative care research and an assessment of their adequacy to inform research governance. Palliat Med. 2010; https://doi.org/10.1177/0269216309352714. (last accessed 17th May 2018)

50. Bloomer MJ, Hutchinson AM, Brooks L, Botti M, et al. Dying persons' perspectives on, or experiences of, participating in research: an integrative review. Palliat Med. 2018;(4):851–60.

51. Nwosu AC, Mayland CR, Mason S, Varro A, Ellershaw JE. At al. Patients want to be involved in end-of-life care research. In: BMJ Supportive & Palliative are; 2013. https://doi.org/10.1136/bmjspcare-2013-000537. Accessed 23rd May 2018.

52. Addington-Hall J. Research sensitivities to palliative care patients. Eur J Cancer Care. 2002;11:220–4.

53. Murray Scott A, Kendall M, Carduff E, Worth A, Harris FM, Lloyd A, Cavers D, Grant L, Sheikh A. Use of serial qualitative interviews to understand patients' evolving experiences and needs. Dig Brit Med J. 2009;339 https://doi.org/10.1136/bmj.b3702.

54. Crowhurst I. The fallacy of the instrumental gate? Contextualizing the process of gaining access through gatekeepers. Int J Soc Res Method. 2013;16:463–75.

55. Leadership Alliance for the Care of Dying People. One chance to get it right: improving People's experience of Care in the Last few Days and Hours of life. 2014 http://tinyurl.com/mad2kql. Accessed 21 Nov 2017.

8

Whose job? The staffing of advance care planning support in twelve international healthcare organizations

Josie Dixon[*] [iD] and Martin Knapp

Abstract

Background: ACP involving a facilitated conversation with a health or care professional is more effective than document completion alone. In policy, there is an expectation that health and care professionals will provide ACP support, commonly within their existing roles. However, the potential contributions of different professionals are outlined only broadly in policy and guidance. Research on opportunities and barriers for involving different professionals in providing ACP support, and feasible models for doing so, is currently lacking.

Methods: We identified twelve healthcare organizations aiming to offer system-wide ACP support in the United States, Canada, Australia and New Zealand. In each, we conducted an average 13 in-depth interviews with senior managers, ACP leads, dedicated ACP facilitators, physicians, nurses, social workers and other clinical and non-clinical staff. Interviews were analyzed thematically using NVivo software.

Results: Organizations emphasized leadership for ACP support, including strategic support from senior managers and intensive day-to-day support from ACP leads, to support staff to deliver ACP support within their existing roles. Over-reliance on dedicated facilitators was not considered sustainable or scalable. We found many professionals, from all backgrounds, providing ACP support. However, there remained barriers, particularly for facilitating ACP conversations. A significant barrier for all professionals was lack of time. Physicians sometimes had poor communication skills, misunderstood medico-legal aspects and tended to have conversations of limited scope late in the disease trajectory. However, they could also have concerns about the appropriateness of ACP conversations conducted by others. Social workers had good facilitation skills and understood legal aspects but needed more clinical support than nurses. While ACP support provided alongside and as part of other care was common, ACP conversations in this context could easily get squeezed out or become fragmented. Referrals to other professionals could be insecure. Team-based models involving a physician and a nurse or social worker were considered cost-effective and supportive of good quality care but could require some additional resource.

Conclusions: Effective staffing of ACP support is likely to require intensive local leadership, attention to physician concerns while avoiding an entirely physician-led approach, some additional resource and team-based frameworks, including in evolving models of care for chronic illness and end of life.

Keywords: Advance care planning, End of life care, Healthcare workforce, Social care

* Correspondence: j.e.dixon@lse.ac.uk
Personal Social Services Research Unit (PSSRU), London School of Economics and Political Science (LSE), Houghton Street, London WC2A 2AE, UK

Background

Advance care planning (ACP) provides an opportunity for people to discuss and record their preferences, goals and decisions for future care. This allows people's wishes to be known in the event that they are unable to speak for themselves, for people and their families to be more prepared for later decision-making and for professionals to be better able to plan ahead so they can provide the most appropriate care. In the United States (US), people can complete an advance directive, which can include a refusal of treatment, a statement of general preferences and assignment of Durable Power of Attorney (DPoA) for health care or finances. Similarly, in England and Wales, people can complete an advance decision to refuse treatment (ADRT), make an advance statement setting out general preferences and assign a Lasting Power of Attorney for health and welfare or property and financial affairs. While legal arrangements and terminology vary, similar frameworks exist in comparable countries such as Canada, Australia and New Zealand. ACP has been associated with improved end of life outcomes including fewer emergency admissions, less time spent in hospital, improved symptom control, increased carer satisfaction and potentially better use of resources [1, 2]. ACP involving a facilitated conversation with a health or care professional has been found to be more effective than document completion alone [1]. In policy, there is an expectation that health and care professionals will provide ACP support within their existing roles [3–7]. ACP support includes making people aware of ACP, facilitating ACP conversations and helping people to record their preferences in ways that can be effectively shared. However, the potential contributions of different professionals are outlined only broadly in policy and guidance, while guidance for specific professional groups and national training have not, in themselves, led to widespread implementation [8, 9]. Without a clear professional lead role, those designing and implementing system-wide strategies for providing ACP support need information about the opportunities and challenges for engaging different health and care professionals and about models for incorporating ACP provision into general care that have proved feasible in practice. Existing evidence is limited. A number of ACP intervention studies have reported on implementation challenges [10], while challenges experienced by a range of professionals in delivering ACP support, including to people with specific conditions, have been explored in a small number of qualitative interview or focus group studies [8, 9, 11–13] and in one national survey of nephrology health professionals involving a non-probability sample [14]. These studies have involved various professionals including general practitioners (GPs), hospital consultants, nurses, social workers, old-age psychiatrists, ambulance staff and physiotherapists, while intervention studies have generally involved staff, commonly clinical nurse specialists, selected and prepared by researchers [10]. Our study adds to the literature by exploring staffing of ACP support from an organizational perspective, drawing on the experiences of twelve healthcare organizations with experience of implementing ACP support across their full range of services. The healthcare organizations that participated in this study are based in four countries with well-developed ACP policy; the United States (US), Canada, Australia and New Zealand. Our research thus also responds to suggestions made in the literature that lessons be identified from international experiences of delivering ACP [15, 16]. Our specific research aims were to:

- provide a descriptive overview of how ACP support is staffed in participating healthcare organizations
- identify opportunities and barriers encountered for involving different types of health and care staff in the provision of ACP support
- identify models for delivering ACP support, with a focus on how health and care staff incorporate ACP support into their existing roles
- identify key themes and ongoing challenges.

Methods

This study is a predominantly exploratory (contextual) qualitative interview study [17] with staff in a sample of twelve international healthcare organizations, each systematically offering ACP support across all of their services. A qualitative approach was adopted to elicit provider perspectives and to explore professionals' first-hand experiences of developing, delivering and staffing ACP support in their organizations.

Sampling and recruitment

A two-stage purposive sampling process was adopted; sampling healthcare organizations and then staff within these organizations. For the first stage, we sought healthcare organizations with 'well-established, system-wide ACP support provision'. 'ACP support provision' was defined as helping patients and members of the public find out about ACP, facilitating ACP conversations and assisting with the completion of ACP documents. 'Well-established' was defined as provision that had been in place for a minimum of 18 months, but longer where possible. 'System-wide provision of ACP' was defined as ACP support being widely and systematically offered across all relevant services and parts of the organization. We also sought diversity against a range of secondary sampling criteria, including different countries and geographies, small and large providers, rural and urban areas, a range of care settings and varied ACP materials and approaches. We estimated that approximately 10 healthcare organizations would provide a sufficient range of experiences and enable diversity against secondary sampling criteria.

Suitable healthcare organizations were identified by drawing upon our own knowledge of relevant practice and literature and through expert, network and snowball sampling (used where sample units are rare, hidden or where there is no available sample frame). While these approaches are prone to identifying sample units within closed systems, we deliberately approached experts with a wide view of international practice, attempted to create different 'start points', took an iterative approach and used multiple sampling strategies [18]. Experts included four members of the International Society of Advance Care Planning and End of Life Care (ACPEL), which organizes a highly-regarded biennial international conference. We additionally asked each organization we approached to identify other suitable healthcare organizations or well-placed informants. Finally, we conducted eight scoping interviews with end of life care experts in the UK, including representatives from the National Council of Palliative Care, Care England and the Association of Directors of Adult Social Services (ADASS). We were able to sample until no more cases likely to add sufficiently new information were identified (e.g. we chose not to sample further organizations using the Respecting Choices approach or allied to the National ACP Cooperative New Zealand) [19]. It is possible that there were relevant organizations outside of our networks. In particular, we may have identified organizations most active in knowledge-exchange networks, including but not limited to ACPEL. However, arguably healthcare systems in these networks may be those with the most developed ACP support. In total, we recruited 12 healthcare organizations, some of which were geographically near to each other. These exhibited a good spread against secondary sampling criteria. Table 1 describes the organizations and indicates how they were identified.

Each organization was approached directly, usually by email, through an appropriate senior member of staff. This was followed with one or more telephone conversations with senior staff to explore eligibility and discuss what participation would involve. All organizations received written information about the study. Once organizational and local ethical approvals were secured we undertook the second stage of sampling.

Stage 2 involved sampling staff within each organization. The key contact person compiled a list of all key personnel with in-depth experience of developing or delivering ACP support, and a range of others with more routine experience, to include a mix of senior managers, dedicated ACP staff, physicians, nurses, social workers, volunteer staff and other clinical and non-clinical staff. These lists were then narrowed, in consultation, with a view to balancing staff with different roles and for reasons of manageability or availability.

All identified staff were sent an introductory letter including information about the study and about what participation would involve. They were informed of the voluntary nature of participation and given the opportunity to opt out of further contact by email or by post, addressed to either the key contact person in the organization or a member of the research team, as preferred. If they did not opt out, they were invited to interview. These were scheduled, for logistic reasons, by the key contact person. Participants were informed that they could withdraw at any time and were also provided contact details for an independent person responsible for research ethics at LSE if they had concerns or queries about the conduct of recruitment or interviews.

Conduct of interviews

We conducted between 3 and 25 (average 13) interviews in each organization [17] during fieldwork visits undertaken between November 2015 and May 2017 (Table 2). Most were individual ($n = 112$) although occasionally, for practicality, group interviews were conducted ($n = 18$). Interviews ranged from 20 to 180 min. Fully informed verbal consent was obtained at the beginning of each interview. Interviews covered various topics, with an over-arching focus on resources used to deliver ACP support. Topic coverage was adapted to reflect the role and expertise of interviewees. In particular, respondents were asked to describe their own role and experiences of providing ACP support and about the staffing of ACP support more generally. All responses were thoroughly probed. Quantitative data about staffing for ACP support were enquired about but availability was limited. Interviews were audio-recorded with permission.

Data analysis and reporting

Audio-recordings were listened back to in full as soon as possible after the interview and a comprehensive written summary produced. This was entirely descriptive and data elements were included in the same order as the original interview. Time-stamps allowed easy reference back to the audio-recording and potential quotes were included verbatim. Recordings were listened to at least once, but longer and more complex interviews were listened to on two or three occasions, with comprehensive summaries written simultaneously. This process of 'data reduction' is appropriate for analyzing large volumes of interview data in thematic analysis and supports the comprehensive and systematic handling of data in analysis [17]. Data management thus also involved several stages, allowing for considerable

Table 1 Participating healthcare organizations

	Description of organization	How organization was identified
United States		
Gundersen Health	A physician-led, not-for-profit healthcare system; birthplace of Respecting Choices, an evidence-based ACP model for person-centered decision making.	Snowball sampling via Wisconsin Medical Society, and known to the authors through the literature
Dartmouth-Hitchcock	A non-profit, academic health system, providing ACP support using the Honoring Care Decisions ACP programme (based on the Respecting Choices model).	Snowball sampling via *Gundersen Health*
Wisconsin Medical Society	A physician member association supporting 32 participating health organizations to implement the Honoring Choices ACP programme (based on the Respecting Choices model).	Known to the authors through an earlier study they led into the economics of ACP
Sharp Healthcare	A not-for-profit, integrated regional health care system, providing ACP support in collaboration with the Coalition for Compassionate Care of California.	An academic expert identified through ACPEL[a] made an introduction to a regional coalition organization that, in turn, made an onward introduction to *Sharp Healthcare. Sharp Healthcare*, and its Transitions program were also known to the authors through the literature
Canada		
Northern Alberta Renal Program (NARP)	Renal programme in Edmonton, Alberta, providing integrated ACP support using an approach based on Conversations Matter.	Identified directly through a clinician, academic and member of ACPEL[a]
Fraser Health	One of six publicly funded health care regions in British Columbia, providing ACP support in community, acute and residential care based on materials developed provincially and at Fraser Health Authority.	*Northern Alberta Renal Program* (NARP) made an introduction to an academic expert in Alberta who, in turn, made an onward introduction to Fraser Health
Australia		
Austin Health	A publicly-funded health service in Melbourne, providing acute, sub-acute, mental health and ambulatory services, providing ACP support using materials developed locally and as part of Advance Care Planning Australia	Identified directly through a clinician and member of ACPEL[a]
Northern Health	A publicly-funded provider of acute, sub-acute and ambulatory specialist services in Melbourne, providing ACP support using the 'A-C-P in three steps' approach developed within Northern Health.	Identified through snowball sampling via *Austin Health*
Barwon Health	A publicly-funded, large regional health service, providing acute, sub-acute, elderly care, community health and mental health services, with ACP support delivered across secondary and primary care using materials, including MyValues, developed in Barwon Health.	Identified through snowball sampling via *Austin Health*
Albany Health	A regional primary and secondary healthcare system, providing ACP support using forms developed by the Western Australian government and piloting systems for communication and access of ACP documents.	Identified through an academic and member of ACPEL[a] and through a contact identified by the authors in an earlier study they led into the economics of ACP

Table 1 Participating healthcare organizations *(Continued)*

	Description of organization	How organization was identified
New Zealand		
The Canterbury Initiative	A District Health Board initiative, delivering change and quality improvement initiatives across community, primary and secondary care and providing ACP support using materials developed by the Canterbury Initiative and by the National ACP Cooperative, New Zealand.	A clinician and member of ACPEL[a] made an introduction to the National ACP Cooperative who, in turn, made an onward introduction to the Canterbury Initiative
Auckland District Health Board	A regional health authority overseeing community, primary and secondary care, providing ACP support using material developed by the National ACP Cooperative, New Zealand	Identified through a clinician and member of ACPEL[a]

[a]The International Society of Advance Care Planning and End of Life Care

familiarization. Analytic notes were also taken. Data were then analyzed thematically using NVivo software [17]. The theoretical orientation employed was pragmatic [20]. Given the requirements of fieldwork, interviews and analysis were conducted primarily by a senior researcher and qualitative specialist (JD). A second senior researcher (MK) read a sample of interview summaries, commented on coding frames and provided regular critical input into evolving and final analyses, with any differences resolved through discussion and consensus. Feedback on coding frames and evolving analyses was also obtained from a project advisory group. Descriptive analyses reported in this paper were checked for accuracy by the key contacts in each system; no substantive changes were proposed. Quotes are identified throughout by country and professional role (with these differing slightly from the categories in Table 2, to provide appropriate context while protecting respondent anonymity.)

Results

Overall, we found many similar experiences and challenges across the twelve healthcare organizations. These are described these from multiple perspectives and with examples from a wide range of settings and contexts, with differences between organizations highlighted as and where relevant. Leadership for ACP support emerged as a key theme and findings on this are described in the first section. The second section describes perceived opportunities and barriers for involving specific types of health and care staff, covering physicians, nurses, social workers, care home staff, spiritual care advisors and volunteers. The third section then describes different models employed by professionals for delivering ACP support, particularly time-intensive ACP conversations, within the context of their existing roles. The implications of these findings are then drawn out in the discussion and conclusion.

Table 2 Interviews by healthcare system and respondent role

	Gundersen	Dartmouth-Hitchcock	Wisconsin Medical	Sharp	NARP	Fraser	Austin	Northern	Barwon	Albany	Canterbury	Auckland	TOTAL
Senior managers/leaders	4	1	2	2	0	1	1	0	2	0	2	2	17
Dedicated ACP staff	2	3	3	3	0	1	4	1	3	0	3	1	27
Physicians	2	2	1	2	1	2	3	2	2	4	3	0	21
Nurses	3	2	5	1	8	6	0	0	1	3	5	3	37
Social workers	4	0	5	2	2	1	0	0	1	0	1	1	17
Other	10	6	1	2	1	5	4	0	2	2	3	2	38
TOTAL	25	14	17	12	12	16	12	3	12	9	16	9	157
Individual	19	1	7	12	12	16	12	1	6	9	10	7	112
Group	3	5	3	0	0	0	0	1	2	0	3	1	18

Respondents sometimes filled more than one role. In these cases, we selected the primary role. For example, physicians with a full time clinical position are categorized as physicians even if they are an ACP lead or hold other leadership roles

The category of physicians includes hospital physicians (including palliative care physicians, geriatricians and other specialists) and general practitioners

Dedicated ACP staff are those whose positions are exclusively or predominantly ACP-related

Other includes spiritual care advisors, volunteers, care home staff, speech therapists and occupational therapists

Leadership for ACP support

All of the organizations placed considerable emphasis on leadership, both strategic and day-to-day, for providing ACP support. The exact way this was provided varied between organizations, reflecting their size, structure, stage of development and individual factors. The range of leaders for ACP support provision included senior managers, ACP leads, dedicated ACP facilitators, physician champions and others.

Senior managers

Senior managers helped to sustain ACP as a strategic organizational priority, supported those leading ACP support day-to-day and provided strategic leadership during periods of ACP support-related development and change. How active senior managers were varied, between organizations and over time, although senior commitment was generally considered high. At the time of the research, one senior manager reported spending around two hours a week supporting strategic developments for ACP support, reviewing structures for day-to-day leadership and facilitating pilots to generate information on resource needs. Senior managers discussed organizational commitment to ACP support in terms of improving patient care, sustainability, overall cost-efficiency, concerns about potential legal challenges associated with unwanted care, organizational reputation and sectoral leadership. Senior managers' personal-level commitments to ACP could also sometimes be important. For example, one Chief Medical Officer in the US attributed his sustained and active commitment to experiences working as an emergency physician and from advocating for his father who had recently died with dementia.

ACP leads

All of the organizations had an ACP lead, or someone in a similar role, responsible for day-to-day coordination and development of ACP support provision. In two systems (in Canada and Australia), coordination was led by a full-time academic physician, while in both New Zealand organizations the provision of ACP support was led by quality improvement teams as sustained improvement projects. More commonly, however, organizations had established ACP programmes or departments with a full-time salaried ACP coordinator or programme manager. These had backgrounds that included nursing, social work, health education and spiritual care. They commonly reported to senior managers, with the majority feeling well-supported. In the two systems led by academic physicians, ACP support was more research-driven than management-driven and, as a result, support from senior management was more arms-length. The content of the ACP lead role was wide-ranging but could include the provision or

facilitation of face-to-face and other training, mentoring and coaching, providing communications and updates, responding to legal and practice queries, networking to secure staff time, developing processes and resources, managing pilots and quality improvement projects, quality control including review of completed documents and working to ensure that ACP is reflected in wider agendas and programmes.

> 'ACP can go off the radar very quickly if you are not present. I sit on a lot of committees; end of life, goals of care document, clinical deterioration, community health.' (ACP lead, Australia)

ACP leads also sometimes facilitated ACP conversations, including more complex ones. Community outreach was also often an important aspect of the role and this could sometimes involve managing volunteers. In two US systems, ACP coordinators also helped to deliver group facilitations, either in disease-specific support groups or in the community. These involved facilitated group discussions with, for those that wished, an opportunity afterwards to complete ACP documents or, potentially, be referred for an ACP conversation.

Dedicated ACP facilitators

Two Australian and two US systems employed dedicated ACP facilitators, specifically to conduct, and support others to conduct, ACP conversations. These were employed part-time, had nursing or social work backgrounds and were acute-sector funded, reflecting that this is where many of the financial and wider benefits of ACP are likely to be realized. Dedicated facilitators were therefore sometimes based in hospitals, conducting conversations at the inpatient bedside and taking referrals from a small number of hospital clinicians or identifying their own clients by consulting patient notes, attending handover meetings and talking with ward staff. In one of the US systems, dedicated facilitators also worked in the community and in one US system and one Australian system, in primary care settings.

A key part of their role was to advise and coach other staff. However, because dedicated facilitators generally had significantly more time available for an ACP conversation than the busy clinicians they were supporting, some respondents believed they were poorly placed to support staff trying to conduct conversations in more time-constrained circumstances. Others thought that having dedicated facilitators gave the impression that ACP was 'someone else's job' and, additionally, could lead to patients experiencing ACP as unintegrated with the rest of their care.

'What they generally do is use that money to put in some management and some facilitators who would actually do the facilitation, and the patient will tend to have a silo experience, separate from the rest of the patient journey.' (Leader, Australia).

However, having dedicated ACP facilitators was thought by some to demonstrate organizational commitment to ACP. They acted as role models and helped to demonstrate that ACP conversations were feasible and acceptable in a clinical context. Their independence was also valued.

'If I've introduced bias, referring on brings in a check, a more independent person. Patients can try to please their doctor.' (Hospital physician, Australia).

However, there was wide agreement that over-reliance on dedicated ACP facilitators to conduct ACP conversations was neither sustainable nor scalable.

'It can't just be shoved off to one or two passionate individuals working separately in a hospital when they are treating 50,000 people a year.' (Hospital physician, Australia).

'Ten facilitators for the number of patients we have, you know, that's not going to be possible.' (Hospital nurse, Canada)

Other leaders
Leadership for ACP support was also provided by a range of other staff. In one organization, a senior staff chaplain founded and coordinated a group of volunteers to provide education about ACP in the community. Physicians also acted as champions, promoting ACP to senior managers and clinical colleagues, for example, by attending meetings, giving talks and contributing to training. In some cases, they were engaged in the development of regional and national ACP policy and were occasionally public figures and educators, writing and speaking on ACP and related issues.

The impacts of leadership for ACP support
Leaders provided a range of support to help health and care staff within the organization, and sometimes in adjoining systems, deliver ACP support within their existing roles. This support was aimed widely at physicians, nurses, social workers and others such as spiritual care advisors, care coordinators and care home staff. Training offerings varied. These were often generic rather than profession-specific, although shorter tailored training for physicians was common. Staff frequently had access to face-to-face training lasting between half-a-day and,

exceptionally, two or three days. Some organizations had also used quality improvement projects, research studies and pilots to help embed ACP support provision and improve processes. As a result of this activity, staff were thought to be widely aware of ACP and its purpose and knew how to access individual support. In organizations with more established programmes, respondents described ACP as a *'familiar concept'* and *'part of the culture'* and identified behaviour changes such as physicians having *'more realistic conversations.'* Senior leaders, especially where ACP support was more established, also stated that it was highly unlikely they would *'turn back'* now. We also found many staff members, from all professional backgrounds, providing ACP support in practice. However, those providing ACP support, particularly facilitated ACP conversations (which was thought to take between 30 and 90 min if completed adequately), remained in a minority overall. Leaders also reported that the lack of professional lead role for ACP support could make it difficult to create ownership and accountability, and to target their support efforts.

'[Quality improvement team] usually kick things off then hand them over to a permanent home, but there is no obvious home for this, so it's staying here right now' (Dedicated ACP staff, New Zealand)

'At the moment, everyone's interested but no one's really accountable. It's all done by everyone's good conscience and their ability to buy in and see the value. It's actually no-one's job to do it.' (Leader, Australia)

Gains also needed to be actively sustained; in two US systems, a sharp decline in awareness and ACP support activity was noted following earlier losses of, respectively, an ACP lead and a highly engaged senior leader.

Opportunities and barriers for involving different types of health and care staff
Physicians
Physicians were seen as key to legitimizing and embedding ACP support provision. They were broadly considered supportive, particularly intensivists and emergency physicians, who worked *'at the sharp end,'* alongside palliative care physicians, geriatricians, some GPs and some respiratory and renal specialists, while surgical specialists were thought to be amongst the least supportive.

'There is no great groundswell of resistance. There are some that are just passive, going along with it, and others are either resisters or, a lot, are champions.' (Leader, Australia)

Nonetheless, even in organizations where ACP support was more established, only a minority of physicians overall were thought to regularly provide ACP support. Reasons were thought to be time constraints; lack of knowledge, skills and confidence; and concerns related to professional autonomy and patient care. Of these, time constraints were considered the most important barrier.

'Typically, physicians say it's our conversation, it's about prognosis etc. but we don't have the time.' (Leader, Canada)

This was thought, by some, to be a particular challenge for hospital physicians.

'To do it well you need time. Busy clinicians don't have this. I think we always feel a bit rushed.' (Hospital physician, Australia).

'The feedback [from a consultation with physicians across the hospital] was unless you are really hammering away at people to do it, it won't get done. People are just too busy.' (Hospital physician, Australia).

GPs were often considered natural leads for ACP, although some respondents thought that they too lacked sufficient time.

'[GPs] can't possibly be doing all the things they are meant to or they would be working 22 hours a day.' (GP, US)

'[As a GP] I do as much as I can. I'm not doing enough though.' (GP, New Zealand)

'There is this view that the GP is the most appropriate place but I'm not sure why. Whenever I go to the GP there's a hundred people in the waiting room and you get five minutes with them.' (Leader, Australia)

Physicians were particularly concerned about the impacts of rushing ACP conversations.

'It's not a quick conversation and they don't want to hurt people by having a quick conversation.' (Physician leader, Australia)

A second set of barriers related to a lack of necessary knowledge, skills and confidence. This included poor communications skills.

'If you are really going to get down to talking about prognosis, about what that illness trajectory is going to look like, they [hospital physicians] actually kind of

suck at it. Whether its ego, whether they feel they are already doing it, there is a real lack of insight as to how poorly trained they are to do this.' (Hospital physician, Canada)

'Physicians [hospital physicians and GPs] are terrible at helping people understand their choices.' (GP, US)

At the same time, when supporting physicians with ACP conversations, it was thought important to recognize and build on physicians' existing communication skills and competencies.

'We say, 'you do a lot of this already.' We mustn't offend people by saying this is new.' (Hospital physician, Australia)

Indeed, one respondent argued that GPs, in particular, often have good communication skills.

They will talk to a 16-year old about whether she will have an abortion, talk, you know, with alcoholics. They talk about difficult stuff every day. They deal with suicidal young people, depressed elderly. There is nothing specific about advance care planning that is harder than anything else they do.' (Physician leader, Australia)

Physicians were also sometimes thought to have poor understanding of the medico-legal aspects of ACP, including medical consent and the extent and nature of physicians' responsibilities to provide treatment. In relation to the above barriers, poor coverage of both communication skills and end of life care in medical training was identified as an important underlying factor.

'We can wait for a new generation of physicians and there is some culture change but we're still not training them properly.' (Hospital physician, US).

'It does seem extraordinary that people who are dealing with really serious illness do not get too much education around end of life. Most people are currently learning on the job, and if you're learning from someone who does it poorly then that's not good.' (Leader, Australia)

Training and other support were widely available in the organizations we visited, although commonly physicians failed to access this or undertook short training activities of relatively limited depth. There was a view, however, that GPs in particular were becoming increasingly aware of their need to develop new knowledge and skills in end of life care and there were examples of ACP training included in well-attended continuing professional education courses.

A final set of barriers involved inter-related concerns around professional autonomy and patient care. Some hospital physicians believed, as a matter of principle, that other professionals should not be having conversations with their patients about prognosis and treatment and were, consequently, reluctant to introduce ACP or refer patients for ACP conversations. In some cases, it was thought that they may have doubted the clinical knowledge and skills of facilitators. Physicians may also sometimes have had concerns that patients were being inappropriately advised against active treatment.

'Maybe they think people are being persuaded to forego treatment. Some think you should do everything possible.' (Hospital physician, Australia).

'There's this idea that the job [of ACP conversations] is to get them to agree to palliative care, but that's not it at all.' (Hospital physician, Australia).

There were also related concerns about the potential for the involvement of other professionals to impact negatively on trust in the physician-patient relationship.

'It potentially plants doubt that the doctors are doing the right thing for you.' (GP, Australia).

'We don't tell people. 'don't trust your healthcare provider', we teach them to ask the right questions.' (ACP lead, US).

However, some hospital physicians were thought to want their patients to have completed ACP prior to coming into their care, often so that they could avoid having to initiate these discussions themselves.

"They can think that someone else should have done advance care planning so they 'know what to do." (Hospital physician, Australia)

Nurses

Nurse practitioners and nurses working in chronic disease management were seen to have a particularly important role in ACP support provision. They commonly saw patients over time, in regular and longer appointments and worked more holistically than physicians, with a focus on prevention and well-being. They were also often embedded in clinical teams, working alongside physicians.

'Nurse practitioners generally aren't 'in the moment' practitioners. They are thinking about

chronic health management. They are thinking about preventative medicine. That's their space. They are already embedded in teams.' (Hospital physician, Australia)

'Nurses write better plans than physicians, bigger picture, not just clinical decisions. Physicians just want the guts. What patients take away from this is that there are things they can't talk about.' (ACP lead, New Zealand)

Nurse-led ACP conversations were also potentially scalable.

'We've 20 trained nurses [currently], but we have hundreds.' (Hospital physician, Canada)

'The nurse practitioner role is still expanding in Australia, developing as a profession, while society is starting to think about these things.' (Physician leader, Australia)

While nurses, particularly clinical nurse specialists, practice nurses, nurse care coordinators and nurse practitioners, constituted a large proportion of those delivering ACP support in the participating organizations, it was still the case that, overall, most nurses did not deliver ACP support. Two barriers were identified; time constraints and concerns about legal aspects.

Lack of time was seen as the most significant barrier. For example, in one US system, trained hospital nurses were asked to commit four hours a month to facilitate ACP conversations. This time was not bought out or protected and, in practice, only about half was realized, with nurses regularly having to be *'chased'*. Competing pressures were a factor, particularly in busy clinical environments. In one US system, one nurse scheduled ACP conversations outside of her normal working hours, taking time off in lieu, to avoid clashes with the responsive commitments of her work role. Other systems faced similar difficulties in involving nursing staff.

'We trained general practice nurses. ACP is chronic disease management but their time is so pressured it doesn't happen in practice.' (ACP lead, Australia).

'They wanted everyone to do one ACP conversation a week. For lots of staff, it was quite unreasonable.' (Hospital nurse, Canada).

'We might just want people to do a conversation a week, but even that makes managers want to run away.' (ACP lead, US).

Occasionally, it was thought that nurses could have concerns about legal aspects.

'Nurses have historically been told not to sign legal documents as there can be conflicts of interest involved.' (Community nurse, Australia)

Social workers

Many systems had health-based social workers and care coordinators with social work backgrounds. Social workers were considered to have an important role in delivering ACP support, since they have a high level of comfort with legal processes and forms, have good facilitation, advocacy and counselling skills and are able to work efficiently with issues such as family conflict and grief.

'We've had a couple of social workers who've been brilliant. They need to sub-contract out the clinical parts of the discussion, but they are really good at bringing it up and really good at facilitation.' (Hospital physician, Australia)

'It needs to be more exploratory, listening for cues. That's not so much in a nurse's scope of practice.' (Social worker, New Zealand)

However, the constraints of some care settings meant that it was often hard for social workers to fully employ these skills and some respondents thought they had become de-skilled.

'We're a busy department, we're also counsellors. It can be hard. What's the priority?' (Social worker, US).

'They don't do any counselling anymore, they're actually not really trained in it. They've really narrowed their scope.' (Hospital physician, Canada).

The large number of social workers and social work-trained care coordinators in some systems was also, as with nurses, thought to allow for scalability. In practice, social workers were well-represented amongst those delivering ACP support. However, overall, social workers offering ACP support, particularly facilitated ACP conversations, remained in the minority. There were two main barriers identified; time constraints and limited clinical knowledge.

Lack of time was, again, the main barrier, particularly in acute settings.

'I do as much ACP as time allows.' (Hospital-based social worker, US)

'I have to protect my time, if it's going to be more than 20 minutes I'll encourage them to read it and do some on their own, and I'll come back.' (Hospital-based social worker, US).

Social workers who engaged patients in longer appointments in primary care and community-based settings were those most likely to be able to find time to facilitate ACP conversations and, occasionally, social workers specialized. For example, in the US, a social worker conducted, and coached others to conduct, ACP conversations with people with dementia.

A second barrier to the greater involvement of social workers was that they have more limited clinical knowledge than physicians or nurses.

'People will tell you what their condition is and you know immediately what kind of issues there might be, and you can ask appropriate questions and advise them about what to ask their doctor. I send people away to ask their doctor further questions. With a non-clinical background, you're going to be doing that a lot more.' (Hospital nurse, Australia)

However, others thought ACP was *'not as clinical as other work'* and, in the US and Canada, social workers reported successfully using leaflets and decision aids to cover key clinical information.

Care home staff

Care homes were widely considered a challenging environment for ACP. Barriers included residents having limited or diminishing capacity, staff with limited formal qualifications, high staff turnover and sometimes weak links to the wider health system. Care homes were thought to commonly produce poor quality plans and make insufficient distinction between ACP and liaison with families concerning best interest decisions. Some systems trained care home staff to conduct ACP conversations, which could raise awareness and potentially increase the amount of ACP undertaken. However, in one Australian organization, an initiative to train care home staff to undertake ACP conversations had resulted in low numbers of completed discussions and poor-quality documentation. Respondents commonly discussed the importance of external clinical input into ACP in care homes.

'The most useless ones are where people completing the forms or the people helping them to complete the forms clearly don't have any idea of what the options are or the likely outcomes of those options.' (Hospital physician, Australia).

'With care home residents, it's good to have a geriatrician come in. They can consider what's feasible and appropriate.' (Hospital physician, Australia).

GP caseloads made it difficult for them to undertake full ACP conversations in care homes. However, in Australia, we found examples of practice-based nurses, GP registrars and inreach teams (comprising geriatricians and palliative specialists) incorporating ACP support into their work in care homes.

Spiritual care advisors
Spiritual care advisors were found mostly in US organizations. They have counselling skills, flexibility to undertake longer ACP conversations and were relatively numerous in some systems. In one organization in particular, spiritual care advisors facilitated a significant proportion of ACP conversations. However, it was occasionally thought that not all patients were necessarily comfortable undertaking ACP with a spiritual care advisor and the demands of providing ACP support could also impinge on their other roles. Spiritual advisors also sometimes held leadership roles, for example, leading community outreach initiatives or, in one case, being employed as a full-time ACP programme coordinator.

Volunteers
Volunteers played an important role in community outreach. They were sometimes faith-based, particularly in the US, or had backgrounds as nurses or social workers. In one US example, links were made between the healthcare organization and a volunteer network for providing education about ACP involving local lawyers, which had pre-existed the healthcare system's own ACP initiative. In another example, in Canada, a Compassionate Communities ACP initiative had been established with provincial funding. This provided seed grants and training for small hospice societies to run ACP workshops, using trialed and tested curricula and teaching materials and with ongoing support from a regional palliative care organization.

Models for delivering ACP support
We identified a broad typology of models used by professionals for delivering ACP support, particularly time-intensive ACP conversations; these were referral models, team-based models and incorporation models. Referral models were those where professionals, usually physicians, identified someone they believed would benefit from an ACP conversation and referred or sign-posted them to another professional, outside of their immediate clinical or professional team. Team-based models were similar to referral models but involved referral to someone within the same team. Incorporation models involved

facilitating ACP conversations in the course of delivering other care, which often required that conversations be broken down into multiple shorter sessions. Occasionally, these different models were not mutually exclusive; for example, where a hospital physician referred to a GP who then incorporated an ACP conversation into other care. However, each of these models had different implications and presented different challenges.

Referral models
Referral models were predominantly, but not exclusively, employed by physicians, with referrals made variously to GPs, dedicated ACP facilitators, social workers, spiritual care advisors, care coordinators and nurses. These could work well where the referral was to a trusted professional with adequate time available to facilitate a conversation. However, such referrals were not always secure. For example, three hospital physicians in New Zealand described referring patients to a GP for an ACP conversation upon discharge.

'We start in hospital but it gets completed at the GP's afterwards.' (Hospital physician, New Zealand)

They identified the benefits as presenting ACP as an integrated part of care and reconnecting the patient and GP prior to subsequent health crises. However, although in this system there was external funding to support GPs to facilitate ACP conversations, GPs were often time-pressured and it was not known if and how GPs responded. Similarly, in Canadian and US-based systems, there were examples of nurse practitioners introducing ACP during home health visits. They encouraged patients to progress their planning with their families and, where possible, their GPs. However, the degree to which GPs were approached or provided this support was unknown. In three organizations in the US, GPs were pro-actively supported to refer patients to dedicated or other trained facilitators. These referrals were mediated through ACP leads and dedicated ACP staff so were more secure, although uptake by GPs varied.

'Primary care physicians feel they are getting more and more tasks dumped on them. Our job is to let them know that, although we need them to open up the conversation, there is another resource that they can refer to.' (Leader, US).

Sometimes physicians referred patients inappropriately in the absence of a suitable resource; for example, in one Australian case, hospital physicians made inappropriate referrals of patients to a hospital-based inreach service, designed to provide palliative care and ACP support to people living in care homes. Professionals also sometimes introduced ACP, with a view to making a later referral; for example, social workers introduced ACP and the prospect of referral to a trained facilitator in introductory meetings with all new patients in a US geriatric clinic.

Another referral route was through outreach activities such as talks, presentations and group facilitations in community settings. Participants could attend these without obligation. Assistance with the completion of documents on the day was sometimes offered, alongside the possibility of referral to a dedicated or other trained ACP facilitator. Many organizations also provided a telephone number that members of the public could use to self-refer. In practice, while community-based events were popular and increased public understanding, referrals to trained facilitators for full ACP conversations were not common.

Team-based models

In team-based models, referrals were more secure and physicians could more readily retain involvement. For example, in New Zealand, the US and Australia there were examples of GPs introducing ACP and referring to a nurse practitioner, care coordinator or dedicated ACP facilitator within their practice with, in one case, the GP regularly coming in for the last 5 min of the meeting to briefly review decisions and agree documentation. These were commonly externally funded positions or otherwise attracted some level of additional funding. In another example, in the US, patients presenting repeatedly or avoidably in the emergency room were referred to a hospital-based Advanced Illness Management (AIM) team, consisting of four specialist nurses (with palliative care and oncology specialisms) and a social worker. The team reviewed existing advance directives and, if needed, introduced and conducted ACP conversations. The team could liaise with the referring consultant, as needed, and if a patient preferred a conversation outside of the hospital, they could be referred on to a dedicated ACP facilitator working in the community.

A key benefit of such models is the ability to offer team-based care, with physicians not facilitating entire ACP conversations but, nonetheless, remaining actively involved. However, some respondents identified the risk of physicians using within-team referrals to avoid difficult discussions with patients.

'Physicians thought, "do I have to do this? Oh no, this is complicated. I am just going to step back and refer." We've had to train the nurse to bring physicians in as needed. It's not something 'someone else' should do. It should be shared for quality of care.' (Hospital physician, Canada)

Both referral and team-based models were seen as more cost-effective than entirely physician-led ACP

support in that they allow for the longer parts of ACP conversations to be conducted by an appropriate but less costly professional.

'Nurses and social workers are so efficient. Physicians don't need to be there for everything.' (GP, US).

Incorporation models

Staff funded to facilitate ACP conversations included dedicated ACP facilitators and some externally-funded practice staff, while others such as care coordinators and Advanced Illness Teams were funded to provide a range of care that centrally included introducing and having ACP conversations. More commonly, however, health and care professionals did not have any protected time to provide ACP support and, if they could not refer on to another professional, needed to incorporate the provision of ACP support into their existing roles. Attempts to do this generally involved breaking the conversation down into shorter sessions. GPs commonly reported doing this to deliver ACP support.

'In my practice, I wrap it up in other consultations. I don't do it all at one time.' (GP, US)

In Australia, one GP introduced ACP when drawing up chronic disease management plans, following this up with a conversation undertaken during a standard 15-min consultation (and sometimes a further consultation, if needed). Similarly, in New Zealand, a GP incorporated ACP into annual planning sessions for patients with complex conditions. He explained how only ten minutes were devoted to ACP, but the intention was for this to accumulate, with patients encouraged to progress their planning in between. Nurses and social workers also commonly used this model. For example, professionals conducting home visits including disease-specific specialist nurses in New Zealand, social workers in a US-based home health programme, a palliative care nurse in Australia and care coordinators in the US and Australia conducted ACP conversations incrementally over the course of a series of home visits. In Australia, a nurse manager in a GP practice spent half the week visiting five care homes, during which she undertook short ACP conversations with residents as part of general care, developing them over time. In Canada, heart failure nurses and dialysis nurses incorporated ACP into regular clinic appointments. A potential benefit of breaking the conversation down in this way was that patients had a chance to reflect and have discussions with family members between sessions. It could work well where there was regular and relatively frequent contact with a trusted professional and time was not unduly pressured (e.g.

during some types of home visit). However, respondents pointed to the risk of the ACP conversation getting squeezed or of the process becoming inconsistent, fragmented and *'gappy.'*

In other cases, professionals managed to facilitate ACP conversations within their existing roles by reducing their scope and/or depth. For example, in one US hospital, social workers conducted ACP conversations in regular outpatient clinics and, in Canada, social workers conducted ACP conversations in pre-dialysis clinics. These were busy, however, limiting how much could be covered. The importance of physician input for nurses and social workers providing ACP support in this way was also repeatedly emphasized.

'A physician needs to be involved; that's hard for us in our setting' (Community nurse, US).

'Where the problems are, [patients] often don't have a good understanding of their illness trajectory. And that's not the nurse's role to explain that. The nurses actually can't. They can help identify where the knowledge gaps are and send them back to the physician.' (Hospital physician, Canada).

Discussion

The healthcare organizations in this study were selected for their diversity and varyied, for example, in terms of their size and in the level and type of resources available to them for the development of ACP support. However, in the absence of significant new funding or a professional group with responsibility for leading ACP support, all of the organizations in our study all placed an emphasis on intensive organizational leadership for promoting and sustaining widespread changes in practice. This included strategic leadership from senior managers to maintain ACP as an organizational priority and provide support for strategic development and change. It also, importantly, included intensive day-to-day leadership and coordination from ACP leads. There were local variations in the qualifications, seniority, scope and specific responsibilities of this role. However, in all cases, the purpose was to create and sustain high awareness of ACP, ensure that heath and care staff across the organization were adequately trained and supported, to motivate staff and create accountability, to develop and maintain ACP-related processes, to help maintain agreed standards and to represent the organization in the community and elsewhere on ACP-related issues. The investments in leadership made by organizations were justified and under-pinned by clearly articulated organizational rationales relating to patient care, sustainability, cost-effectiveness, possible legal challenge, reputational

benefit and sectoral leadership. Senior managers and ACP leads often worked closely and evidence suggested that organizational awareness and provision of ACP support was significantly increased as a result and that it slipped back when either strategic or day-to-day leadership was absent. Other important leadership for ACP support included support from physician champions, who had a particular role in promoting ACP support to physician and other clinical colleagues. In many organizations, community outreach and public engagement, undertaken as part of a 'whole system' approach, was also considered key, as a way of raising public awareness, stimulating interest and demand and creating accountability directly to users and local communities.

While there were various barriers to involving wider health and care staff in the provision of ACP support, there was not thought to be significant resistance to the provision of ACP support in any organization and we heard of numerous professionals, across a wide range of professional groups, delivering ACP support to patients and the wider public. However, professionals providing ACP support, particularly the facilitation of ACP conversations, remained in the minority. From the perspective of leaders, the lack of a clear professional lead group made it difficult to create accountability or target support. For wider health and care staff, the most significant barrier was a lack of protected time, particularly for ACP conversations. However, even introducing ACP could be difficult, especially in busy acute environments or in 15-min general practice appointments. Longer appointments such as annual chronic care management reviews, nurse appointments or some types of home visit presented more opportunity. However, it was commonly considered unrealistic to expect most health and care staff to find the time needed to facilitate ACP conversations routinely within their existing roles. Within organizations, this resulted in variability in the reach, scope and depth of facilitated ACP conversations and also in what one respondent referred to as a *'significant gap between introducing it and doing it'*. Lack of time is not a novel barrier; the *'pressure of competing demands',* for example, is identified as one of the main barriers to implementation in a systematic review of ACP intervention studies [10], while finding time to have adequate conversations is identified as a key barrier to implementation of the RESPECT ACP initiative currently being developed in the UK [21].

Time constraints, however, were not the only barrier. Physician leadership and involvement in the provision of ACP support was universally considered vital; to legitimize the role of ACP in clinical care, to provide clinical input into wider conversations about values and care preferences, to ensure that ACP is well-integrated with day-to-day clinical care and to help ensure the effectiveness of ACP processes. However, physicians experienced the widest range of barriers and concerns. As well as lack of time, physicians sometimes had insufficient communication skills for more values-based discussions, a factor that has been previously identified in the literature as an important barrier in the provision of ACP support and in shared decision-making more generally [22]. Perhaps notably, however, physicians believing that patients would be reluctant to engage in these conversations was not identified as a barrier [9, 10]. This possibly reflects the level to which ACP conversations were normalized within these organizations and the, sometimes extensive, organizational experience gained of patients, members of the public and families finding ACP support acceptable. A barrier we found that is less commonly identified in the existing literature involved physicians having misunderstandings about medico-legal issues, including around the role of ACP in processes of medical consent and the extent of physicians' responsibilities to treat. Nurses sometimes also had concerns about legal forms, while social workers were considered to be more confident with legal documents and processes. Physicians were also thought to tend towards having conversations of limited scope, late in the disease trajectory. Other concerns arose for some physicians where other professionals initiated and facilitated ACP conversations with their patients. These encompassed potential concerns about facilitators' clinical skills and knowledge, the possibility that patients may be being persuaded to inappropriately forego treatments, professional autonomy with regard to discussions about prognosis and goals of care and the potential for negative effects on trust in the patient-physician relationship. While the majority of physicians were thought to be supportive of ACP in principle, it also remained the case that most physicians were not engaged actively in the provision of ACP support and the barriers and concerns identified were frequently considered important implementation challenges. One physician and leader in the US noted that *physicians have the power to undo everything that has been achieved*, a viewpoint that is also reflected in the literature about the role of physicians in promoting innovation and practice change more widely [23]. On one hand, these challenges suggest the need for a supportive and sustained approach that works with physicians' concerns with an emphasis on physician champions and educators. However, there is a need to balance this with the competing concern, also reflected in the existing literature [9, 11, 24], that if ACP becomes predominantly the responsibility of physicians it may become what one physician in our study described as *just another treatment decision*, limited in scope, occurring late in the illness trajectory and with insufficient recognition given to potential risks and burdens.

Models for delivering ACP support were driven primarily by the resource-intensiveness of facilitating ACP conversations, with few staff able to routinely deliver full ACP conversations within their roles. The widespread employment of dedicated ACP facilitators was not considered scalable or sustainable, nor necessarily desirable as it was commonly thought that over-reliance on dedicated staff could lead to lead to poorly integrated care. In one US organization, uniquely, a group of spiritual care advisors were able to find substantial time in their roles to facilitate ACP conversations, although this sometimes impinged on their other responsibilities. In other cases, external sources of funding were sometimes available. For example, in one organization in New Zealand, there was separate District Health Board incentive funding for GPs, usually working with other practice staff, to facilitate ACP conversations and complete plans. This was associated with increased levels of ACP [25]. In other organizations, separate funding streams, including for care coordination and reducing the risk of hospital admission, helped to fund professionals' time to conduct ACP conversations with relevant target groups. Furthermore, during our fieldwork, the Centers for Medicare and Medicaid Services (CMS) in the US introduced the potential for including ACP conversations in Medicare wellness exams (for people aged 65 and over) as well as ACP-specific Medicare billing codes for an ACP conversation of 30 min and an additional 30 min (for people of any age). Although the level of funding is modest, this development represents the first funding at scale of these longer conversations, with the result that around 575,000 Medicare beneficiaries received an ACP conversation in 2016, twice as many as anticipated by the American Medical Association [26].

More commonly, however, health and care professionals had to find ways of incorporating the provision of ACP support into their existing roles with no additional resource. One model, most commonly used by physicians, was the referral model, which involved introducing ACP and then referring on to other staff for a longer ACP conversation. A number of organizations actively encouraged physicians to use this approach, focusing efforts on encouraging and supporting them to introduce ACP. This could work well where there was a trusted professional with protected time for facilitating ACP conversations to refer on to. However, many referrals appeared insecure, for example, in the case of referrals to GPs who themselves may lack the time to conduct full ACP conversations. Incorporation models were those where ACP support was provided by a single professional alongside and as part of other care. Because of time pressures, this generally involved breaking the conversation down into multiple shorter sessions. If appropriately systematized so that the evolving conversation did not become too fragmented, the merits of this approach included it being easier to incorporate into routine appointments and that it allowed patients and families to reflect and develop their preferences over time. However, this approach could mean that ACP conversations got squeezed out or became too fragmented and, in much shorter sessions, it is possible that facilitators and patients may have felt less able to prompt or raise more complex questions and concerns. For nurses, social workers, care staff and others, the use of an incorporation model was also often associated with insufficient physician input.

Team-based models potentially allowed nurses, social workers and others, to undertake the most time-consuming aspects of providing ACP support, but with physicians retaining active involvement. This shared approach was thought to be the most cost-effective as well as supportive of good quality care. It was also thought to be a good fit with new models of care such as Patient-Centered Medical Homes in the United States and Australia [27] or multi-specialty community providers or primary care homes in England [28, 29]. However, even where facilitation of conversations could be somewhat absorbed into other care, there often remained a need for some additional resource. As noted by one leader in New Zealand, 'It takes time, but lots of things to do with chronic illness take time.' Finally, it is worth noting that the challenges of providing ACP in care homes could mean that care home residents have inequitable access to ACP support. Strengthening links with external healthcare providers able to assist in the delivery of ACP support is, therefore, also important [30].

Conclusion

The emphasis on ACP in national policy is important but not sufficient, on its own, to ensure widespread provision of ACP support in health and care settings locally. This research highlights the need, in the absence of significant new funding or a professional lead role, for intensive and committed organizational leadership, both at a strategic and day-to-day level. The intractability of time constraints, however, remains a significant challenge, particularly for facilitating ACP conversations and, while there may be some scope for absorbing ACP support into existing health and care provision, there is likely to remain a need for some new resource. Physician leadership and involvement are key, and approaches to developing ACP need to work with physicians' concerns while, at the same time, balancing this against the risk of ACP becoming entirely physician-led, with ACP limited in scope and occurring late in the illness trajectory. Team-based frameworks embedded in evolving models of care for chronic illness and end of life are likely to

help to achieve this balance, manage costs and maximize quality of care. The importance of ensuring strong links with external healthcare providers in care homes is emphasized for equity of care. While the full consideration of transferability issues is beyond the scope of this study, the consistency of findings across the four countries provides some confidence that lessons drawn may have relevance in a range of socio-economically similar countries.

Abbreviations
ACP: Advance care planning; GP: General practitioner; US: United States

Acknowledgments
The authors would like to extend their most sincere thanks to all of the healthcare leaders and key staff who facilitated access and for their work helping to organize fieldwork visits and set up interview schedules, as well as to all of the staff and stakeholders who agreed to participate in the research interviews and share their experiences and views. We would also like to thank the many people who contributed information and advice at different stages throughout the project, including in initial scoping interviews and by participating in a project advisory group.

Funding
This article presents independent research funded by the National Institute for Health Research School for Social Care Research (NIHR SSCR). The views expressed in this publication are those of the author(s) and not necessarily of NIHR SSCR, or the Department of Health, NIHR or the NHS.

Authors' contributions
JD initiated and developed the idea for this research project and is the primary investigator. She led the design of topic guides, conducted fieldwork, undertook data management, conducted analysis and was the primary author of this article. MK was involved at all stages of the project. He provided important critical input into the design of the study and is a co-investigator. He contributed towards the design of topic guides, participated in analysis by reading a selection of interview summaries, commented on coding frameworks as they developed, met with JD to discuss evolving and final analyses and provided helpful critical input into, and editing of, the final manuscript. Both authors read and approved the final manuscript.

Competing interests
The authors declare that they have no competing interests.

References
1. Brinkman-Stoppelenburg A, Rietjens JA, van der Heide A. The effects of advance care planning on end-of-life care: a systematic review. Palliat Med. 2014;28(8):1000–25.
2. Dixon J, Matosevic T, King D, Knapp M. The economic case for advance care planning: a systematic review. Palliat Med. 2015;29(10):869–84.

3. Carr D, Luth E. Advance care planning: contemporary issues and future directions. Innovation in Aging. 2017;1(1):1–10.

4. Victorian Department of Health. Advance care planning: have the conversation. A strategy for Victorian health services 2014–2018. Victorian Department of Health. 2014.

5. Ministry of Health. Advance care planning: a guide for the New Zealand health care workforce. Wellington: Ministry of Health; 2011.

6. National Health Service. National End of Life Care Programme. Capacity, care planning and advance care planning in life limiting illness: a guide for health and social care staff. 2011.

7. NHS Improving Quality. Routes to success series. 2008-2014. http://endoflifecareambitions.org.uk/route-to-success/. Accessed 18 May 2018.

8. Gott M, Gardiner C, Small N, Payne S, Seamark D, Barnes S, Halpin D, Ruse C. Barriers to advance care planning in chronic obstructive pulmonary disease. Palliat Med. 2009;23(7):642–8.

9. Pollock K, Wilson E. Care and communication between health professionals and patients affected by severe or chronic illness in community care settings: a qualitative study of care at the end of life. Health Services and Delivery Research. 2015;3:31.

10. Lund S, Richardson A, May C. Barriers to advance care planning at the end of life: an explanatory systematic review of implementation studies. PLoS One. 2015;10:2.

11. Robinson L, Dickinson C, Bamford C, Clark A, Hughes J, Exley C. A qualitative study: professionals' experiences of advance care planning in dementia and palliative care, 'a good idea in theory but …'. Palliat Med. 2012;27(5):401–8.

12. Boddy J, Chenoworth L, McLennan V, Daly M. It's just too hard! Australian health care practitioner perspectives on barriers to advance care planning. Aust J Prim Health. 2013;19(1):38–45.

13. Sharp T, Malyon A, Barclay S. GP's perceptions of advance care planning with frail and older people: a qualitative study. Br J Gen Pract. 2017; bjgp17X694145. Available from: http://bjgp.org/content/early/2017/12/18/bjgp17X694145. Accessed 18 May 2018.

14. Luckett T, Spencer L, Moreton R, Pollock C, Lam L, Sylvester W, Sellars M, Detering K, Butow P, Tong A, Clayton J. Advance care planning in chronic kidney disease: a survey of current practice in Australia. Nephrol (Carlton). 2017;22(2):139–49.

15. Henry C, Seymour J. Advance care planning: a guide for health and social care staff. National Health Service (NHS)/ University of Nottingham. 2008.

16. Harrison-Dening K, Jones L, Sampson E. Advance care planning for people with dementia: a review. Int Psychogeriatr. 2011;23(10):1535–51.

17. Ritchie J, Lewis J, editors. Qualitative research practice: a guide for social science students and researchers. London: Sage Publications; 2003.

18. Cresswell JW, Plano Clark VL. Designing and conducting mixed method research. Third Edition. Sage Publications Inc: Thousand Oaks. 2017.

19. Miles MB, Huberman AM. Qualitative data analysis: an expanded sourcebook. Thousand Oaks: Sage Publications Inc; 1994.

20. Cresswell J. Chapter 1: The selection of a research approach in Cresswell J. Research design: qualitative, quantitative, and mixed methods approaches (5th edition). Los Angeles: Sage Publications Inc; 2018.

21. Fritz Z, Slowther AM, Perkins GD. Resuscitation policy should focus on the patient, not the decision. BMJ. 2017;356(j813(February)):1–6.

22. Tuller D. Medicare coverage for advance care planning: just the first step. Health Aff. 2016;35(3):390–3.

23. Black N. From cutting costs to eliminating waste: reframing the challenge. J Health Serv Res Policy. 2017;22(2):73–5.

24. Hoeffer D, Johnson S, Bender M. Development and preliminary evaluation of an innovative advanced chronic disease care model. Chronic Disease Care. 2013;20(9):408–18.

25. Duckworth S, Thompson, A. Evaluation of the Advance Care Planning Programme. Prepared for Health Quality and Safety Commission. Litmus. March 29, 2017.

26. Aleccia J. End-of-life advice: more than 500,000 chat on Medicare's dime. Kaiser Health News. 2017. http://khn.org/news/end-of-life-advice-more-than-500000-chat-on-medicares-dime/. Accessed 18 May 2018.

27. Royal Australian College of General Practitioners. Standards for Patient-Centred Medical Homes: Patient-centred, comprehensive, coordinated, accessible and quality care. 2016.

28. Collins B. New care models: emerging innovations in governance and organisational form. London: Kings Fund; 2016.

29. Kumpunen S, Rosen R, Kossarova L, Sherlaw-Johnson C. Primary care homes: evaluating a new model of primary care. Nuffield trust. 2017. https://www.nuffieldtrust.org.uk/files/2017-08/pch-report-final.pdf.

30. Detering KM, Carter RZ, Sellars M, Lewis V, Sutton EA. Prospective comparative effectiveness cohort study comparing two models of advance care planning provision for Australian community aged care clients. BMJ Support Palliat Care. 2017;7(4):486–94.

9

Unmet care needs of advanced cancer patients and their informal caregivers

Tao Wang[1], Alex Molassiotis[1*], Betty Pui Man Chung[1] and Jing-Yu Tan[1,2]

Abstract

Background: This systematic review aimed to identify the unmet care needs and their associated variables in patients with advanced cancer and informal caregivers, alongside summarizing the tools used for needs assessment.

Methods: Ten electronic databases were searched systematically from inception of each database to December 2016 to determine eligible studies. Studies that considered the unmet care needs of either adult patients with advanced cancer or informal caregivers, regardless of the study design, were included. The Mixed Methods Appraisal Tool was utilized for quality appraisal of the included studies. Content analysis was used to identify unmet needs, and descriptive analysis was adopted to synthesize other outcomes.

Results: Fifty studies were included, and their methodological quality was generally robust. The prevalence of unmet needs varied across studies. Twelve unmet need domains were identified in patients with advanced cancer, and seven among informal caregivers. The three most commonly reported domains for patients were psychological, physical, and healthcare service and information. The most prominent unmet items of these domains were emotional support (10.1–84.4%), fatigue (18–76.3%), and "being informed about benefits and side-effects of treatment" (4–66.7%). The most commonly identified unmet needs for informal caregivers were information needs, including illness and treatment information (26–100%) and care-related information (21–100%). Unmet needs of patients with advanced cancer were associated with their physical symptoms, anxiety, and quality of life. The most commonly used instruments for needs assessment among patients with advanced cancer were the Supportive Care Needs Survey ($N = 8$) and Problems and Needs in Palliative Care questionnaire ($N = 5$). The majority of the included studies investigated unmet needs from the perspectives of either patients or caregivers with a cross-sectional study design using single time-point assessments. Moreover, significant heterogeneity, including differences in study contexts, assessment methods, instruments for measurement, need classifications, and reporting methods, were identified across studies.

Conclusion: Both advanced cancer patients and informal caregivers reported a wide range of context-bound unmet needs. Examining their unmet needs on the basis of viewing patients and their informal caregivers as a whole unit will be highly optimal. Unmet care needs should be comprehensively evaluated from the perspectives of all stakeholders and interpreted by using rigorously designed mixed methods research and longitudinal studies within a given context.

* Correspondence: alex.molasiotis@polyu.edu.hk

[1]School of Nursing, The Hong Kong Polytechnic University, Hung Hom, Hong Kong

Full list of author information is available at the end of the article

Background

According to the World Health Organization (WHO), more than 15 million people will be diagnosed with cancer by 2020 [1]. With the advances in cancer treatments, the illness trajectory and prognosis of cancer have changed, and patients diagnosed with advanced cancer can live for a relatively long period [2, 3]. However, lengthy cancer experience and anticancer treatments make patients suffer from a wide range of problems, such as physical, psychological, emotional, and practical issues [4]. Cancer-related symptoms and patients' experiences during cancer treatment vary across different cancer stages, and patients at advanced stage commonly experience different symptoms from those with early-stage cancer [5, 6]. Such 'chronic and uncertain' conditions pose a challenge to not only the cancer services but also to their informal caregivers [7]. Informal caregivers commonly take care of their loved ones for a long period [8]. The long-term caregiving process is physically and psychologically challenging, particularly when taking care of patients with advanced cancer [9]. Many informal caregivers, including those who do not regard caregiving as a burden, suffer from a wide range of problems, such as sleep disturbance, anxiety, depression, and practical and financial difficulties [10, 11]. Informal caregivers are usually regarded as fellow sufferers alongside patients [12]. Unmet needs of patients can increase the level of caregiver burden [13]. In turn, caregivers' problems are closely linked with patients' well-being [14], and unsolved problems or unmet needs of caregivers will not only decrease their own quality of life [15] but also affect the patients' health outcomes negatively [15]. Informal caregivers and patients with advanced cancer are considered a whole unit in fighting the illness [10].

High-quality and patient-and-family-centered care is needed to address the problems of both the advanced cancer patients and their informal caregivers, including symptom and side effect management, as well as emotional, psychosocial, and spiritual support. All these aspects of support are typically categorized under palliative care [16]. Mismatched healthcare that is inconsistent with patients and caregivers' needs can increase healthcare expenditure and lead to harmful effects [17]. Therefore, the unmet care needs of patients and informal caregivers should be comprehensively assessed prior to designing and providing tailored palliative care services [18, 19]. Care needs are defined as "the requirement of some action or resource in care that is necessary, desirable, or useful to attain optimal well-being" (Foot, 1996, as cited in Sanson-Fisher, et al., 2000, p.227) [20]. Unmet needs assessment is designed to identify how well and how much their needs have been satisfied or not [21]. An early review [17] summarized the instruments for needs assessment; however, a majority of these instruments have been designed for general patients

with cancer (e.g., Supportive Care Needs Survey, SCNS [17]). After the publication of that review, several tools that were specifically designed for advanced cancer patients (e.g., Needs Assessment of Advanced Cancer Patients, NA-ACP [22]) have been developed and used.

An early systematic review [21] published in 2009 analyzed the unmet needs of patients with advanced cancer with nine included studies. Another systematic review [7] with 23 studies reported eight unmet need domains. These two systematic reviews only focused on patients, with limited literature searches in only four databases. Meanwhile, the inclusion criteria were relatively ambiguous in the second review because studies with mixed samples (patients at different cancer stages) were included; moreover, the definition of advanced cancer was not presented [7]. Moreover, neither of the two reviews summarized and reported detailed information regarding the needs assessment tools used, which is important information to allow readers to appreciate the quality and reliability of study results. Furthermore, to date, no systematic review has been conducted to explore the unmet needs of informal caregivers of patients with advanced cancer. Therefore, the current systematic review was carried out to update evidence from previous reviews and provide a more comprehensive picture regarding the unmet needs among patients with advanced cancer and informal caregivers. An intensive literature search was performed on 10 electronic databases, and the inclusion criteria were more specific for advanced cancer diagnosis than those of the previous reviews. This current systematic review also included informal caregivers on the basis of the following concepts: fellow sufferers [12], a whole unit [10], and patient-and-family-centered care that is emphasized by the WHO [16]. Specific objectives of this review included: (1) to identify the unmet care needs and their associated factors in patients with advanced cancer and their informal caregivers, and (2) to summarize needs assessment tools that were used in the included studies.

Methods

Search strategies

With consideration of the language expertise of the review authors, English and Chinese databases were included. Ten databases, including PubMed, Cumulative Index to Nursing and Allied Health Literature (CINAHL), EMBase, Cochrane Central Register of Controlled Trials (CENTRAL), PsycINFO, Web of Science, Wan Fang Data, China National Knowledge Infrastructure (CNKI), Chongqing VIP (CQVIP), and Chinese Biomedical Literature Database (CBM), were searched systematically from inception of each database to December 2016. Restrictions regarding study design were not set. The used MeSH terms, key words, and free words included needs assessment, assessment of healthcare needs, unmet needs,

neoplasms, advanced cancer, terminal cancer, metastatic cancer, and the forth. Manual searches were
also conducted by examining the reference lists of the
included studies. Three representative search strategies of this systematic review are listed in Table 1.

Study identification and data extraction

Duplications were identified and eliminated through a
reference management software (NoteExpress). Titles
and abstracts of the remaining studies were screened independently by two review authors (WT and TJY), and
full text of potentially eligible studies were subsequently
located for further screening. Studies satisfying the following inclusion criteria were included: (1) studies that included either adult (≥18 years old) patients with advanced
cancer[1] or adult informal caregivers of patients with advanced cancer; (2) studies that reported data in terms of
unmet care needs[2] or concerns that are directly linked to
the unmet care needs of patients with advanced cancer
and/or their informal caregivers, regardless of the study
design; and (3) accessible full texts were published in
peer-reviewed journals. Exclusion criteria were: (1) studies
with mixed sample of patients with cancer at any cancer
stage (except those patients with advanced cancer who
were analyzed separately); (2) studies solely focusing on
quality of life [21], satisfaction with healthcare services,
care service utilization, or presence of symptoms/prob-
lems; (3) studies focusing on instrument development,
translation, or evaluation; and (4) conference articles with
only abstracts, editorial comments, guidelines, policies, or
treatment recommendations. Data were extracted by two
independent review authors. These data included information regarding the first author of the study, year of publication, country of origin, research setting, research design,
sampling approach, sample size, need assessment methods
(interview or other instruments), prevalence of unmet
needs, and related factors for unmet needs. Any disagreement was settled and discussed by the two other review
authors (CPM and AM).

Methodological quality appraisal

The methodological quality of included studies was
assessed by two review authors (WT and TJY) independently with the Mixed Methods Appraisal Tool (MMAT)
[25]. This tool is highly efficient; it takes approximately
14 min to evaluate one study [25] with robust
consistency among reviewers (intraclass correlation =
0.72 [25]); MMAT is specifically designed to assess the
quality of either quantitative or qualitative studies. Four
different quality criteria for qualitative studies and different types of quantitative studies, including randomized
control trials, quantitative nonrandomized trials, and
quantitative descriptive studies, were used [25]. Each criterion was graded as 0 (unmet) or 1 (meet), and the

Table 1 Selected Search Strategies

PubMed

#1   Search (((("needs assessment"[MeSH Terms]) OR "needs
     assessment"[Title/Abstract]) OR "assessment of healthcare
     needs"[Title/Abstract]) OR "assessment of health care needs"[Title/
     Abstract]) OR "unmet needs"[Title/Abstract]

#2   Search (((((("palliative care"[MeSH Terms]) OR "palliative
     medicine"[MeSH Terms]) OR "hospice care"[MeSH Terms]) OR
     "supportive care"[Title/Abstract]) OR "palliative nursing"[Title/
     Abstract]) OR "palliative care nursing"[Title/Abstract]) OR "terminal
     care"[Title/Abstract]) OR "hospice nursing care"[Title/Abstract]

#3   Search ((((("neoplasms"[MeSH Terms]) OR "advanced cancer"[Title/
     Abstract]) OR "terminal cancer"[Title/Abstract]) OR "metastatic
     cancer"[Title/Abstract]) OR "tumor"[Title/Abstract]) OR "cancer"[Title/
     Abstract]

#4   #1 AND #2 AND #3

CINAHL

#1   TI needs assessment OR TI assessment of healthcare needs OR TI
     assessment of health care needs OR TI unmet needs

#2   AB needs assessment OR AB assessment of healthcare needs OR
     AB assessment of health care needs OR AB unmet needs

#3   AB palliative care OR AB palliative medicine OR AB hospice care
     OR AB supportive care OR AB palliative nursing OR AB palliative
     care nursing OR AB terminal care OR AB hospice nursing

#4   TI palliative care OR TI palliative medicine OR TI hospice care OR TI
     supportive care OR TI palliative nursing OR TI palliative care
     nursing OR TI terminal care OR TI hospice nursing

#5   TI neoplasms OR TI tumor OR TI cancer OR TI advanced cancer OR
     TI terminal cancer OR TI metastatic cancer

#6   AB neoplasms OR AB tumor OR AB cancer OR AB advanced cancer
     OR AB terminal cancer OR AB metastatic cancer

#7   #1 OR #2

#8   #3 OR #4

#9   #5 OR #6

#10 #7 AND #8 AND #9

EMBase

#1   'needs assessment'/exp

#2   'needs assessment':ab,ti OR (assessment:ab,ti AND of:ab,ti AND
     healthcare:ab,ti AND needs:ab,ti) OR (assessment:ab,ti AND of:ab,ti
     AND health:ab,ti AND care:ab,ti AND needs:ab,ti) OR 'unmet
     needs':ab,ti

#3   #1 OR #2

#4   'palliative care':ab,ti OR 'palliative medicine':ab,ti OR 'hospice
     care':ab,ti OR 'supportive care':ab,ti OR 'palliative nursing':ab,ti OR
     'terminal care':ab,ti OR 'hospice nursing':ab,ti

#5   'palliative nursing'/exp

#6   #4 OR #5

#7   'advanced cancer'/exp

#8   'neoplasm'/exp

#9   'advanced cancer':ab,ti OR (terminal:ab,ti AND cancer:ab,ti) OR
     (metastatic:ab,ti AND cancer:ab,ti) OR neoplasm:ab,ti OR cancer:ab,ti
     OR tumor:ab,ti

#10 #7 OR #8 OR #9

#11 #3 AND #6 AND #10

global score of each study was calculated from 0 to 4 (0 = no criterion satisfied, 1 = satisfied one criterion, 2 = satisfied two criteria, 3 = satisfied three criteria, and 4 = satisfied all four criteria). When any disagreement occurred, the review authors conducted a group discussion to reach final agreement.

Data analysis

Content analysis [26] was used to identify the unmet need domains of patients with advanced cancer and informal caregivers across quantitative and qualitative studies. A priori content categories of patients with advanced cancer were determined on the basis of previous studies; these categories included health system and information, patient care and support, activities of daily living (ADL), physical, psychological, financial, and spiritual [7]. With regards to informal caregivers, five content categories were determined on the basis of a previous review [10]; these categories included cancer care services, informational, psychological, spiritual, and social needs. Data of the included studies were compared, combined, and clustered with respect to those domains for patients and informal caregivers. Terms, such as instrumental and personal care, were included in the

ADL domain because they were frequently mentioned in several North American studies [21]. Summative content analysis was used to identify and extract new categories within content not covered by previous domains. The approach of descriptive analysis was used for the prevalence of unmet needs due to the significant heterogeneity of the included studies [27]. Variables associated with patients and informal caregivers' needs and used instruments were analyzed through descriptive approach.

Results[3]

Characteristics of included studies

Among the 4277 potentially eligible studies, 45 studies were included. After screening the reference lists, five other eligible studies were retrieved. Finally, 50 studies [6, 9, 28–75] (5 published in Chinese and 45 in English language) were included in this review (Fig. 1). The majority of the studies (43/50) used quantitative study designs, with 42 surveys (1 longitudinal survey [75] and 41 cross-sectional surveys) and 1 [6] pre-post intervention study (only baseline data were used in this review). The seven other studies [48, 49, 57, 62, 71–73] were qualitative designs with individual in-depth interviews and/or focus group. Among the 50 included studies, 33 studies investigated the unmet needs of

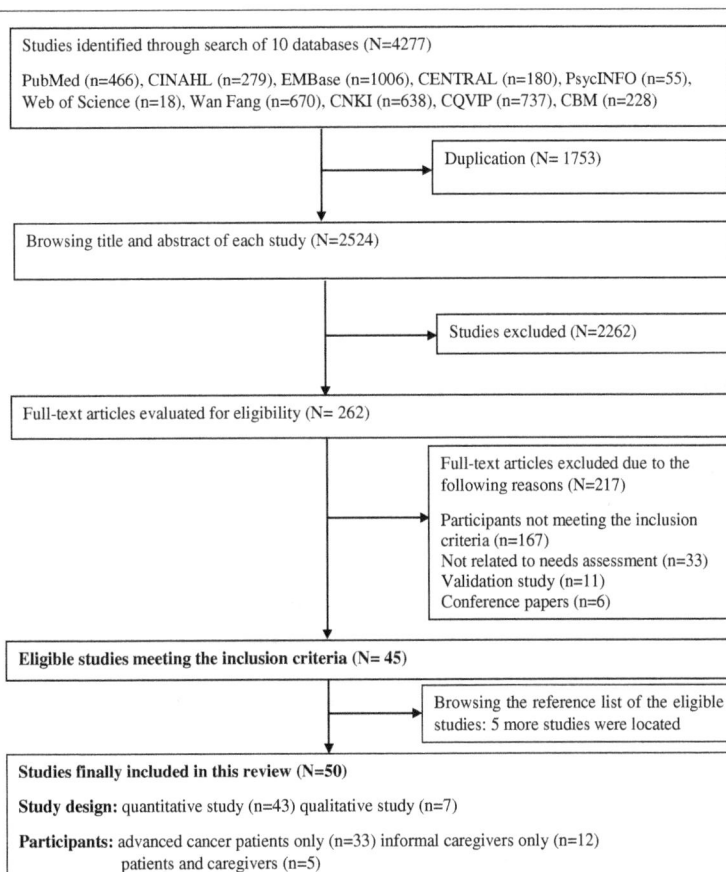

Fig. 1 Flow chart of study selection

patients with advanced cancer only, with 31 out of 33 studies from the perspective of patients, one study from the perspective of informal caregivers, and one from the perspectives of both patients and informal caregivers. Twelve studies [9, 30, 32, 35, 39, 40, 49, 51, 52, 57, 62, 64] explored the unmet needs of informal caregivers, and five other [48, 56, 59, 63, 67] studies investigated the unmet needs of patients with advanced cancer and their informal caregivers. With regards to sample sources, six studies [32, 40, 45, 46, 49, 61] reported no information regarding the recruitment setting, while in the remaining studies patients, and/or caregivers were mainly recruited from outpatient departments ($n = 16$), inpatient departments ($n = 11$), home/home-based care units ($n = 10$), and mixed settings ($n = 7$). In terms of cancer sites, 29 studies focused on patients with mixed cancer site and/or their caregivers, 11 studies focused on specific patients with cancer and/or caregivers (3 studies on prostate cancer [57, 69, 73], 5 studies on breast cancer [41, 48, 58, 60, 75], and three on lung cancer [35, 42, 71]), while 10 other studies [47, 50, 51, 53, 59, 64, 66, 68] reported no information about cancer types. The diagnostic criteria of advanced cancer were presented in 13 studies (13/50), with five studies [6, 30, 31, 60, 61] adopting the criteria of cancer with metastasis, and seven studies [9, 41, 42, 45, 58, 63, 75] using the stage III/IV criterion according to TNM staging system. With regards to geographic distribution, nine studies were conducted in the USA [38, 40, 46, 49, 52, 57, 59, 70, 74], seven were in mainland China (six of which were conducted in Shanghai) [9, 53, 63–67], five in Australia [6, 54, 55, 60, 68], five in the Netherlands [29–31, 34, 44], four in Canada [47, 50, 56, 73], three in Japan [33, 39, 41], three in Taiwan [35, 42, 62], two in the UK [69, 71], two in Denmark [45, 72], two in Hong Kong [58, 75], and one each in Italy [28], France [61], South Korea [32], Spain [37], Indonesia [36], Czech Republic [43], India [51], and Bangladesh [48]. Characteristics and main findings of all included studies are presented in Table 2.

Quality of the included studies

The methodological quality of the included studies was generally robust, with 17 and 18 studies satisfying all four criteria (34%) and three of the four criteria (36%), respectively. The prominent weaknesses of 43 quantitative studies were poor sampling strategy and low response rate. The response rates of 16 studies [32, 33, 37, 39, 40, 43, 47, 52–56, 61, 63, 68, 74] were lower than 60%, and 14 studies [30–32, 38, 42, 43, 51–54, 67, 68, 70, 74] failed to report the sampling method, sampling procedure, or sample size justification. Among the seven other qualitative studies, three studies (3/7, 42.9%) [49, 62, 73] failed to interpret how findings were related to the study context, and two studies (2/7, 28.6%) [57, 73] provided no

explanation on how the research process was influenced by the researchers. The overall quality score of each study is presented in the first column of Table 2.

Descriptions of unmet needs in patients with advanced cancer

A total of 12 domains of unmet needs were identified from 34 quantitative and 4 qualitative studies. These domains included physical, ADL, psychological, health system and information, patient care and support, social, communication, financial, spiritual, autonomy, sexuality, and nutritional needs.

Unmet patient needs based on quantitative studies

Study sample sizes ranged from 40 to 977, with the average sample size being 165 and the response rate ranging from 36 to 100%. Physical needs were reported in 24 studies, and the most prominent physical unmet need was fatigue [6, 31, 33, 34, 42, 43, 45, 47, 50, 54, 56, 63]. In terms of ADL, 11 studies were included, and the most highlighted item was "not being able to do the things you used to do" [6, 33, 50, 58, 60]. Twenty-eight studies reported psychological needs, and the most common item was "emotional support" [6, 28, 29, 31, 33, 36, 41, 45, 46, 50, 70, 72, 73]. In terms of health system and information, "being informed about benefits and side-effects of treatment" was the most common one [31, 41, 42, 44, 54, 61, 63, 66, 69, 75]. With regards to patient care and support needs, two prominent unmet needs, namely, "reassurance by medical staff that the way you feel is normal" [33, 41] and "doctor acknowledges and shows sensitivity to your feelings and emotional needs" [33, 42], were identified. "Family and friends' support" was the most common social unmet need [29, 45, 54, 55, 63, 65, 67]. Communication and financial support needs were also reported [28, 29, 31, 36, 43, 46, 54, 56, 63, 66, 55, 70]. "Meaning of death" [31, 36] was the most commonly mentioned spiritual need. "I can do less than before" [31, 34, 43] was the most prominent unmet autonomy need. Detailed unmet needs and their prevalence are presented in Table 3.

Unmet patient needs extracted from qualitative studies

According to four qualitative studies [48, 71–73], several unmet needs that were similar to those identified in quantitative studies were extracted and categorized. For instance, patients commonly expressed "pain, fatigue or side effects of treatment, such as urinary incontinence and loss of sexual function" (p. 191–192) (physical needs) [73], "feelings of fear, hopelessness and uncertainty about the future" [48, 71] or "feelings of sadness, anger, anxiety, frustration and desperation" [48, 71, 73] (psychological and spiritual needs), "insufficient information

Table 2 Characteristics and Main Findings of the Included Studies

Author, Year & QS	Country/ Region	Setting	Study Design	Participant	Diagnosis	Response Rate	Data Collection Method/ Instrument & Findings
Studies Regarding Advanced Cancer Patients (n = 33)							
S1 [28]: Morasso G, et al., 1999, QS:3	Italy	Inpatients	Semi-structured interview survey	Sampling: Random sampling Sample size: 94 Age (yr): 64.8 ± 11.1 Gender: 38/89 (F)	Terminal cancer patients (mixed cancer sites)	89/94 (94.7%)	Interviews guide: 5 domains and 41 items: "physiological needs", "safety needs", "loved and belonging needs", "self-esteem needs" and "self-fulfillment needs" (p.404)
							Unmet needs (p.406): 1) symptoms control (62.8%), 2) occupational functioning (62.1%), 3) emotional support (51.7%), 4) Nutrition (43.2%), 5) sleep (37.1%), 6) self-fulfillment (32.5%), 7) communication (27.7%), 8) information (25.0%), 9) personal care (14.6%), 10) financial support (14.1%) and 11) emotional closeness (13.8%)
S2 [6]: Waller, et al., 2012, QS: 4	Australia	Outpatients	Multiple time points pre-post intervention study [a]	Sampling: unclear (219/613) Sample size: 219 Age (yr): 66.1 ± 10.7 Gender: 91/ 195 (F)	Advanced cancer patients (extensive local, regional or metastatic) (mixed cancer sites)	195/219 (89.0%)	Supportive Care Needs Survey (SCNS-SF34): 5 domains and 34 items Needs Assessment for Advanced Cancer Patients (NA-ACP): only used 6 items on spiritual needs
							Moderate-to-high unmet needs: 1) "not being able to do the things you used to do" (33.0%), 2) "concerns about the worries of those close to you" (27.9%), 3) "lack of energy, tiredness" (26.2%), 4) "work around the home" (23.0%), 5) "uncertainty about the future"(21.4%), 6) "pain" (20.9%), 7) "worry that results of treatment are beyond your control" (19.4%), 8) "fears about the cancer spreading" (18.8%), 9) "felling unwell a lot of the time"(17.3%), and 10) "anxiety" (15.3%)
S3 [29]: Teunissen, SC, et al., 2006 QS: 3	Netherla-nds	Inpatients	Structured interview survey	Sampling: unclear Sample size: 181 Age (median, yr): 18–79 Gender: 101/ 181 (F)	Advanced cancer patients (mixed cancer sites)	181/181 (100%)	Structured interview with a standard list: 4 domains: emotional needs, social needs, spiritual needs, and functional needs. (p.153) Each item including 2 parts: 1) if the issue is a "problem"; 2) actual wishes to receive professional support were labelled as palliative care needs. (p. 153)
							Unmet needs: 1) functional support (62.4%), 2) support in coping (57.5%), 3) emotional support (53.1%), 4) support of informal caregivers (34.3%), 5) spiritual support (7.7%), 6) co-ordination of care (9.9%), 7) relational support (9.9%), and 8) support in communication (7.7%).
S5 [31]: Osse BHP, et al., 2005, QS: 3	Netherla-nds	Home-based	Questionnaire survey	Sampling: unclear? Sample size: 112 Age (yr): 58 ± 12.3 (30–87)	Distant metastatic cancer (mixed cancer sites)	94/112 (84.0%)	Problems and Needs in Palliative Care questionnaire (PNPC): 10 domains and 90 items
							Top 10 unmet needs: 1) "difficulty coping with the unpredictability of the future" (25%), 2) "fear of metastases" (25%), 3) "fear of

Table 2 Characteristics and Main Findings of the Included Studies *(Continued)*

Author, Year & QS	Country/ Region	Setting	Study Design	Participant	Diagnosis	Response Rate	Data Collection Method/ Instrument & Findings
				Gender: 66/94 (F)			physical suffering" (24%), 4) "experiencing difficulties in remembering what was told" (24%), 5) "difficulties to accept the disease" (23%), 6) "extra expenditure because of disease" (23%), 7) "fear of death" (21%), 8) "frustrations because I can do less than before" (20%); 9) "experiencing loss of control over one's life" (19%); 10) "fear of treatments" (19%)
S7 [33]: Hasegawa, et al., 2016 QS: 3	Japan	Inpatients	Questionnaire survey	Sampling: random sampling Sample size: 45 Age (yr): 66.6 ± 9.8 Gender: 21/45 (F)	Advanced cancer patients (mixed cancer sites)	NR	Supportive Care Needs Survey (SCNS-SF34): 5 domains and 34 items Hospital Anxiety and Depression Scale (HADS) Functional Independence Measure (FIM) Top 10 Moderate-to-high unmet needs: 1) "Being informed about things you can do to help yourself to get well" (51.1%); 2) "Having one member of hospital staff with whom you can talk to about all aspects of your condition, treatment, and follow-up" (51.1%); 3) "Concerns about the worries of those close to you"(44.1%); 4) "Anxiety"(41.8%); 5) "Not being able to do the things you used to do" (37.2%); 6) "Feeling down or depressed" (37.2%); 7) "Being treated like a person not just another case" (34.8%); 8) "Hospital staff acknowledging, and showing sensitivity to, your feelings and emotional needs" (34.8%); 9) "Hospital staff attending promptly to your physical needs" (34.8%); 10) "Feelings of sadness" (32.5%); 11) "Feelings about death and dying"; (32.5%); 12) "Reassurance by medical staff that the way you feel is normal" (32.5%); 13) "Learning to feel in control of your situation" (32.5%);
S8 [34]: Uitdehaag MJ et al., 2015 QS: 4	Netherlands	Outpatients	Questionnaire survey	Sampling: consecutive sampling Sample size: 57 Age (yr): EC: 65 ± 11.8 PBC: 64 ± 12.2 Gender: EC: 2/24 (F) PBC:10/33 (F)	Incurable EC or PBC cancer patients	57/90 (63%), with 24 EC and 33 PBC	Problems and Needs in Palliative Care questionnaire (PNPC): 9 domains and 90 items EORTC QLQ-OES18 EORTC QLQ-PAN26 Unmet needs: EC: 1) "fatigue" (21%); 2) "frustration can do less than usual" (21%); 3) "shortness of breath" (17%) PBC: 1) "fear of physical suffering" (34%), 2) "lack of written information" (28%), 3) "fatigue" (22%).
S10 [36]: Effendy, C, et al., 2014	Indonesia	Outpatients	Questionnaire survey	Sampling: unclear	Advanced cancer (mixed cancer sites)	NR	Revised Problems and Needs in Palliative Care questionnaire-short version (PNPC-sv,24 items):

Table 2 Characteristics and Main Findings of the Included Studies *(Continued)*

Author, Year & QS	Country/ Region	Setting	Study Design	Participant	Diagnosis	Response Rate	Data Collection Method/ Instrument & Findings
QS: 2				Sample size: 180 Age (yr): Indonesian: 49.3 ± 10.7 Netherlands: 58 ± 12.3 Gender: Indonesian: 133/180 (F) Netherlands: 66/94 (F)			adjusted within Indonesian context and deleted 9 items, and 24 items were maintained

Unmet needs: Physical: sweating (76.2%), sexuality (75%), short of breathless (67.3%), pain (66.4%) Autonomy: "difficulties in finding someone to talk to" (82.8%); Psychological: "difficulties showing emotions" (84.4%) Spiritual: "difficulties about the meaning of death" (85.4%) Financial: "extra expenses because of the disease" (72%) |
| S11 [37]: Vilalta, A, et al., 2014 QS: 3 | Spain | Outpatients | Questionnaire survey | Sampling: unclear Sample size: 50 Age (yr): Mean 60.9 (33–81) Gender: 19/50 (F) | Advanced cancer (mixed cancer sites) | NR | Self-designed questionnaire for spiritual needs:11 domains and 28 items

Top 10 spiritual needs (p. 594): 1) "to be recognized as a person until the end of life" (8.6 ± 1.3); 2) "the need for truth" (8.3 ± 2.7); 3) "to reinterpret life" (6.2 ± 1.9); 4) "to look for a meaning to existence" (5.7 ± 2.5); 5) "the need for hope" (5.7 ± 3.5); 6) "to see life beyond the individual" (5.2 ± 2.5); 7) "the need for religious expression" (4.9 ± 2.5); 8) "the needs for continuity and an afterlife" (4.0 ± 2.0); 9) "the need for freedom and to be free" (3.8 ± 3.4); 10) "to be free blame and to forgive others" (1.5 ± 2.0). |
| S12 [38]: Schenker Y. et al., 2014 QS: 3 | USA | Outpatients | Questionnaire survey | Sampling: unclear Sample size: 169 Age (yr): 62.3 ± 11.6 Gender: 107/ 169 (F) | Advanced cancer (mixed cancer sites) | 169/272 (62.1%) | Adapted Needs Assessment of Advanced Cancer Patients (NA-ACP): 32 items and 6 domains, without reporting psychological properties

Unmet needs: 1) symptom (62%); 2) psychological (62%); 3) medical communication/information (39%); 4) daily living (27%); 5) spiritual (23%); 6) social (20%) |
| S16 [41]: Uchida M, et al., 2011 QS: 4 | Japan | Outpatients | Questionnaire survey | Sampling: random sampling Sample size: 85 Age (yr): 58.6 ± 11.9 Gender: 85/87 (F) | Advanced breast cancer patients (stage IV) | 85/87 (97.7%) | Supportive Care Needs Survey (SCNS-SF34): 5 domains and 34 items Hospital Anxiety and Depression Scale (HADS) EOERC-QLQ-C30

Top 10 moderate-to-high unmet needs: 1) "Fears about the cancer spreading" (78.8%); 2) "Worry that the results of treatment are beyond your control" (71.8%); 3) "Concerns about the worries of those close to you" (68.2%); 4) "Having one member of hospital staff with whom you can talk to about all aspects of your condition, treatment and follow-up" (67.1%); 5) "Being informed about things you can do to help yourself to get |

Table 2 Characteristics and Main Findings of the Included Studies *(Continued)*

Author, Year & QS	Country/ Region	Setting	Study Design	Participant	Diagnosis	Response Rate	Data Collection Method/ Instrument & Findings
							well" (65.9%); 6) "Anxiety" (65.9%); 7) "Feeling down or depressed" (62.4%); 8) "Uncertainty about the future" (62.4%); 9) "Feeling about death and dying" (62.4%); 10) "Having access to professional counseling if you, family or friends need it" (57.6%);
S17 [42]: Liao YC, et al., 2011 QS: 3	Taiwan	Mixed	Questionnaire survey	Sampling: unclear Sample size: 152 Age (yr): 60.2 ± 11.0 Gender: 73/ 152 (F)	Advanced lung cancer patients (95.4% stage III-IV or extensive metastasis)	152/188 (80.9%)	Cancer Needs Questionnaire (CNQ)-Chinese version: 5 domains and 32 items Hospital Anxiety and Depression Scale (HADS) Symptom Severity Scale (SSS)
							Items of highest unmet needs by each domain: 1) "things helping self get well" (65.8%), 2) "cancer remission" (63.8%), 3) "benefit and side-effects of treatment" (63.8%), 4) "test results as soon as possible" (62.5%); 5) "dealing with fears about disease spreading and return" (40.2%), 6) "doctor acknowledges and shows sensitivity to your feelings and emotional needs" (39.5%), 7) "dealing with lack of energy and tiredness" (28.3%)
S18 [43]: BUŽGOVÁ, et al., 2014 QS: 2	Czech Republic	Inpatients	Questionnaire survey	Sampling: unclear Sample size: 93 Age (yr): 61.6 ± 16.8 Gender: 41/93 (F)	Advanced cancer (mixed cancer sites)	NR	Patient Needs Assessment in Palliative Care (PNAP): 5 domains and 42 items Hospital Anxiety and Depression Scale (HADS) EOERC-QLQ-C30
							Items of highest unmet needs by each domain: 1) Spiritual: "attending religious services or other ceremonies" (44%); 2) Autonomy: "continue my usual activities" (38%); 3) Social: "being financially secure" (27%); 4) psychological: "fear of dependence on help from others" (30%); 5) physical: "fatigue" (30%);
S19 [44]: Voogt E, et al., 2005 QS: 4	Netherlands	Home-based	Questionnaire survey	Sampling: unclear Sample size: 128 Age (yr): 63.6 ± 10.5 Gender: 66/ 128 (F)	Advanced cancer (mixed cancer sites)	128/192 (66.7%)	Problems and Needs in Palliative Care questionnaire (PNPC): used the 12 items on information needs Hospital Anxiety and Depression Scale (HADS) Utrecht Coping List to measure disease-specific coping
							Unmet information: 1) complementary care (93%); 2) alternative medicine (86%); 3) euthanasia: (83%); 4) care settings (78%); 5) Sexuality and cancer (72%); 6) psychological care (71%); 7) cause of cancer (65%); 8) food and diet (44%); 9) helpful devices (33%); 10) organizations that offer help (32%); 11) expected physical (20%); 12) treatment options and side effects (4%)

Table 2 Characteristics and Main Findings of the Included Studies *(Continued)*

Author, Year & QS	Country/ Region	Setting	Study Design	Participant	Diagnosis	Response Rate	Data Collection Method/ Instrument & Findings
S20 [45]: Johnsen AT, et al., 2013 QS: 4	Denmark	NR	Questionnaire survey	Sampling: random sampling Sample size: 977 Age (yr): mean 64 Gender: 547/ 977 (F)	Advanced cancer with mixed sites (95% at stage III/ IV)	977/1630 (60%)	3-Levels-of-Needs Questionnaire (3LNQ):12 items Unmet needs: 1) fatigue (35%); 2) physical activities (32%); 3) work and daily activities (29%); 4) worry (31%); 5) sexuality (28%); 6) pain (23%); 7) concentration (25%); 8) depression (24%); 9) dyspnea (19%); 10) nausea (12%); 11) lack of appetite (13%); 12) difficulties with family life and contact with friends (11%)
S21 [46]: Houts P, et al., 1988 QS: 4	USA	NR	Semi-structured interview survey (retrospective)	Sampling: stratified random sampling Sample size: 433 Age (yr): ≥20y Gender: unclear	Caregivers of terminal cancer (mixed cancer sites)	433/515 (84.0%)	Self-designed questionnaire of needs in cancer patients, including 14 areas: physical, activities of daily lives, reaction to treatment, nutrition, emotional, life purpose, social, family, financial, insurance, getting health care, medical staff, home health care, and transportation (p. 629) Unmet needs: 1) activities of daily lives (42%); 2) emotional (21%); 3) physical (21%); 4) insurance (19%); 5) financial (15%); 6) medical staffs (20%)
S22 [47]: Khan L, et al., 2012 QS: 3	Canada	Outpatients	Questionnaire survey	Sampling: unclear Sample size: 40 (patients = 20, caregivers = 20) Age (yr): Patients: unclear Caregivers: unclear Gender: unclear	Advanced cancer patients and their caregivers (cancer site unclear)	NR	Problems and Needs in Palliative Care- short version (PNPC-sv): 8 domains and 33 items Patients' unmet needs from their own perspectives: 1) "doing light housework" (25%); 2) "pain" (25%), 3) "fatigue" (25%), 4) "personal transportation" (22.2%); 5) "sleeping problems" (21.1%); 6) "body care, washing, dressing, or toilet" (20%); 7) "fear of metastases" (17.6%); 8) "pricking or numb sensation" (16.7%); 9) "experiencing loss of control over one's life" (16.7%), 10) "fear of physical suffering" (16.7%) Patients' unmet needs from caregivers' perspectives: 1) "sexual dysfunction" (100%);2) "problems in relationship with life companion" (100%); 3) "finding others not receptive to talking about the disease" (100%); 4) "difficulties to show emotions" (100%), 5) "difficulties to be of avail for others" (100%), 6) "difficulties to accept the disease" (100%), 7) "extra expenditures because of the disease" (100%), 8) "loss of income because of the disease" (100%), 9) "pain"(35%), 10) "fear of physical suffering" (29.4%)
S25 [50]: Fitch MI, 2012 QS: 4	Canada	Outpatients	Questionnaire survey	Sampling: convenience sampling Sample size: 69	Advanced cancer patients (cancer sites unclear)	69/106 (65.1%)	Adapted Supportive Care Needs Survey (SCNS): 7 domains and 61 items: information, physical symptoms, psychological, emotional, spiritual, social, and practical, Cronbach's α = 0.35–0.81

Table 2 Characteristics and Main Findings of the Included Studies *(Continued)*

Author, Year & QS	Country/ Region	Setting	Study Design	Participant	Diagnosis	Response Rate	Data Collection Method/ Instrument & Findings
				Age (yr): mean 65y (35-84y) Gender: 34/69 (F)			Unmet needs in terms of issues reported by 50% patients: 1) "pain" (63.5%); 2) "fear of pain" (62.9%); 3) "lack of energy" (52.8%); 4) "fear about physical disability or deterioration" (50%); 5) "fear about cancer spreading" (51.4%;); 6) "not being able to do things you used to" (46.9%); 7) "decreased appetite" (47.4%); 8) "feeling unwell" (44.7%); 8) "feeling down or depressed" (30%), 9) "not being able to work around at home" (44.2%); 10) "concerns about the worries of those close to you"(29.4%)
S28 [53]: Deng D, et al. 2015 QS: 2	China	Home-based	Interview survey	Sampling: unclear Sample size: 107 Age (yr): mean 57y (18-87y) Gender: 58/107 (F)	Advanced cancer patients (cancer sites unclear)	NR	Guided life review (2–3 times in-depth interview) Three expectations (spiritual needs) (p.728): 1) have a nice day without pain (14.3%) 2) wish family health and happiness (37.6%) 3) fulfill patients' dreams (witness future family events, company of their families, etc.)(45.8%)
S29 [54]: Rachakonda K, et al., 2015 QS: 1	Australia	Inpatients	Questionnaire survey	Sampling: unclear Eligible sample: unclear Sample size:75 Age (yr): 68 ± 12 Gender: 32/75 (F)	Advanced cancer patients (mixed cancer sites)	NR	Needs Assessment of Advanced Cancer Patients (NA-ACP): 7 domains and 132 items Items of highest unmet needs by each domain: 1) symptom "dealing with lack of energy or tiredness" (30.7%); 2) psychological "coping with frustration at not being able to do the things you used to do" (24.3%); 3) daily livings "getting assistance with preparing meals" (12%); 4) social "receiving emotional support from friends and family" (12.2%); 5) medical information and communication (9.3–14.9%), "getting information about non-conventional treatments" (14.9%); 6) financial "paying the non-medical costs of your illness"; (17.3%); 7) spiritual "being able to choose the place where you want to die" (11%).
S30 [55]: Rainbird K, et al. 2009 QS: 3	Australia	Home-based	Questionnaire survey	Sampling: unclear Sample size: 246 Age (yr): 61 ± 11.9 Gender: 131/246 (F)	Advanced cancer patients (mixed cancer sites)	246/418 (59%)	Needs Assessment of Advanced Cancer Patients (NA-ACP): 7 domains and 132 items Items of highest unmet needs by each domain: 1) symptom (15–22%)' "dealing with loss of appetite" (22%); 2) psychological (39–40%), "coping with fears about the caner spreading" (40%) and "coping with frustration at not being able to do the things you used to do" (40%); 3) daily livings (10–30%), "dealing with doing work around the house" (30%); 4) social (10–13%),

Table 2 Characteristics and Main Findings of the Included Studies *(Continued)*

Author, Year & QS	Country/ Region	Setting	Study Design	Participant	Diagnosis	Response Rate	Data Collection Method/ Instrument & Findings
							"being able to express feeling with friends and/or family" (13%); 5) medical information and communication (31–35%), "getting information about factors, which could influence the course of the cancer" (35%); 6) financial (11–12%), "dealing with concerns about your financial situation" (12%); 7) spiritual (11–15%), "being able to choose the place where you want to die" (15%)
S33 [58]: Au A, et al., 2013, QS: 4	Hong Kong	Outpatients	Questionnaire survey	Sampling: consecutive sampling Sample size: 198 Age (yr): 53.4 ± 9.74 Gender: 198/ 198 (F)	Advanced breast cancer patients (stage III/IV)	198/220 (90%)	Chinese version of Supportive Care Needs Survey (SCNS-SF33-C): 4 domains and 33 items: physical and daily living, psychological, sexuality, health system, information and patient support (HSIPS) Hospital Anxiety and Depression Scale (HADS) Memorial Symptom Assessment Scale Short-Form (MSAS-SF) Chinese Patient Satisfaction Questionnaire
							Top 10 moderate-to-high unmet needs: 1) "Having one member of hospital staff with whom you can talk to about your concerns" (63.7%); 2) "informed about cancer is under control or diminishing" (61.6%); 3) "Informed about things you can do to get well" (58.6%); 4) "Informed about your test results" (51%); 5) "Given written information" (46.9%); 6) "given information about aspects of managing illness and side-effects at home" (39.9%); 7) "adequately information about the benefits and side-effects of treatments" (39.3%); 8) "given explanations of those tests for which you would like explanations" (36.9%); 9) "being treated like a person" (35.4%); 10) "more choice about cancer specialists" (31.8%)
S35 [60]: Aranda S, et al., 2005 QS: 4	Australia	Outpatients	Questionnaire survey	Sampling: consecutive sampling Sample size: 105 Age (yr): (34–85, median 57) Gender: 105/ 105(F)	Metastatic breast cancer	105/172 (61%)	Supportive Care Needs Questionnaire (SCNQ): 5 domains and 59 items
							Moderate to high unmet needs: 1)Psychological needs (24–41%): "concerns about the worries of those close to you" (41%), "uncertainty about the future" (38%), etc. 2)Information needs (26–41%): "informed about things you can do to help yourself get well" (41%), "one member of hospital staff with whom you can talk" (32%), etc. 3)Physical and daily living needs (25–28%): "pain" (28%), "not being

Table 2 Characteristics and Main Findings of the Included Studies *(Continued)*

Author, Year & QS	Country/ Region	Setting	Study Design	Participant	Diagnosis	Response Rate	Data Collection Method/ Instrument & Findings
							able to do the things you used to" (25%).
S36 [61]: Lelorain S, et al., 2015 QS: 2	France	NR	Questionnaire survey	Sampling: consecutive sampling Sample size: 201 Age (yr): mean 62 Gender: 146/ 201 (F)	Metastatic cancer (mixed cancer sites)	NR	Adapted Supportive Care Needs Survey (SCNS): 2 domains and 13 items: psychological dimension, and staff-related dimension. Seven-point scale (1–7): 1 = no need at all, 7 = a total need of help
							Unmet needs: 1) psychological needs: "being informed about things you can do to help yourself to get well" (3.83 ± 2.24), etc. 2) staff-related needs: "being informed about your test results as soon as feasible"(3.44 ± 2.27), etc.
S40 [65]: Gu WJ, et al., 2015 QS: 3	Shanghai, China	Inpatients	Questionnaire survey	Sampling: convenience sampling Sample size: 134 Age (yr): 75.9 ± 10.5 Gender: 62/ 134 (F)	Advance cancer (mixed cancer sites)	134/134 (100%)	Self-designed questionnaire for needs including 4 parts (26 items) (p. 2656): basic information, quality of life, health care service needs and attitudes towards disease and death
							Needs: 1) psychological (47%); 2) daily living (31.3%); 3) spiritual (13.4%); 4) families' support and accompany (67.9%); 5) needs of volunteers (18.7%); 6) friends' support and accompany (59%)
S41 [66]: Huang J, et al., 2008 QS: 3	Shanghai, China	Home-based	Questionnaire survey	Sampling: random sampling Sample size: 113 Age (yr): 58.31 ± 8.7 Gender: 54/ 113 (F)	Advance cancer (cancer sites unclear)	113/116 (97.4%)	Self-designed questionnaire for needs including (items: not described)
							Needs on community wards: (pp. 34–35) 1) treatment care like transfusion, injection (77%); 2) pain (46.9%); 3) constipation, nausea (45.1%); 4) information about disease (37.2%) and rehabilitation (32.7%), psychological like anxiety (38.9%), sense of fear (20.4%). Needs on home-based care: 1) treatment care like transfusion, injection (71.7%); 2) regular health assessment (43.4%); 3) knowledge about nutrition (31.0%) and care skills (23.9%), pain (36.3%), communication (28.3%). Needs on day care center: 1) treatment care like transfusion, injection (69%); 2) regular health assessment (42.5%); 3) information and education (28.3%); 4) communication (18.6%); 5) nutrition (38.9%)
S43 [68]: Waller A, et al., 2012 QS: 2	Australia	Mixed	Multi-center questionnaire survey	Sampling: unclear Sample size: 219 patients NAT: PD-Cs were completed on 120 patients	Advance cancer (cancer sites unclear)	36%	Needs Assessment Tool: Progressive Disease-Cancer (NAT: PD-C): 4 sections and 18 items (significant)
							Overall: 80% had at least one concern Patients' well-being: 1) physical:58%

Table 2 Characteristics and Main Findings of the Included Studies *(Continued)*

Author, Year & QS	Country/ Region	Setting	Study Design	Participant	Diagnosis	Response Rate	Data Collection Method/ Instrument & Findings
				Age (yr): 66.1 ± 10.7 Gender: 90/ 198 (F)			2) daily living: 29% 3) psychological:19%
S44 [69]: Templeton, H, et al., 2003 QS: 4	UK	Home-based	Structured interview survey	Sampling: unclear Sample size: 90 Age (yr): 71–80 (48.9%) Gender: 90 (M)	Advance prostate cancer	79%	Adapted Toronto Information Needs Questionnaire (TINQ-BC): 5 domains and 29 items Unmet needs: 82.2% of the patients need more information: 1) "side effects of treatment" (66.7%); 2) "how to ease side effects of treatment" (64.4%)
S45 [70]: Hwang, S, et al., 2004 QS:3	USA	Mixed	Questionnaire survey	Sampling: consecutive sampling Sample size: 296 Age (yr): median 68 (29–96) Gender: 296 (M)	Advance cancer (mixed cancer sites)	296/312 (94.9%)	14-item unmet needs questionnaire: 5 domains and 14 items Unmet needs: 1) physical: 46.1–80%; 2) emotional/social: 10.1–32.5%; 3) economic: 6.6–17.3% 4) medical: 12.5–13.6% 5) community: 0–14.3%
S46 [71]: Murray, SA, et al., 2004 QS: 4	UK	Outpatients	Semi-structured interview	Sampling: purposive sampling Sample size: 20 Age (yr): median 65 Gender: unclear	Advance lung cancer	NA	Semi-structured interview, 40mins-2 h, tape recorded Unmet needs: 1) "fear, distress and uncertainty" (p. 41) 2) review "what they had achieved, what still needed to be done before death" (p. 42), and establish themselves as they 'really' are (p. 41) 3) "feeling of loss of control" (p. 42) 4) "hard to find hope," and "questioned their faith wonder why God had not heeded their prayers" (p.42)
S47 [72]: Soelver L, et al., 2014 QS: 4	Denmark	Inpatients	Semi-structured interview	Sampling: open and strategic sampling Sample size: 11 Age (yr): median 71.3 (54–86) Gender: 7/11 (F)	Advance cancer (mixed cancer sites)	NA	Semi-structured interview, 30mins-1 h Unmet needs (pp. 177–180): 1) professionals failed to provide patients timely information; 2) patients experienced that "professionals failed to give much help in terms of physical and emotional burden"; 3) Not being regarded as a person: "lack of dialogue with professionals make patients feel neglected and uncertain in the sense of belonging"; 4) autonomy: "patients wanted to be proactive in problem solving, but did not know how to do"; 5) lack of help for their physical and emotional problem
S48 [73]: Cater N, et al., 2011 QS: 2	Canada	Outpatients	Semi-structured focus group and in-depth interview	Sampling: unclear Sample size: 29	Advance prostate cancer	NA	Semi-structured focus group (90–120 min) and in-depth interview (30–60 min), tape recorded Unmet needs (pp. 191–193):

Table 2 Characteristics and Main Findings of the Included Studies *(Continued)*

Author, Year & QS	Country/ Region	Setting	Study Design	Participant	Diagnosis	Response Rate	Data Collection Method/ Instrument & Findings
				Age (yr): mean 75 (59–88) Gender: 29 (M)			1) function issues: pain, fatigue, side (e. g., urinary incontinence issues, loss of sexual function, etc.); 2) information needs of treatment, medication, side effects and health care service etc.; 3) emotional distress: sadness, anger, frustration and regret which associated with some unsolved issues about diagnosis and treatment decisions.
S49 [74]: Christ G, et al., 1990 QS: 1	USA	Outpatients	Interview survey	Sampling: unclear Sample size: 200 Age (yr): 45–64 (54%) Gender: 62% (F)	Advance cancer (mixed cancer sites)	NR	Structured in-depth telephone interview (30 min) Unmet needs (p. 762): 1) personal: 6%; 2) instrumental: 43%; 3) administrative: 38%; 4) medical:18%
S50 [75]: Lam W. W.T, ET AL., 2014 QS: 4	Hong Kong	Outpatients	Questionnaire survey (longitudinal)	Sampling: consecutive sampling Sample size: 228 Age (yr): 53.4 ± 9.79 Gender: 228 (F)	Advance breast cancer (stage III/IV)	228/262 (87.0%)	Supportive Care Needs Survey-Chinese version (SCNS-SF33): 4 domains and 33 items Hospital Anxiety and Depression scale (HADS): 14 items Memorial Symptom Assessment Scale Short-form (MSAS-SF)- Chinese version: 32 items Top 10 Moderate-to-high unmet needs: 1) "Having one member of staff with whom you can talk to about all aspects of your condition" (64.5%), 2) "Being informed about cancer which is under control" (60.4%), 3) "Being informed about things you can do to help yourself to get well" (57.4%), 4) "Being informed about your test results as soon as feasible" (50.8%), 5) "Being given written information about the important aspects of your care" (42.3%), 6) "Being adequately informed about the benefits and side effects of treatments before you choose to have them" (42.3%), 7) "Being given explanations of those tests for which you would like explanations" (37.6%), 8) "Being treated like a person not just another case" (34.5%), 9) "Being given information about aspects of managing your illness and side effects at home" (34.2%), 10) "More choice about which cancer specialists you see" (30.5%).

Studies Regarding Informal Caregivers (*n* = 12)

Author, Year & QS	Region	Setting	Study Design	Participants	Diagnosis	Response Rate	Data Collection Method/ Instrument
S4 [30]: Osse BHP, et al., 2006 QS: 3	Netherlands	Home-based	Questionnaire survey	Sampling: unclear? Sample size: 81 Age (yr): mean 54y (28-78y)	Informal caregivers of mixed advanced cancer patients (distant metastasis)	76/81 (93.8%)	Problems and Needs in Palliative Care questionnaire-caregiver form (PNPC-c): 67 items Unmet needs (top 10): 1) "knowing physical signs what I should notice" (25%), 2) "lacking of

Table 2 Characteristics and Main Findings of the Included Studies *(Continued)*

Author, Year & QS	Country/ Region	Setting	Study Design	Participant	Diagnosis	Response Rate	Data Collection Method/ Instrument & Findings
				Gender: 30/76 (F)			information in writing" (23%); 3) "fear of an unpredictable future" (22%), 4) "difficulty in coordinating the care of different professionals" (22%), 5) "difficulty in getting access to help from agencies/ professional organizations" (22%); 6) "difficulty in getting a second opinion from another doctor" (21%), 7) "how I should handle the patient's pain" (21%), 8) "extra expenditure because of the disease" (17%), 9) "insufficient adjustment of hospital care to the home situation" (17%), 10) "the possibility to choosing another care provider" (14%) Information needs: information on 1) "the physical problems" (69%), 2) "expectations for the future" (59%), 3) "the possibilities of treatment and side effects" (52%); 4) "euthanasia" (41%); 5) "cause on cancer"(39%), 6) "on nourishment" (37%); 7) "on places and agency that provide help" (30%); 8) "aids to help me" (29%)
S6 [32]: Park SM, et al., 2010 QS: 1	South Korea	NR	Questionnaire survey (retrospective)	Sampling: unclear? Sample size: 1662 Age (yr): not report Gender: 1099/ 1662 (F)	Informal caregivers of mixed advanced cancer patients (patients died)	1662/4042 (41.4%)	Self-designed needs questionnaire: including 5 domains: 1) symptom management, 2) psychosocial support, 3) financial support, (4) community support, including volunteer assistance, and 5) religious support.. (p.701)
							Unmet needs (p. 703): 1) symptom support (42.8%), 2) financial support (42.7%), 3) psychological support (20.6%), 4) community support (19.7%), and 5) religious support (3.8%)
S9 [35]: Chen SC, et al., 2016 QS: 4	Taiwan	Mixed	Questionnaire survey	Sampling: consecutive sampling Sample size: 166 Age (yr): 49.6 ± 12.0 Gender: 71/ 166 (F)	Informal caregivers of advanced lung cancer patients	166/190 (87.4%)	1) Partners and Caregivers supportive care needs survey (SCNS-P&C):6 domains and 44 items 2) Numerical rating scale (NRS) (0–10, 0 = no fatigue or sleep disturbance, 10 = worst imaginable): fatigue or sleep disturbance
							Top 10 unmet needs: 1) "Managing concerns about the cancer coming back" (78.3%); 2) "Addressing fears about the person with cancer's physical or mental deterioration" (72.3%); 3) "Ensuring there is an ongoing case manager to coordinate services for the person with cancer" (71.1%); 4) "Accessing information on what the person with cancer's physical needs are likely to be" (68.7%); 5) "Accessing information about the person with cancer's prognosis, or likely outcome" (65.1%); 6) "Accessing information about the

Table 2 Characteristics and Main Findings of the Included Studies *(Continued)*

Author, Year & QS	Country/ Region	Setting	Study Design	Participant	Diagnosis	Response Rate	Data Collection Method/ Instrument & Findings
							benefits and side-effects of treatments so you can participate in decision making about the person with cancer's treatment" (62.1%); 7) "Obtaining adequate pain control for the person with cancer" (61.5%); 8) "Finding out about financial support and government benefits for you and/or the person with cancer" (60.9%); 9) "Understanding the experience of the person with cancer" (58.5%); 10) "Reducing stress in the person with cancer's life" (56.1%)
S13 [9]: Cui J, et al., 2014 QS: 4	Shanghai, China	Inpatients	Questionnaire survey	Sampling: convenience sampling Sample size: 649 Age (yr): 49.2 ± 13.18 Gender: 369/ 649 (F)	Family caregivers of mixed advanced cancer patients (stage IV)	649/700 (95.6%)	Self-designed needs questionnaire: 7 dimensions and 36 items (p. 567) Cronbach's α = 0.902 Scores of Needs (p. 567): 1) "maintaining health" (3.48 ± 1.04); 2) "support from professionals" (4.11 ± 0.84); 3) "knowledge about disease and treatment" (4.37 ± 0.81); 4) "funeral support" (2.85 ± 1.30); 5) "information for hospice care" (3.01 ± 1.14); 6) "psychological support from patients" (3.08 ± 1.18); 7) "symptom control for patients" (4.26 ± 0.95); 8) overall (3.6 ± 0.75)
S14 [39]: Fukui S,2004 QS: 2	Japan	Inpatients	Questionnaire survey	Sampling: convenience sampling Sample size: 66 Age (yr): 55.6 ± 12.1 Gender: 46/66 (F)	Family caregivers of mixed advanced cancer patients	66/125 (52.8%)	Self-designed information needs questionnaire: 7 items Information needs (p. 32): Disease-related Information 1) Information on disease (54, 82%); 2) Information on treatment (48, 73%); 3) Information on prognosis (43,65%) Care-related information 1) Patients' physical care (40, 61%); 2) Patients' psychological care (33,56%); 3) Family care (31,47%)
S15 [40]: Dubenske LL, et al., 2008 QS: 3	USA	NR	Questionnaire survey	Sampling: convenience sampling Sample size: 159 Age (yr): 50.28 ± 12.91 Gender: 159/ 159 (F)	Informal female caregivers of mixed advanced cancer patients	NR	Self-designed Cancer Caregiver Needs Checklist: 9 domains and 104 items Information needs (p. 269): 1) Disease/ medical (0.59 ± 0.29); 2) Caregiving (0.56 ± 0.27); 3) Relating with the patient (0.59 ± 0.31) 4) Caregiver well-being (0.41 ± 0.30); 5) Financial/legal (0.28 ± 0.35); 6) Family and close others (0.42 ± 0.33) 7) Future outlook (0.42 ± 0.39); 8) Dying (0.48 ± 0.33); 9) Spirituality (0.19 ± 0.27)
S24 [49]: Mangan PA, et al. 2003 QS: 3	USA	NR	Qualitative study (focus group)	Sample size: 32 Active caregivers (n = 17)	Informal caregivers of mixed advanced cancer patients (metastasis)	56/60 (93.3%)	Semi-structured focus groups interview (audiotaped) and constant-comparative for analysis Unmet needs (p. 247): 1) Medical care such as provision of information, coordination of care; 2) quality of life (caregiver

Table 2 Characteristics and Main Findings of the Included Studies *(Continued)*

Author, Year & QS	Country/ Region	Setting	Study Design	Participant	Diagnosis	Response Rate	Data Collection Method/ Instrument & Findings
				Bereaved caregivers (*n* = 15) Sampling: unclear			well-being including physical and emotional, caregivers roles); 3) help from others (practical assistance and social support) 4) unsolicited needs such as non-professional information needs, impacts on their family
S26 [51]: Joad ASK, et al., 2011 QS: 2	India	Mixed	Interview survey with semi-structured questionnaire	Sampling: unclear Sample size: 56 Age (yr): 36 caregivers aged 30–60 Gender: unclear	Family caregivers 3–6 months after the death of patients (cancer sites unclear)	NR	Semi-structured questionnaire Unmet needs (pp. 192–193): 1) Medical needs: "lack of home -care services" (17%); "training in "care giving"" (71%); "need for an admission to a hospice/hospital" (40%). 2) Psychological needs: 1) "felling of tense" (39%); 2) "anxious" (17%); 3) "depressed" (32%); 3) Financial needs: "need financial help from other families or friends" (55.6%); 4) Information needs: "help in communicating disease status and prognosis with their loved one" (35%); 5) Social needs: "lack of social life" (71.4%); "affected the relationships and interactions with others" (42.9%)
S27 [52]: Buck HG, et al., 2008 QS: 2	USA	Home-based	Questionnaire survey	Sampling: unclear Sample size: 110 Age (yr): 64.7 ± 14.6 Gender: 83/ 110 (F)	Informal caregivers of mixed advanced cancer patients	NR	Spiritual Needs Inventory (SNI): 17 items Top 10 unmet needs of each item: 1) "be with family" (20%); 2) "laugh"(16%); 3) "be with friends"(12%); 4) "see smiles of others"(12%), 5) 'think happy thoughts'(11%), 6) "be around children" (10%); 7) "go to religious services" (10%); 8) "talk about day-to-day things" (8%); 9) "read inspirational materials" (8%), 10) "talk with someone about spiritual issues" (6%)
S32 [57]: Carter N, et al., 2010 QS: 3	USA	Mixed	Qualitative study (semi-structured in-depth interview and focus group)	Sampling: unclear Sample size: 19 (16 wives, 3 children) Gender: unclear	Family caregivers of advanced prostate cancer	NA	Semi-structured in-depth interview (40–90 min) and focus group (60–90 min), audiotaped Needs (pp. 167–168): 1) informational needs regarding disease, treatment, side effects and care services, etc. 2) "uncertainty about the future" 3) caregiver burden including supporting the physical, functional and emotions needs of patients 4) "practical assistance needs like household chores" 5) "feelings of isolation as lack of social activities"
S37 [62]: Lee HT, et al., 2013 QS: 3	Taiwan	Home-based	Qualitative study (in-depth interview)	Sampling: consecutive sampling Sample size: 44	Family caregivers of terminal cancer patients (mixed cancer sites)	44/49 (89.8%)	In-depth interview with open-ended questionnaire (30–40 min) (tape recorded) Needs: 1) Emotional support from families and professionals including listening, encouragement, etc. 2) Information needs regarding "symptom management, nutrition,

Table 2 Characteristics and Main Findings of the Included Studies *(Continued)*

Author, Year & QS	Country/ Region	Setting	Study Design	Participant	Diagnosis	Response Rate	Data Collection Method/ Instrument & Findings
							concerns about dying, medication and nursing aids" (p. 633).
S39 [64]: Chen HY, et al.,2008 QS: 2	Shanghai, China	Inpatients	Questionnaire survey	Sampling: convenience sampling Sample size: 89 Age (yr): (23–72, median 52.1) Gender: 58/89 (F)	Family caregivers of advanced cancer patients (cancer sites unclear)	89/100 (89.0%)	Self-designed questionnaire (unclear items) Needs (p. 19): 1) prognosis of disease (100%); 2) help to realize patient's wishes(100%); 3) continuous support after discharge from hospital(100%); 4) knowledge of self-care(100%); 5) relevant knowledge of disease(98.9%); 6) regular counseling service (84.3%); 7) emotional support(69.7%); 8) pain management of patients(59.6%); 9) accompany (50.6%)

Studies Regarding Both Advanced Cancer Patients and their Informal Caregivers (*n* = 5)

Author, Year & QS	Region	Setting	Study Design	Participants	Diagnosis	Response Rate	Data Collection Method/ Instrument & Findings
S23 [48]: Dehghan R, et al., 2012 QS: 4	Bangladesh	Outpatients	Qualitative study (in-depth interview)	Sampling: convenience sampling Sample size: 20 Patients (n = 3), Family members (*n* = 9), Clinical staffs (n = 8)	Advanced breast cancer and family members	NA	Semi-structured in-depth interview with open-ended questions (tape recorded) and qualitative description for analysis Needs (pp. 147–148): 1) "social needs of patients and families" due to financial impact, economic uncertainty and needs for social security; 2) "psychological and spiritual needs of patients and families": feeling of sadness, anxiety, anger, abandonment, fear and hopeless; 3) "need for information among patients and families". 4) "Access to and receipt of care from professional systems and providers"
S31 [56]: Wong RK, et al., 2002 QS: 2	Canada	Outpatients	Questionnaire survey	Sampling: unclear Sample size: 144 Patients: *n* = 71 Caregivers: *n* = 73 Age (yr): Patients: unclear Caregivers: unclear Gender: unclear	Mixed advanced cancer patients and their caregivers	144/264 (55%)	Advanced Cancer Information Needs Survey (ACIN): 22 items Needs for patients: 1) "pain control" (75%), 2) "weakness and fatigue" (58%), 3) "shortness of breath" (52%), 4) "what cause cancer" (48%), 5) "home care services" (46%), 6) "communicating with loved ones" (46%) Needs for caregivers: 1) "pain control" (82%), 2) "weakness and fatigue" (66%), 3) "home care services" (58%), 3) "what cause cancer" (53%), 4) "how can we prevent cancer" (58%), 5) "why are some cancers not curable" (56%)
S34 [59]: Hwang SS, et al., 2003 QS: 4	USA	Mixed	Questionnaire survey	Sampling: consecutive sampling Sample size: 100	Informal caregivers of advanced cancer patients (cancer sites unclear)	100/ 149 (67.1%)	The Family Inventory of Needs (FIN): 20 items Caregiver's Perception of Patients' Unmet Needs (PPUN): 14 items Perception of Patients' Unmet Needs (PPUN):

Table 2 Characteristics and Main Findings of the Included Studies *(Continued)*

Author, Year & QS	Country/ Region	Setting	Study Design	Participant	Diagnosis	Response Rate	Data Collection Method/ Instrument & Findings
				Age (yr): (27–85, median 62) Gender: unclear			1) physical (80%), 2) nutritional (51%), 3) daily living (44%), 4) emotional (33%). Caregiver unmet needs (FIN): 1) "having information about what to do for the patient at home" (37%); 2) "knowing when to expect symptoms to occur" (31%); 3) "being told about people who could help with problems" (26%); 4) "knowing the probable outcome of the patient's illness" (26%)
S38 [63]: Liu Y, 2008 QS: 3	Shanghai, China	Home-based	Questionnaire survey	Sampling: convenience sampling Sample size: 400 Age (yr): Patients:60.61 ± 12.67 Caregivers: 56.04 ± 12.57 Gender: Patients:63/ 115(F) Caregivers:29/ 113(F)	Mixed cancer patients at stage III/ IV and their caregivers	228/400 (57%) (patients:115, caregiver:113)	Self-designed needs questionnaire for advanced cancer patients and their caregivers Needs for patients (pp. 30–31): 1) psychological: families' understanding and support(96.5%), etc. 2) Physical care: information of treatment, rehabilitation (80.9%), etc. 3) Social: peer activities and support (54.8%), etc. Needs for caregivers (p. 38): 1) psychological: communication with families and professionals (76.1%), etc. 2) social: information about treatment and prognosis(81.4%) etc. 3) educational: medication guidance(80.5%) etc.
S42 [67]: Miu J, et al., 2016 QS: 2	Shanghai, China	Inpatients	Questionnaire survey	Sampling: unclear Sample size: 42 (42 patients and 42 family caregivers) Age (yr): Patients:72.9 ± 11.6 Caregivers: 55.9 ± 13.45 Gender: Patients:18/42 (F) Caregivers:23/ 42 (F)	Mixed advanced cancer patients and their caregivers	42/45 (93.3%)	Self-designed needs questionnaire for advanced cancer patients and their caregivers [63] Needs for patients (p. 2387): 1) "families' understanding and support" (2.43 ± 0.59); 2) "relieving constipation" (2.38 ± 0.62) 3) "psychological support for caregivers after the death of themselves" (2.36 ± 0.66); 4) "pain assessment" (2.33 ± 0.61); 5) "pain management" (2.31 ± 0.64); 6) "improving appetite" (2.31 ± 0.6) Needs for caregivers: 1) "dietary and nutrition" (2.38 ± 0.66); 2) "guidance about how to help patients do activities" (2.38 ± 0.66); 3) "pain assessment" (2.38 ± 0.73); 4) "communication between families and professionals" (2.36 ± 0.58); 5) "information about treatment and prognosis" (2.33 ± 0.65)

Notes 1: QS: overall quality score; ADL: Activities of daily living; M: male; F: female; G1: group1; G2: group2; G3: group3; EC: Esophageal; PBC: Pancreaticobiliary; EORTC QLQ-OES18: EORTC QLQ-Esophagus (OES) 18 (Esophagus cancer module) questionnaire; EORTC QLQ-PAN26: EORTC QLQ-Pancreatic (PAN) 26 (Pancreatic cancer module) questionnaire; EORTC QLQ-C30: European Organization for Research and Treatment of Cancer Quality of Life Core 30; a: only the baseline data was used in this review

Notes 2: in the "Data Collection Method/ Instrument & Findings" column, direct quotations from several included quantitative studies using commonly utilized research scales with documented psychometric properties were details of each of the used research questionnaire items. Thus, information regarding page numbers was not provided, but that for direct quotations from studies using self-designed semi-structured questionnaires and/or qualitative methods, as well as page numbers for such quotations, was provided

Table 3 Overall unmet needs domains and prevalence ranges of prominent items by each domain (Patients)

Domains	Number of studies	Subdomains/ items	Prevalence ranges
Physical	22	Fatigue	18–76.3% [6, 31, 33, 34, 42, 43, 45, 47, 51, 54, 56, 63]
		Pain	18–75% [6, 31, 33, 36, 45, 47, 50, 60, 66]
		Sleep problems	21.1–37.1% [28, 47]
		Dyspnea	19–67.3% [36, 45, 56]
		Lack of appetite	13–80% [45, 50, 55, 63]
		gastrointestinal symptoms	12–45.1% [45, 66]
		"Felling unwell a lot of the time"	17.3–44.7% [6, 33, 50]
Activities of Daily Living (ADL)	11	"not being able to do the things you used to do"	19–46.9% [6, 33, 50, 58, 60]
		"Work around the home"	18.6–44.2% [6, 33, 50, 55]
Psychological	25	"Uncertainty about the future"	21.4–62.4% [6, 31, 33, 41, 60]
		Emotional Support	10.1–84.4% [6, 28, 29, 31, 33, 36, 41, 45, 46, 50, 70, 72, 73] (Anxiety [6, 33]: 15.3–41.8%; Depression [31, 33, 41, 50]:15–62.4%)
		"worry that the results of treatment are beyond your control"	19–71.8% [6, 41, 50, 58, 60]
		"Feeling about death and dying"	32.5–62.4% [33, 41]
		"Fears about the cancer spreading"	17.6–78.8% [6, 31, 41, 42, 47, 50, 55]
		"concerns about the worries of those close to you"	27.9–68.2% [6, 33, 41, 50, 60]
		"Support in coping"	24.3–57.5% [29, 54, 55]
		"Learning to feel in control of your situation"	32.5–56.5% [33, 41]
		"Fear of physical suffering"	16.7–62.9% [31, 34, 36, 47, 50]
Social	9	family and friends' support	9.9–96.5% [29, 45, 54, 55, 63, 65, 67]
		volunteers	18.7% [65]
Communication	5	Communication	7.7–87.9% [28, 29, 56, 63, 66]
Financial	8	Financial	6.6–72% [28, 31, 36, 43, 46, 54, 55, 70]
Spiritual	5	Meaning of death	15–85.4% [31, 36]
		Religious	44% [43]
		"being able to choose the place where you want to die"	11–15% [54, 55]
Autonomy	5	"I can do less than before"	17–83% [31, 34, 43]
		"experiencing loss of control over one's life"	16–19% [31, 47]
Patients care and support	3	"Reassurance by medical staff that the way you feel is normal"	32.5–56.5% [33, 41]
		"doctor acknowledges and shows sensitivity to your feelings and emotional needs"	34.8–39.5% [33, 42]
Healthcare service and information	14	"Being informed about things you can do to help yourself to get well"	41–65.9% [33, 41, 42, 60, 75]
		"Having one member of hospital staff with whom you can talk to"	32–72% [33, 41, 75, 58, 75]
		"Being informed about your test results as soon as feasible"	50.8–62.5% [41, 42, 75]
		"benefit and side-effects of treatment"	4–66.7% [31, 41, 42, 44, 54, 63, 66, 69, 75]
		"Being given written information about the important aspects of your care"	42.3–52.9% [41, 75]
		"Being treated like a person not just another case"	34.5–54.1% [37, 41, 61, 75]
		"Being informed about cancer which is under control"	54.1–60.4% [41, 75]
Sexuality	4	Sexuality	5–75% [31, 36, 45, 58]

Table 3 Overall unmet needs domains and prevalence ranges of prominent items by each domain (Patients) *(Continued)*

Domains	Number of studies	Subdomains/ items	Prevalence ranges
Nutrition	2	Nutrition	38.9–43.2% [28, 66]
Counseling	1		17–24% [31]

Notes: Needs items (sentences or phrases) which were put in the quotation marks were directly extracted from the corresponding included studies

from professional staff" (information needs) [48, 72, 73], "*need more social security*" (social needs) [48], and "not being regarded as a person" (p. 178) (healthcare service and information needs) [72]. However, the needs in qualitative studies were more detailed than those in quantitative studies, and the specific causes of unmet needs were identified. For example, patients elaborated that "lack of dialogue with the professionals led some patients to feel neglected and uncertain in their sense of belonging" (p. 178) [72] was the cause of "not being regarded as a person" (p. 178). Additionally, "*sadness, anger, frustration and regret*" resulted from "*some unsolved issues about diagnosis and treatment decisions*" [73]. Several unmet needs identified from the qualitative data were not identified in quantitative studies. For instance, subjects expressed "what they had achieved in their lives and what still needed to be done before death" (p. 42), "establish themselves as they 'really' are" (p. 41) (spiritual needs) [71], and "patients want to *be proactive* in problem solving" (p. 179), but they did not know how to do it (autonomy needs) [72].

Descriptions of unmet needs in informal caregivers

Seven unmet need domains were extracted on the basis of qualitative (*n* = 4) and quantitative (*n* = 13) studies.

In terms of the quantitative studies, the sample size ranged from 42 to 1662, with the mean sample size being 259. The response rates ranged from 41.4 to 95.6%. Seven domains, including information, physical, psychological, financial, cancer care service, spiritual, and social needs, were identified. Information domain included two subdomains, namely, illness and treatment and care-related information. Unmet needs regarding illness and treatment information were mentioned in nine studies, and the prevalence ranged from 26 to 100% [9, 30, 35, 39, 40, 51, 56, 67, 63]. Care-related information was reported in 10 studies with the prevalence rate in the range of 21–100% [9, 30, 35, 39, 40, 51, 59, 63, 64, 67]. With regard to cancer care services, 21–72.3% of the informal caregivers presented unmet needs in terms of quality of care [29, 30, 35], and 14–100% reported unmet needs on transitional care services [30, 32, 51, 64]. The percentages of the five other domains, including physical, psychological, financial, spiritual, and social unmet needs, were 42.8% [32], 17–78.3% [32, 35, 51, 63, 64], 17–67.3% [30, 32, 35, 51], 3.8–100% [30, 32, 52, 64], and 42.9–71.4% [51], respectively. Furthermore, "managing concerns about the cancer coming back" (78.3%) [35],

"finding out about financial support and government benefits for you and/or the person with cancer" (60.9%) [35], "help to realize patient's wishes" (100%) [64], and "lack of social life" (71.4%) [51] were reported as the most common psychological, financial, spiritual, and social needs.

According to four qualitative studies [48, 49, 57, 62], three similar unmet need domains, namely, informational, psychological, and social needs, were identified through summative content analysis. Informal caregivers commonly stated about "*unmet information needs in terms of disease, treatment, side effects, care services, symptom management, nutrition, medication and nursing aids*" (informational) [48, 57, 62], "*feelings of sadness and loneliness, as well as a sense of abandonment, fear and helplessness*" (p. 147) [48] or "*insufficient listening and encouragement from other family members and professionals*" [62] (psychological), and "*feelings of isolation due to the lack of social activities*" (social) [57]. Several specific unmet needs, including the manner of communication between professional staff and caregivers or patients, the administration and function of the healthcare system, and some practical assistance, such as cleaning the house and walking the dog [49], were also identified in qualitative studies [49].

Variables associated with the unmet needs of patients with advanced cancer

Variables associated with the unmet needs of patients with advanced cancer are summarized in Table 4. Relevant variables were categorized as patient-related variables (demographics, disease-related, physical, and psychological) and informal caregiver-related variables (age, gender, and psychological distress of informal caregivers).

In several studies, age, gender, marital status, education level, and income level were insignificantly associated with patients' unmet needs. Although a significant relationship was reported, results were inconsistent across studies in terms of age and marital status. With regards to gender, three studies [28, 33, 63] reported that female patients indicated more physical and psychological unmet needs than those of male patients. Patients who were living alone experienced high psychological needs [28], and patients with high educational level presented considerable unmet needs in physical [42], ADL [42], information [44], community service [46], and sexuality [58] domains. Moreover, financial needs were less reported in patients with high income [46, 63].

Table 4 Summary of the variables associated with advanced cancer patients' unmet needs

Study	Demographics						Physical		Disease-related			Psychosocial			Caregiver		
	Older	Female	Living alone	Married	High education	High income	Physical	ADL (dependent)	Cancer sites	Stage	Treatment	Anxiety	Depression	High QOL	Distress (anxiety/ depression)	Older	Female
[28]	+ (phy)	+ (psy, com)	+ (psy)	- (psy, com)	↔			+ (info, com, psy, occup)	↔								
[29]	- (phy, psys, com)																
[31]	-(fin, psys,)																
[33]	↔	+ (phy, ADL)		+ (phy, psys, ADL)								+(phy, psys, ADL)					
[41]	↔											+ (psy, phy, ADL, HSIPS)		-(psy, phy, ADL, HSIPS)			
[42]	-(psy)	↔			+ (phy ADL)		+ (phy, psys, ADL)			↕	↕	+ (psy, ADL,phy, HSIPS)	-(HSIPS) +(psy)				
[43]														- (phy, psy, spiri)			
[44]	↔	↔		-(info)	+(info)						↕	+(info)	↕				
[46]	- (phy, psys, fin)	↔		↕	+ (comm- unity)	- (fin)			+/↔ *	↕	↕		↕				
[58]	↔			- (phy, ADL) +(sex)	+ (sex)	↕	+ (phy, ADL, psy, HSIPS)			↕	-(HSIPS)	+ (psy)	↕				
[63]	-(phy)	+ (phy)		-(phy, soc)		–			+/↔ *	+					+		
[70]	-(phy, fin,med)						+(phy,psy fin,med)		↕	+			+(psy,fin,med)			-(psy)	-(psy)
[75]							+ (HSIPS, psy, phy, ADL)			↕	+ (psy)						

Notes: "-": negative relationship; "+": positive relationship; "↔": no significant relationship; "*": relationship variable across different types of cancer; "fin": financial needs; "PM": pain management; "soc": social needs; "phy": physical needs; "psy":psychological needs; "psys": psychosocial needs; "occup": occupational needs; "HSIPS": health system, information, and patient care support; "med": medical needs; "spiri": spiritual needs

Four studies [42, 58, 70, 75] explored the relationships between symptom distress and unmet needs, and all these studies showed that patients with symptom distress experienced more unmet needs in the psychological, physical, and ADL domains. Patients with poor ability in daily living [28] indicated more unmet needs than those of independent patients, especially in terms of information, communication, psychological, and occupational needs.

Two studies [28, 70] showed that no relationships were observed between cancer site and their unmet needs, but two other [46, 63] studies showed opposite results. Two [42, 75] out of five studies reported that no relationship was observed between cancer stage (only stages III and IV) and unmet needs, and three ones [58, 63, 70] indicated that patients with stage IV cancer presented more unmet needs than those with stage III cancer. Results were inconsistent across studies for cancer treatment, with two studies showing no relationship [42, 44] and two other studies suggesting either positive [75] or negative [58] relationship.

Patients with anxiety experienced high levels of physical, psychological, healthcare, and information, as well as ADL unmet needs, which was confirmed across several studies [33, 41, 42, 44, 58]. Patients with depression [42, 44, 58, 70] demonstrated varied results. Patients with low quality of life showed high unmet needs, especially in physical and psychological domains [41, 43]. Patients reported more unmet needs when their caregivers were male [28], young people [28], or those who suffered from psychological distress [28].

Variables associated with the unmet needs of informal caregivers

Older caregivers [30, 35] showed less unmet needs in terms of financial, social, and care-related information needs than those of younger caregivers. Caregivers in different caregiving settings reported different levels of unmet needs (home>general hospital>hospice care unit) [32, 39]. Caregivers with many physical problems experienced many unmet needs [35, 63]. Caregivers had higher levels of unmet needs when patients suffered from anxiety [35], depression [35], or low physical performance [35]. Results varied across studies in terms of gender [30], length of caregiving [9, 63], and education level of caregivers [63] (Table 5). Similarly, results were conflicting with regard to the relationships between caregivers and patients. One study [39] showed that spousal caregivers presented many information needs, and another study [63] indicated that non-spousal caregivers reported many unmet needs.

How their unmet needs were assessed in the included studies

For patients with advanced cancer, the most commonly used multidimensional instruments were Supportive Care Needs Survey (SCNS, $n = 8$) [6, 33, 41, 50, 58, 60, 61, 75], Problems and Needs in Palliative Care questionnaire (PNPC, $n = 5$) [31, 34, 36, 44, 47], and Needs Assessment of Advanced Cancer Patients (NA-ACP, $n = 3$) [38, 54, 55]. Other multidimensional instruments that were adopted included Cancer Needs Questionnaire [42], Patient Needs Assessment in Palliative Care [43], 3-Levels-of-Needs Questionnaire [45], Needs Assessment Tool: Progressive Disease–Cancer [68], Caregiver's Perception of Patients' Unmet Needs [59], and other instruments without reporting their psychometric properties. Among studies that focused on one specific need domain ($n = 4$), three explored information needs [44, 56, 69], and one investigated spiritual needs [37]. The unidimensional

Table 5 Summary of the variables associated with informal caregivers' unmet needs

Study	Demographics of caregivers					Caregivers' physical symptom	Relationship	Patients-related		
	Older	Female	Education level	Length of caregiving	Care setting		Spousal caregivers	Patients' anxiety	Patients' depression	Lower physical performance
[30]	-(fin, PM, soc.,)	F (+phy) M (+ inf)								
[32]					Conventional hospital care > hospice care (symptom management, psy support, religious support)					
[35]						+ (overall)		+(overall)	+(overall)	+(overall)
[9]				—						
[39]	–				Home > hospital (inf)		+			
[63]	-(soc,psy,inf)		-(psy) +(soc)	+(soc)		+	-(inf)			

Notes: "-": negative relationship; "+": positive relationship; "fin": financial needs; "PM": pain management; "soc": social needs; "phy": physical needs; "inf": information needs; "overall": overall needs instruments adopted included the following: Toronto Information Needs Questionnaire [69], Advanced Cancer Information Needs [56], PNPC (only used the items of the information domain) [44], and an instrument [37] for spiritual needs assessment without specifying its psychometric properties. Overall, more than half of the quantitative studies (20/34) adopted instruments with acceptable validity and reliability.

Among the 13 quantitative studies reporting unmet needs of informal caregivers, comprehensive unmet needs (multiple domains) were explored in 10 studies [9, 30, 32, 35, 40, 51, 59, 63, 64, 67]. Different quantitative studies used different measures, which included PNPC questionnaire-caregiver form [30], Family Inventory of Needs [59], Partners and Caregivers SCNS [35], needs of family caregivers of patients with advanced cancer [9], and other self-designed instruments [32, 40, 51, 63, 64, 67]. Among the three other studies that focused on unidimensional needs assessment, two [39, 56] measured information needs, and one [52] explored spiritual needs. The scales used were Spiritual Needs Inventory [52] and two other self-designed instruments, namely, with [56] or without [39] psychometric property testing. Among all the 13 studies, only four studies used scales with documented psychometric properties.

Discussion

The included studies highlighted that both advanced cancer patients and their informal caregivers possess a wide range of unmet needs. Psychological and physical unmet needs are two areas of focus for patients with advanced cancer; this result is consistent with a previously published review [7]. Among informal caregivers who had experience in managing patients' negative emotions, more than 30% of them reported that emotional management is the most challenging part of caregiving [76]. Three other unmet needs, namely, the need for autonomy, communication, and nutrition, were identified in this review compared with the previous review [7]. These needs may be related to the differences in cultural contexts, healthcare systems, and economic levels because several included studies in this review were conducted in eastern and developing countries. For instance, the need for autonomy is commonly culture-related [36]. Family members usually make decisions for patients in eastern cultures because family-collective decision-making is much more popular there than in other cultures [77]. This result showed the importance of developing tailored healthcare services or interventions based on context-specific unmet needs. Disease-related information needs were the most commonly reported unmet needs of informal caregivers. Considerably fewer studies reported unmet needs that are associated with the caregivers' own well-being, as

they generally focus more on the patients' well-being than their own [30]. The prominent care needs of each domain were identified for patients with advanced cancer and informal caregivers in this review provide useful information and evidence for the development and implementation of tailored healthcare services. For example, emotional support was identified as the most commonly unmet need in the psychological domain for patients, thereby indicating that emotional distress (e.g., anxiety and depression) management should be a priority when providing mental health services. In addition, patients with advanced cancer and informal caregivers' unmet need domains involved multiple disciplines, which indicated that healthcare services should be multidisciplinary. The value of multidisciplinary care for patients with cancer has been well recognized [78]. Support for informal caregivers is suboptimal in many instances [79]. The unmet needs of informal caregivers are often ignored and excluded from healthcare planning [80, 81].

The prevalence of unmet needs varied across the quantitative studies for both patients and caregivers. This variability may be caused by the heterogeneity of the included studies, which were conducted within different cultural contexts, healthcare systems, and economic levels that may be associated with unmet needs. High-income countries or regions generally present well-established healthcare service systems, which can facilitate the timely identification and resolution of healthcare problems (several physical symptoms particularly require high-quality professional support [28]). Different study designs, especially the diverse instruments used, for unmet needs assessment also contribute to this heterogeneity. The highlighted heterogeneity makes it difficult to gauge and pool the percentages of unmet needs by domains. SCNS was the most commonly used instrument, which was used in eight studies. However, these eight studies adopted five different variants of the same scale, with 13 [61], 33 [58], 34 [6, 33, 41], 59 [60], and 61 items [50] for each of the five versions. Different methods of need classification are also a major barrier in gauging unmet needs by domains. For instance, in SCNS, several items were classified as spiritual needs (e.g., [50]). In other studies, the same items were coded as psychological needs (e.g., [41]). Moreover, approaches in defining unmet needs were inconsistent. Among studies that utilized the SCNS, several of them regarded moderate and high levels of need as unmet needs (e.g., [41]. In other studies, low need level was calculated as an unmet need (e.g., [50]). Different reporting methods also caused heterogeneity. Several studies reported the prevalence of unmet needs by domains without specifying the percentage of items within each domain. Some studies (e.g., [33]) only listed the prevalence of the top 10 or 20 items without reporting the prevalence by domain. Thus, directly combining the prevalence of reported items within a domain may increase the risk of overestimating the actual unmet need level [21].

Although consistent results across studies showed that patients with advanced cancer with symptoms of distress and anxiety and low quality of life are more likely to report high demands of unmet needs, the conclusion must be interpreted with caution. Causality cannot be established because almost all of the included studies were cross-section in design. Other patient-related variables with inconsistent results, (e.g., gender, marital status, education level, cancer site, and depression) may be caused by cultural differences and/or methodological flaws (e.g., insufficient sample size to explore relationships between two factors) of the included studies. Hence, more longitudinal studies with rigorous study designs should be adopted. In addition, whether caregivers' health outcomes were associated with the unmet needs of patients is still unclear because of the limited evidence that can be drawn from current studies. Therefore, more studies should focus on caregiver-related variables. Relevant studies regarding variables associated with informal caregivers' unmet needs are limited, and no conclusion can be drawn from the current findings.

Patients with cancer at an advanced stage commonly experience fluctuating unmet needs over time due to rapid disease progression [6]. Nevertheless, little is known about how patients with advanced cancer and/or their informal caregivers' unmet needs change across the illness trajectory. Almost all the included quantitative studies investigated unmet needs at a single time point with cross-sectional study designs. Unmet care needs assessment in the majority of the included studies is also mainly problem-oriented from a biomedical lens. Few studies considered contextual issues (sociocultural and healthcare service provisions) when assessing and interpreting results in a given context although it will be of benefit to the development and implementation of tailored interventions at a local level. Accordingly, qualitative studies are an appropriate approach because it can explore participants' in-depth experience and subjective feelings that cannot be measured by quantitative methods; additionally, the scope can be much broader than those of quantitative methods [82, 83]. Deeper understanding of unmet needs can be extracted from the qualitative studies than from quantitative findings. However, limited studies adopted qualitative study designs, and only few studies utilized mixed methods. Care needs should be comprehensively evaluated from all stakeholders, including patients, caregivers, and healthcare providers [84]. A comprehensive understanding of both patients with advanced cancer and informal caregivers' unmet needs can enable healthcare providers to develop evidence-based and tailored interventions

[18]. Nevertheless, the majority of the included studies assessed patients' unmet needs only, and almost all included studies examined unmet needs from the participants' own perspective rather than from the perspectives of all relevant stakeholders. Despite that the concept of patient-and-family-centered care is advocated by the WHO [16], structured unmet needs assessment of informal caregivers is still an uncommon practice. Only a few studies assessed the unmet needs of patients and informal caregivers, and their unmet needs were assessed separately. The mechanism of integrating the data of patients and caregivers should be considered to further embody the conceptualization as a whole unit. Focused group with mixed samples, including patients and informal caregivers in the same group, may be an appropriate approach. Finally, research instruments used for needs assessment in several included studies were inappropriate. Some scales are generic ones used for supportive care needs assessment. Several items, such as "fear about the cancer spreading," may be unsuitable for patients with advanced cancer.

A strength of this systematic review is that a large number of studies with considerable information were assimilated and analyzed through a systematic method, which can minimise biases and facilitate reliable conclusions. This work is the first systematic review conducted by considering patients with advanced cancer and their informal caregivers as a whole unit. However, this review also presents several limitations. First, subgroup analysis in terms of contexts and economic levels was not conducted. Second, given the confounding factors and insufficient number of studies in each subgroup, meta-analysis was also not performed to compare the prevalence of each identified need domain. Third, language bias cannot be excluded because only papers that were published in English or Chinese language were included. Finally, instruments for needs assessments were only summarized from the included studies, and studies in terms of instrument development were excluded.

Conclusions

A wide range of unmet care needs existed in both advanced cancer patients and informal caregivers. Given the context-bound feature, their unmet needs should be comprehensively assessed and interpreted from the perspectives of all stakeholders within a given context by using rigorous mixed methods research and longitudinal research with prospective study designs. Assessing unmet care needs by viewing patients with advanced cancer and their informal caregivers as a whole unit is highly desirable. Associated factors of their unmet needs should not be ignored, which can provide evidence for decision-making with regards to healthcare resource allocation. The value of better examining unmet needs and their associated factors in advanced cancer patients and informal caregivers ultimately depends on how well it could inform the development and implementation of tailored healthcare service or intervention.

Endnotes

[1]In this review, patients with advanced cancer are defined as follows: patients with advanced, secondary, metastatic, or terminal cancer [23, 24] or patients with cancer at stage III or IV according to TNM Staging System or Dukes' D according to Dukes' staging system [23, 24]).

[2]In this review, when external help for patients and informal caregivers' existing problems was inadequate, any level of need for addressing the unsolved problems was regarded as unmet care needs, which included low, moderate, and high needs.

[3]In this paper, direct quotations from several included quantitative studies using commonly utilized research scales with documented psychometric properties were details of each of the used research questionnaire items. Thus, information regarding page numbers was not provided, but that for direct quotations from studies using self-designed semi-structured questionnaires and/or qualitative methods, as well as page numbers for such quotations, was provided.

Abbreviations

3LNQ: 3-Levels-of-Needs Questionnaire; ACIN: Advanced Cancer Information Needs; ADL: Activities of Daily Living; FIN: The Family Inventory of Needs; MMAT: Mixed Methods Appraisal Tool; NA-ACP: Needs Assessment of Advanced Cancer Patients; NAT: PD-C: Needs Assessment Tool: Progressive Disease-Cancer; PNAP: Patient Needs Assessment in Palliative Care; PNPC: Problems and Needs in Palliative Care questionnaire; PPUN: Caregiver's Perception of Patients' Unmet Needs; SCNS: Supportive Care Needs Survey; SCNS-P&C: Partners and Caregivers supportive care needs survey; SNI: Spiritual Needs Inventory; TINQ-BC: Toronto Information Needs Questionnaire

Authors' contributions

Study conception and design, literature search, data extraction and checking, data synthesis and interpretation, and manuscript drafting and revision: TW; Study conception and design, and manuscript revision: AM and BPMC. Data extraction and checking, and manuscript revision: JYT. All authors read and approved the final manuscript.

Competing interests

The authors declare that there is no any conflict of interests regarding the publication of this paper.

Author details
[1]School of Nursing, The Hong Kong Polytechnic University, Hung Hom, Hong Kong. [2]College of Nursing and Midwifery, Charles Darwin University, Darwin, Australia.

References

1. World Health Organization. Global cancer rates could increase by 50% to 15 million by 2020. Available at: http://www.who.int/mediacentre/news/releases/2003/pr27/en/. Last accessed 20 March 2017.
2. Thorne SE, Oliffe JL, Oglov V, Gelmon K. Communication challenges for chronic metastatic cancer in an era of novel therapeutics. Qual Health Res. 2013;7(23):863–75. https://doi.org/10.1177/1049732313483926.
3. Kim Y, Schulz R, Carver CS. Benefit finding in the cancer caregiving experience. Psychosom Med. 2007;69(3):283–91.
4. Gysels M, Higginson IJ, Rajasekaran M, et al. Improving supportive and palliative care for adults with cancer: research evidence. London: National Institute for Health and Clinical Excellence; 2004.
5. Okediji PT, Salako O, Fatiregun OO. Pattern and Predictors of Unmet Supportive Care Needs in Cancer Patients. Cureus. 2017;9(5):e1234.
6. Waller A, Girgis A, Johnson C, et al. Improving outcomes for people with progressive cancer: interrupted time series trial of a needs assessment intervention. J Pain Symptom Manag. 2012;43(3):569–81.
7. Moghaddam N, Coxon H, Nabarro S, et al. Unmet care needs in people living with advanced cancer: a systematic review. Support Care Cancer. 2016;24(8):3609–22.
8. Chen MC, Chen KM, Chu TP. Caregiver burden, health status, and learned resourcefulness of older caregivers. West J Nurs Res. 2015;37(6):767–80.
9. Cui J, Song LJ, Zhou LJ, et al. Needs of family caregivers of advanced cancer patients: a survey in shanghai of China. Eur J Cancer Care. 2014;23(4):562–9.
10. Lambert SD, Harrison JD, Smith E, et al. The unmet needs of partners and caregivers of adults diagnosed with cancer: a systematic review. BMJ Support Palliat Care. 2012;2(3):224–30.
11. Grunfeld E, Coyle D, Whelan T, et al. Family caregiver burden: results of a longitudinal study of breast cancer patients and their principal caregivers. Can Med Assoc J. 2004;170(12):1795–801.
12. Proot IM, Abu-Saad HH, Ter Meulen RH, et al. The needs of terminally ill patients at home: directing one's life, health and things related to beloved others. Palliat Med. 2004;18(1):53–61.
13. Sharpe L, Butow P, Smith C, et al. The relationship between available support, unmet needs and caregiver burden in patients with advanced cancer and their carers. Psycho-Oncology. 2005;14(2):102–14.
14. Milbury K, Badr H, Fossella F, et al. Longitudinal associations between caregiver burden and patient and spouse distress in couples coping with lung cancer. Support Care Cancer. 2013;21(9):2371–9.
15. Hodgkinson K, Butow P, Hunt GE, et al. Life after cancer: couples' and partners' psychological adjustment and supportive care needs. Support Care Cancer. 2007;15(4):405–15.
16. World Health Organization. WHO definition of palliative care, 2012. Available at: http://www.who.int/cancer/palliative/definition/en/. Last Accessed 20 March 2017.
17. Wen KY, Gustafson DH. Needs assessment for cancer patients and their families. Health Qual Life Outcomes. 2004;2(1):11.
18. Valery PC, Powell E, Moses N, et al. Systematic review: unmet supportive care needs in people diagnosed with chronic liver disease. BMJ Open. 2015;5(4):e007451.
19. Lam WW, Au AH, Wong JH, et al. Unmet supportive care needs: a cross-cultural comparison between Hong Kong Chinese and German Caucasian women with breast cancer. Breast Cancer Res Treat. 2011;130(2):531–41.
20. Sanson-Fisher R, Girgis A, Boyes A, Bonevski B, Burton L, Cook P. The unmet supportive care needs of patients with cancer. Supportive Care Review Group. Cancer. 2000;88(1):226–37.
21. Harrison JD, Young JM, Price MA, et al. What are the unmet supportive care needs of people with cancer? A systematic review. Support Care Cancer. 2009;17(8):1117–28.

22. Rainbird KJ, Perkins JJ, Sanson-Fisher RW. The needs assessment for advanced Cancer patients (NA-ACP): a measure of the perceived needs of patients with advanced, incurable cancer. A study of validity, reliability and acceptability. Psycho-Oncology. 2005;14(4):297–306.

23. Cancer Council. Living with advanced Cancer 2016. http://www.cancervic.org.au/about-cancer/advanced-cancer. Last accessed 30 Dec 2016.

24. Cancer Research UK. What is advanced bladder cancer? Available at: http://www.cancerresearchuk.org/about-cancer/type/bladder-cancer/treatment/advanced/what-is-advanced-bladder-cancer. Last accessed 30 Dec 2016.

25. Pace R, Pluye P, Gillian B, et al. Testing the reliability and efficiency of the pilot Mixed Methods Appraisal Tool (MMAT) for systematic mixed studies review. Int J Nurs Stud. 2012;49:47–53.

26. Hsieh HF, Shannon SE. Three approaches to qualitative content analysis. Qual Health Res. 2005;15(9):1277–88.

27. Ryan R; Cochrane Consumers and Communication Review Group. 'Cochrane Consumers and Communication Review Group: data synthesis and analysis'. http://cccrg.cochrane.org/author-resources, Last accessed 20 March 2017.

28. Morasso G, Capelli M, Viterbori P, et al. Psychological and symptom distress in terminal cancer patients with met and unmet needs. J Pain Symptom Manag. 1999;17(6):402–9.

29. Teunissen SC, de Haes HC, Voest EE, et al. Does age matter in palliative care? Crit Rev Oncol Hematol. 2006;60(2):152–8.

30. Osse BH, Vernooij-Dassen MJ, Schadé E, et al. Problems experienced by the informal caregivers of cancer patients and their needs for support. Cancer Nurs. 2006;29(5):378–88.

31. Osse BH, Vernooij-Dassen MJ, Schadé E, et al. The problems experienced by patients with cancer and their needs for palliative care. Support Care Cancer. 2005;13(9):722–32.

32. Park SM, Kim YJ, Kim S, et al. Impact of caregivers' unmet needs for supportive care on quality of terminal cancer care delivered and caregiver's workforce performance. Support Care Cancer. 2010;18(6):699–706.

33. Hasegawa T, Goto N, Matsumoto N, et al. Prevalence of unmet needs and correlated factors in advanced-stage cancer patients receiving rehabilitation. Support Care Cancer. 2016;24(11):4761–7.

34. Uitdehaag MJ, Verschuur EM, van Eijck CH, et al. Problems and needs in patients with incurable esophageal and Pancreaticobiliary Cancer. Gastroenterol Nurs. 2015;38(1):42–54.

35. Chen SC, Chiou SC, Yu CJ, et al. The unmet supportive care needs-what advanced lung cancer patients' caregivers need and related factors. Support Care Cancer. 2016;24(7):2999–3009.

36. Effendy C, Vissers K, Osse BH, et al. Comparison of problems and unmet needs of patients with advanced cancer in a European country and an Asian country. Pain Practice. 2015;15(5):433–40.

37. Vilalta A, Valls J, Porta J, et al. Evaluation of spiritual needs of patients with advanced cancer in a palliative care unit. J Palliat Med. 2014;17(5):592–600.

38. Schenker Y, Park SY, Maciasz R, et al. Do patients with advanced cancer and unmet palliative care needs have an interest in receiving palliative care services? J Palliat Med. 2014;17(6):667–72.

39. Fukui S. Information needs and the related variables of Japanese family caregivers of terminally ill cancer patients. Nurs Health Sci. 2004;6(1):29–36.

40. DuBenske LL, Wen KY, Gustafson DH, et al. Caregivers' differing needs across key experiences of the advanced cancer disease trajectory. Palliative and Supportive Care. 2008;6(03):265–72.

41. Uchida M, Akechi T, Okuyama T, et al. Patients' supportive care needs and psychological distress in advanced breast cancer patients in Japan. Jpn J Clin Oncol. 2011;41(4):530–6.

42. Liao YC, Liao WY, Shun SC, et al. Symptoms, psychological distress, and supportive care needs in lung cancer patients. Support Care Cancer. 2011;19(11):1743–51.

43. Bužgová R, Hajnová E, Sikorová L, et al. Association between unmet needs and quality of life in hospitalised cancer patients no longer receiving anti-cancer treatment. Eur J Cancer Care. 2014;23(5):685–94.

44. Voogt E, van Leeuwen AF, Visser AP, et al. Information needs of patients with incurable cancer. Support Care Cancer. 2005;13(11):943–8.

45. Johnsen AT, Petersen MA, Pedersen L, et al. Do advanced cancer patients in Denmark receive the help they need? A nationally representative survey of the need related to 12 frequent symptoms/problems. Psycho-Oncology. 2013;22(8):1724–30.

46. Houts PS, Harvey HA, Hartz AJ, et al. Unmet needs of persons with cancer in Pennsylvania during the period of terminal care. Cancer. 1988;62(3):627–34.

47. Khan L, Chiang A, Barnes E, et al. Needs assessment of patients and their caregivers at the rapid response radiotherapy program. J Pain Manag. 2012;5(2):153–62.

48. Dehghan R, Ramakrishnan J, Uddin-Ahmed N, et al. 'They patiently heard what we had to say... this felt different to me': the palliative care needs and care experiences of advanced cancer patients and their families in Bangladesh. BMJ Support Palliat Care. 2012;2(2):145–9.

49. Mangan PA, Taylor KL, Yabroff KR, et al. Caregiving near the end of life: unmet needs and potential solutions. Palliat Support Care. 2003;1(03):247–59.

50. Fitch MI. Supportive care needs of patients with advanced disease undergoing radiotherapy for symptom control. Can Oncol Nurs J. 2012; 22(2):84–91.

51. Joad AS, Mayamol TC, Chaturvedi M. What does the informal caregiver of a terminally ill cancer patient need? A study from a cancer Centre. Ind J Palliat Care. 2011;17(3):191–6.

52. Buck HG, McMillan SC. The unmet spiritual needs of caregivers of patients with advanced cancer. J Hosp Palliat Nurs. 2008;10(2):91–9.

53. Deng D, Deng Q, Liu X, et al. Expectation in life review: a term of spiritual needs easily understood by Chinese hospice patients. Am J Hosp Palliat Care. 2015;32(7):725–31.

54. Rachakonda K, George M, Shafiei M, et al. Unmet supportive Cancer care needs: an exploratory quantitative study in rural Australia. World J Oncol. 2015;6(4):387–93.

55. Rainbird K, Perkins J, Sanson-Fisher R, et al. The needs of patients with advanced, incurable cancer. Br J Cancer. 2009;101(5):759–64.

56. Wong RK, Franssen E, Szumacher E, et al. What do patients living with advanced cancer and their carers want to know? -a needs assessment. Support Care Cancer. 2002;10(5):408–15.

57. Carter N, Bryant-Lukosius D, DiCenso A, et al. The supportive care needs of family members of men with advanced prostate cancer. Canadian oncology nursing journal/revue canadienne de soins infirmiers en. Oncologie. 2010; 20(4):166–70.

58. Au A, Lam W, Tsang J, et al. Supportive care needs in Hong Kong Chinese women confronting advanced breast cancer. Psycho-Oncology. 2013;22(5):1144–51.

59. Hwang SS, Chang VT, Alejandro Y, et al. Caregiver unmet needs, burden, and satisfaction in symptomatic advanced cancer patients at a veterans affairs (VA) medical center. Palliat Support Care. 2003;1(04):319–29.

60. Aranda S, Schofield P, Weih L, et al. Mapping the quality of life and unmet needs of urban women with metastatic breast cancer. Eur J Cancer Care. 2005;14(3):211–22.

61. Lelorain S, Brédart A, Dolbeault S, et al. How does a physician's accurate understanding of a cancer patient's unmet needs contribute to patient perception of physician empathy? Patient Educ Couns. 2015;98(6):734–41.

62. Lee HT, Melia KM, Yao CA, et al. Providing hospice home care to the terminally ill elderly people with cancer in Taiwan: family experiences and needs. Am J Hosp Palliat Med. 2014;31(6):628–35.

63. Liu Y. The status of the needs and service utilization wills of advanced cancer patients and their informal caregivers and service contents of some community health service centers delivery in Shanghai. 2008. The Second Military Medical University, Master Thesis. (in Chinese).

64. Chen HY, Ju BB, Lu BQ, et al. Investigation and intervention of nursing demand and emotional state of family members of patients with advanced neoplasm. Shanghai Nurs. 2008;8(6):18–20.

65. Gu WJ, Shi YX, Yuan W, et al., Health service needs of terminal inpatients with advanced malignant tumor in community hospice care pilot settings in shanghai. Chinese General Practice 2015., 18 (22):2655–2661. (in Chinese).

66. Huang J, Xu Y, Peng P, et al. A survey of advanced cancer patients' community health service needs. Nurs J Chinese People's Liberation. 2008; 25(4A):33–5.

67. Miu J, Cao WQ, Wang XY, et al. Investigation on community care needs of patients with cancer and their family members in a community in shanghai. Chin Nurs Res. 2016;30(7A):2386–90.

68. Waller A, Girgis A, Johnson C, et al. Implications of a needs assessment intervention for people with progressive cancer: impact on clinical assessment, response and service utilisation. Psycho-Oncology. 2012; 21(5):550–7.

69. Templeton H, Coates V. Informational needs of men with prostate cancer on hormonal manipulation therapy. Patient Educ Couns. 2003;49(3):243–56.

70. Hwang SS, Chang VT, Cogswell J, et al. Study of unmet needs in symptomatic veterans with advanced cancer: incidence, independent

predictors and unmet needs outcome model. J Pain Symptom Manag. 2004;28(5):421–32.

71. Murray SA, Kendall M, Boyd K, et al. Exploring the spiritual needs of people dying of lung cancer or heart failure: a prospective qualitative interview study of patients and their carers. Palliat Med. 2004;18(1):39–45.

72. Soelver L, Rydahl-Hansen S, Oestergaard B, et al. Identifying factors significant to continuity in basic palliative hospital care—from the perspective of patients with advanced cancer. J Psychosoc Oncol. 2014; 32(2):167–88.

73. Carter N, Bryant-Lukosius D, DiCenso A, et al. The supportive care needs of men with advanced prostate cancer. Oncol Nurs Forum. 2011;38(2):189–98.

74. Christ G, Siegel K. Monitoring quality-of-life needs of cancer patients. Cancer. 1990;65:760–5.

75. Lam WW, Tsang J, Yeo W, et al. The evolution of supportive care needs trajectories in women with advanced breast cancer during the 12 months following diagnosis. Support Care Cancer. 2014;22(3):635–44.

76. Deshields TL, Rihanek A, Potter P, et al. Psychological aspects of caregiving: perception of cancer patients and family caregivers. Support Care Cancer. 2012;20:349–56.

77. Gu X, Chen M, Liu M, et al. End-of-life decision-making of terminally ill cancer patients in a tertiary cancer center in shanghai, China. Support Care Cancer. 2016;24(5):2209–15.

78. Health Care Guideline- Palliative Care for Adults (Fifth Edition, November 2013). Available at: https://www.icsi.org/guidelines_more/catalog_guidelines_and_more/catalog_guidelines/catalog_palliative_care_guidelines/palliative_care/. Last accessed 1 Nov2016.

79. Hudson P, Remedios C, Zordan R, et al. Guidelines for the psychosocial and bereavement support of family caregivers of palliative care patients. J Palliat Med. 2012;15(6):696–702.

80. Halkett GK, Lobb EA, Miller L, et al. Protocol for the care-IS trial: a randomised controlled trial of a supportive educational intervention for carers of patients with high-grade glioma (HGG). BMJ Open. 2015; 5(10):e009477.

81. Sealey M, Breen LJ, O'Connor M, et al. A scoping review of bereavement risk assessment measures: implications for palliative care. Palliat Med. 2015;29(7):577–89.

82. Grypdonck MH. Qualitative health research in the era of evidence-based practice. Qual Health Res. 2006;16(10):1371–85.

83. Britten N, Campbell R, Pope C, et al. Using meta ethnography to synthesise qualitative research: a worked example. J Health Serv Res Policy. 2002;7(4):209–15.

84. Field D, Clark D. Researching palliative care; 2001. p. 146–51.

10

Key features of palliative care service delivery to Indigenous peoples in Australia, New Zealand, Canada and the United States

Shaouli Shahid[1,2]*(iD), Emma V. Taylor[2], Shelley Cheetham[2,3], John A. Woods[2], Samar M. Aoun[4,5] and Sandra C. Thompson[2]

Abstract

Background: Indigenous peoples in developed countries have reduced life expectancies, particularly from chronic diseases. The lack of access to and take up of palliative care services of Indigenous peoples is an ongoing concern.

Objectives: To examine and learn from published studies on provision of culturally safe palliative care service delivery to Indigenous people in Australia, New Zealand (NZ), Canada and the United States of America (USA); and to compare Indigenous peoples' preferences, needs, opportunities and barriers to palliative care.

Methods: A comprehensive search of multiple databases was undertaken. Articles were included if they were published in English from 2000 onwards and related to palliative care service delivery for Indigenous populations; papers could use quantitative or qualitative approaches. Common themes were identified using thematic synthesis. Studies were evaluated using Daly's hierarchy of evidence-for-practice in qualitative research.

Results: Of 522 articles screened, 39 were eligible for inclusion. Despite diversity in Indigenous peoples' experiences across countries, some commonalities were noted in the preferences for palliative care of Indigenous people: to die close to or at home; involvement of family; and the integration of cultural practices. Barriers identified included inaccessibility, affordability, lack of awareness of services, perceptions of palliative care, and inappropriate services. Identified models attempted to address these gaps by adopting the following strategies: community engagement and ownership; flexibility in approach; continuing education and training; a whole-of-service approach; and local partnerships among multiple agencies. Better engagement with Indigenous clients, an increase in number of palliative care patients, improved outcomes, and understanding about palliative care by patients and their families were identified as positive achievements.

Conclusions: The results provide a comprehensive overview of identified effective practices with regards to palliative care delivered to Indigenous populations to guide future program developments in this field. Further research is required to explore the palliative care needs and experiences of Indigenous people living in urban areas.

Keywords: American native continental ancestry group, Oceanic ancestry group, Aboriginal, Indigenous, Palliative care, Terminal care, End-of-life care, Hospice care, Model of care

* Correspondence: s.shahid@curtin.edu.au
[1]Centre for Aboriginal Studies (CAS), Curtin University, Kent Street, Bentley, WA 6102, Australia
[2]Western Australian Centre for Rural Health (WACRH), School of Population and Global Health, The University of Western Australia, Geraldton, WA 6530, Australia
Full list of author information is available at the end of the article

Background

Palliative care services aim to improve quality of life (QoL) among patients with life-threatening illnesses and their families [1]. These services provide relief from pain and other distressing symptoms, incorporate psychological and spiritual aspects of patients' end-of-life (EOL) needs [1], and can support terminally ill patients to die at or close to home [2]. Referral to palliative care early in the course of illness is important for optimal QoL, and also reduces unnecessary hospitalisations and use of health-care services [3]. Growing evidence confirms financial savings associated with palliative care [4]. In 2014, the first ever resolution to integrate hospice and palliative care services into national health services for all people was endorsed by the World Health Assembly [5]. Since then, palliative care has been explicitly recognised under human rights to health. The World Health Organisation (WHO) has endorsed the importance of palliative care to be provided in accordance with the principles of universal health coverage: all people, irrespective of income, disease type or age, should have access to a nationally determined set of basic health services, including palliative care [1]. It has been reinforced that palliative care should be provided through person-centred and integrated health services that pay special attention to the specific needs and preferences of individuals, especially through primary health care and community/home-based care. It is hoped that this endorsement will promote international action to reduce barriers to the accessibility and availability of palliative care.

In developed countries, palliative care now warrants attention as a priority for Indigenous people (the term 'Indigenous' refers to First Nation peoples or original inhabitants prior to colonisation in Australia, Canada, NZ and the USA), given their disproportionate burden from chronic diseases and higher mortality rates compared with non-Indigenous people [6]. However, Indigenous populations are among those least likely to receive adequate services [7]. Palliative care service data suggest low rates of utilisation by Indigenous people [8, 9], who often experience multiple episodes of acute hospitalisation for life-limiting conditions [10]. Lack of access to acceptable and appropriate palliative care services among Indigenous populations is a major concern [11]. Furthermore, there are 'profound cultural dissonances' [12, 13] between Indigenous and non-Indigenous beliefs in relation to death, disease management, health and health care. Therefore, ensuring cultural respect and sensitivity is of central importance for effective health care delivery to Indigenous peoples [14]. Although priorities have been set, service providers and policymakers face considerable uncertainty over ways to provide appropriate palliative care to Indigenous peoples, and seek research-based insights to guide practice [14].

The objective of this review was to learn from experiences and inform ways to improve palliative care service delivery for the Indigenous peoples of Australia, Canada, NZ, and the USA, recognising that the Indigenous peoples of these four developed countries share similar histories of colonisation and marginalisation. We aimed to highlight what is known of the needs and preferences of Indigenous patients at the EOL, any barriers to quality care at this time, but primarily the focus was to identify the key features of specific models of care and innovative strategies developed to address these needs, preferences and barriers. We adopted the Agency for Clinical Innovation's definition of Model of Care (MOC) which is broadly defined as 'the way health services are delivered. It outlines best practice care and services for a person or population group or patient cohort as they progress through the stages of a condition, injury or event. It aims to ensure people get the right care, at the right time, by the right team and in the right place' [15] p.3. Innovation in service delivery has been defined as a 'novel set of behaviours, routines, and ways of working that are directed at improving health outcomes, administrative efficiency, cost effectiveness, or users' experience, and that are implemented by planned and coordinated actions' [16] p.582. We combined these two concepts and defined the innovative model of care in EOL for Indigenous populations as: a novel set of behaviours, activities, approaches, initiatives, ways of working that are directed at improving access to, take up and quality of palliative care for Indigenous peoples. This definition was used to identify the key strategies and/ or services that have been applied to deliver EOL care among the Indigenous populations.

Methods

The review of studies was conducted in accordance with the principles of the Preferred Reporting Items for Systematic Review and Meta-Analysis (PRISMA) statement [17], with the aim of minimising methodological bias, and to ensure accurate and consistent reporting of the review. However, unlike conventional systematic reviews, which are often restricted to specific forms of evidence that are inadequate to explain complex social phenomena, we aimed to synthesise all forms of evidence, including qualitative and quantitative data, an approach similar to that taken by Dixon-Woods (2006) [18].

Search strategy

The search was from the year 2000 and was conducted in November 2016 across the following databases: PubMed, CINAHL, Embase, PsycInfo, InfoRMIT, Global Health, ScienceDirect, Web of Science and Scopus. The key concepts of 'palliative care' and 'Indigenous' were searched using a combination of prescribed subject headings and free text keywords. (The search string is presented in Additional file 1: Appendix 1.)

Screening process: Inclusion and exclusion criteria

The screening process is illustrated below using the PRISMA Flow Diagram (Fig. 1). Three authors (SS, ET and JW) independently screened titles and abstracts of publications identified in the search in relation to prede-termined inclusion criteria: (i) publication in English lan-guage; (ii) publication from the year 2000 onwards (selected to ensure that studies were relatively current); (ii) peer-reviewed articles or full-conference papers; (iv) related to palliative care; and (v) based on findings from Australia, Canada, New Zealand, or the USA.

Four authors (SS, ET, SC and JW) independently reviewed the full text of articles, and conferred in pairs to confirm whether articles met the selection criteria. Any remaining uncertainties were discussed and resolved by the entire team. A publication was excluded following full text examination if it: (i) included no findings on the provision of palliative care to Indigenous patients (such as articles on the delivery of rural-based palliative care with-out Indigenous-specific findings); (ii) included findings only on advance care planning and EOL care within aged-care services; (iii) had a primary focus on cultural or ceremonial EOL practices; iv) focused on pre and post bereavements rather than on the patients care (covering topics such as the grieving process, bereavement rituals or

support); (v) described palliative care education programs, or (vi) was an opinion or reflection piece without research findings.

Multiple papers from the same authors reporting on the same study population were included only if different findings were reported.

Quality assessment through grading

The methodological quality of the selected publications was assessed using Daly's hierarchy of evidence-for-practice in qualitative research [Level I: Generalizable Studies; Level II: Conceptual Studies; Level III: Descriptive Studies; Level IV: Single Case Study] [19]. Only 17 key articles that described and explored different models of care were included for grading. Although the use of such tools helps to assess the quality of evidence, it was difficult to grade the included published studies using the traditional taxonomies for levels of evidence [20]. Most publications were descriptive studies (evidence level III) as per Daly's hierarchy of evidence-for-practice, and many reported findings from program and/or project evaluations where a participatory action research approach was used in designing and developing the pro-gram. The heterogeneity in data collection and reporting of findings made it difficult to rate these articles. No article was excluded on the grounds of not meeting a quality standard as our focus was to review papers relevant to the topic, rather than particular study types that met strict methodological standards [18].

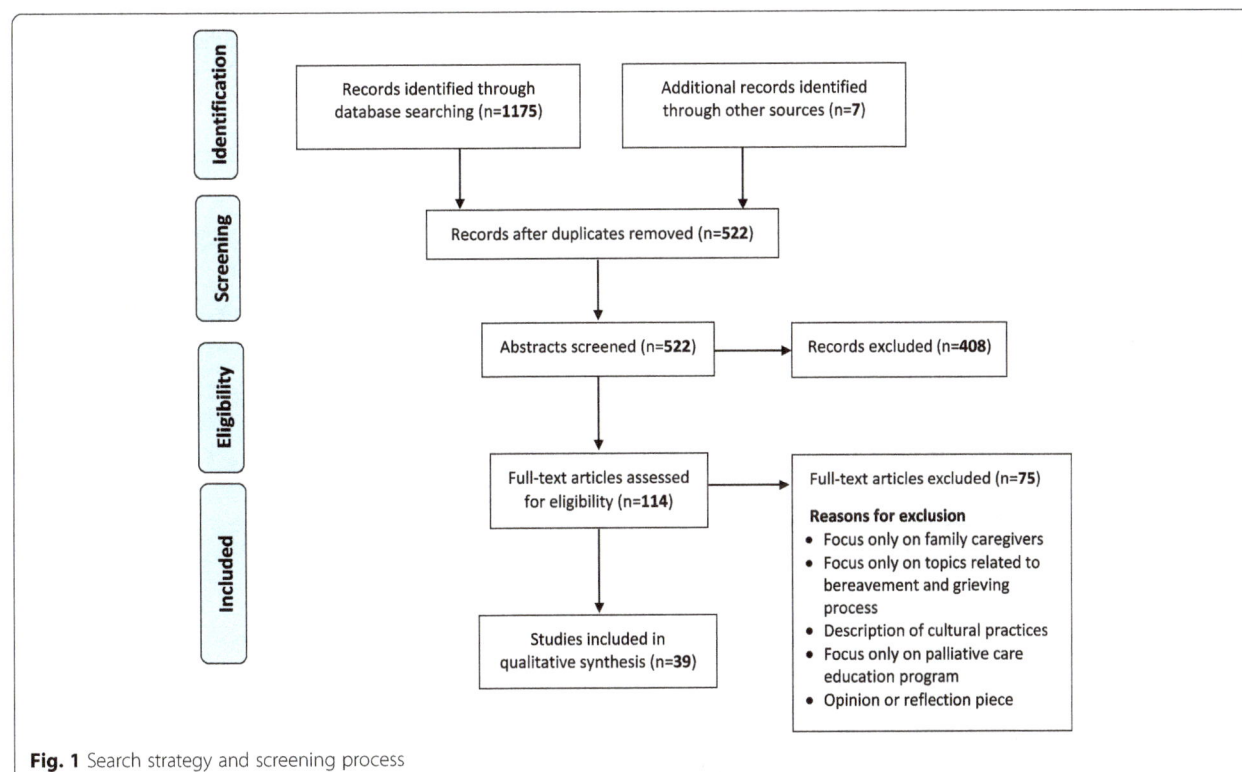

Fig. 1 Search strategy and screening process

Data extraction

A data extraction pro-forma was developed in Microsoft Excel to assist identifying the details of the study design, aims, sample, study context, analytical framework and key findings, including needs, preferences, barriers, opportunities, and also critical elements of approaches/ initiatives/ models of palliative care service delivery to Indigenous peoples. Data extraction was performed by the authors (SS, ET and SC), initially individually, then working in pairs to confirm the themes. Thematic synthesis [21] was used to analyse the findings. Due to the large volume of data, two clusters of studies were separated: one cluster focused mainly on the barriers, needs and preferences for Indigenous palliative care, and the other one on models of care. Findings related to the needs, preferences, barriers and opportunities have been summarised in tables according to similarity of themes. Themes relating to the primary objective of this review (the models of care) have been inductively derived, interpreted and presented [18].

Results

Once duplicates (*n* = 660) had been discarded, 515 potentially relevant articles were identified through our search, and an additional 7 through citation snowballing. Of the 522 publications, 408 were excluded during title and abstract screening. Full text review of the remaining 114 publications eliminated a further 75 that did not meet the inclusion criteria, leaving 39 articles to be included in the systematic review.

Overview of included articles

The 39 papers included were from Australia (9), New Zealand (10), Canada (8), and the USA (12). In 11 studies, the study population consisted of both Indigenous peoples and clinical staff (both Indigenous and non-Indigenous), 17 studies included Indigenous peoples only and three comprised service providers only (both Indigenous and non-Indigenous). Four studies comprised diverse ethnic groups including Indigenous peoples, and five studies did not specifically mention the study population as two of them were literature reviews, and three described specific models for Indigenous populations. The Indigenous populations studied included Aboriginal and Torres Strait Islander Australians, Māori and Samoans, Canadian First Nations (including Cree, Saulteaux/ Anishinaabe, and Lakota/Dakota), Métis, Alaska Natives (including Tlingit/ Haida, Yup'ik Eskimo, Inupiaq, Athabascan, Aleut and Alutiiq/Sugpiaq), Native Americans (including Pueblo, Navajo, Hopi and Zuni), and Native Hawaiians.

Most articles (*n* = 33 [85%]) focused on the provision of general palliative care with no terminal condition specified, three focused on palliative care for cancer patients, and one on palliative care for patients with a chronic disease other than cancer. Most studies (29) used qualitative methods

only, five were based on mixed methods, two were quantitative, two were literature reviews and one described a palliative care model.

The majority of the articles (30) contributed to findings about the palliative care needs and preferences of Indigenous people and the barriers they face in this context. Only 17 papers described actual approaches (presented in Table 4) to making palliative care more accessible to Indigenous peoples, either through the development of a model for delivering palliative care to Indigenous people (conceptual model) or a description of a palliative care service that had been implemented for Indigenous people (service model). These two categories were not mutually exclusive, as eight articles had components relevant to both (Fig. 2).

The first section of the results presents an overview and describes the preferences, barriers and needs of Indigenous people at the EOL identified from the literature. Five main themes on models of care were extracted, with sub-themes identified and supported by several exemplar statements. These will be presented in the final section.

Needs, preferences and barriers

Tables 1, 2 and 3 present a summary of the key needs, preferences and barriers of Indigenous populations in relation to EOL care.

Needs

Throughout the literature, the need to collaborate and to engage meaningfully with communities [6, 14, 22–28] and families [14, 24, 25, 29–34] before designing and implementing any program was highlighted as a fundamental prerequisite for progress. Most of the studies

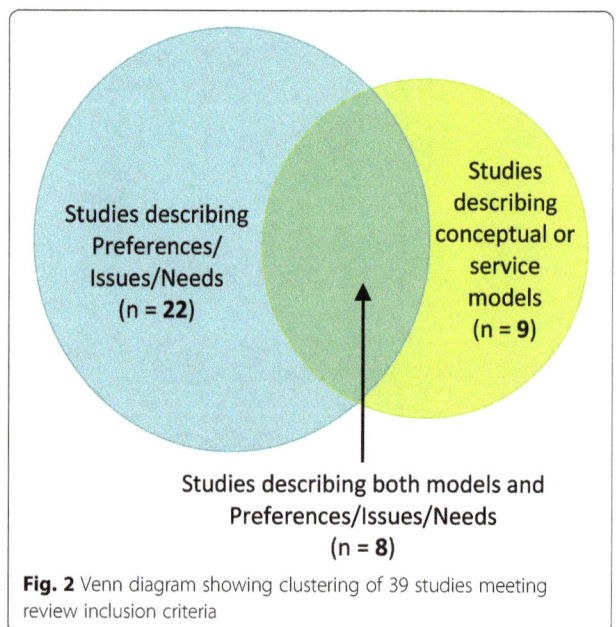

Fig. 2 Venn diagram showing clustering of 39 studies meeting review inclusion criteria

Studies describing Preferences/Issues/Needs (n = 22)

Studies describing conceptual or service models (n = 9)

Studies describing both models and Preferences/Issues/Needs (n = 8)

Table 1 Needs of Indigenous populations at the end-of-life

Needs		Australia	Canada	NZ	USA	No. of articles
Collaboration	Community Engagement	X [14, 28]	X [22]	X [24, 26]	X [6, 23, 25, 27]	9
	Family Engagement	X [14, 31]	X [32–34]	X [24, 30]	X [25, 27, 29]	10
	Health Care Provider Collaboration	X [28]	None identified	None identified	X [25]	2
Service Delivery	Funding	X [14, 37]	None identified	None identified	X [6, 23, 25]	5
	Communication	X [14, 31, 37]	X [33, 34, 42]	X [24, 26, 65]	X [6, 23]	11
	Policy Change	X [37]	X [32, 34, 35]	X [26, 65]	X [6, 23, 25, 27]	10
	Staff	X [14, 56]	X [22, 33]	X [24, 26, 36, 65]	X [2, 25, 27, 29, 39]	13
	Built Environment	X [14, 37]	X [22, 33, 35]	X [24, 26, 36, 41]	None identified	9
	Service Delivery, Provision of Care, Capacity of Care	X [14, 28, 31, 40]	X [32, 33, 66]	X [26, 30, 36, 41]	X [2, 6, 25, 27, 29]	16
	Cultural & Spiritual	X [14, 28, 37]	X [22, 32–35, 42, 66]	X [26]	X [25, 27]	13
Education & Training	Training for Health Care Providers	X [14]	X [22, 32, 35]	X [24, 26]	X [2, 6, 23, 25, 39]	11
	Education for Patient, Family and Community	X [40]	X [32]	X [24, 30, 36]	X [6, 27, 38, 39]	9

were conducted in rural or remote locations where EOL care provisions were often not well-developed or well-understood. Better communication, commitment around EOL care at the policy level, staff capacity building, and improved physical environment and access to services were identified as key service delivery needs.

Furthermore, the need for more education and training for both the Indigenous communities and the health care staff in palliative care was identified repeatedly [2, 6, 14, 22–27, 30, 32, 35–40]. Health service providers (HSPs) need to be committed and spend sufficient time to gain the confidence of Indigenous patients and their families.

Preferences

There was a strong preference for living with family and within the community at EOL [23, 29, 31, 33, 35–37, 39, 41–43]. Family members generally wanted to be with their loved ones and to fulfil their wishes, including

finding ways of enabling care and support to die at home. EOL care was regarded as a process that should involve the entire family, with several studies reporting that families should be at the centre of any decision-making process [24, 26, 27, 30, 31, 44]. Community and/or extended family members gathering was regarded as significant and part of the process for how a dying person is prepared for death [35].

The importance of dying at home or being cared for at home was a common theme for Indigenous people across the four countries [2, 26, 29, 31, 32, 39–41, 43, 44]. Special cultural ceremonies and rituals practiced at the EOL were regarded as important. Dying people benefit from both Western physicians and traditional healers. Elders in one particular study suggested that non-Indigenous HSPs should ask for assistance from 'elders, priests, spiritual leaders, women who are very strong in their medicine' (p. 11) if they are unsure of what to do [35]. Thus, in the

Table 2 Preferences of Indigenous populations at the end-of-life

Preferences		Australia	Canada	NZ	USA	No. of articles
Family and Community	Community Support	None identified	X [32, 35]	X [11]	X [2, 29, 39]	6
	Presence of Families	X [40]	X [32]	X [9, 11, 24, 26]	X [27, 29]	8
	Families Involved in Decision-making	X [14, 31]	X [42]	X [24, 26, 30]	X [27]	7
	Families Involved in Care	X [14]	X [32]	X [9, 11, 26, 41]	X [23, 29, 39]	9
Spiritual and Cultural	Die at Home	X [14, 31, 40]	X [32, 33, 42]	X [11, 26, 41]	X [2, 23, 27, 29, 39, 43]	15
	Ceremonies	X [14, 40]	X [32, 33, 35, 42]	X [26]	X [29, 43]	9
	Language	X [14]	None identified	X [26]	X [39]	3
	Spiritual	X [28, 31, 40]	X [32, 35, 42]	X [41]	X [27]	8
	Pass on Knowledge	X [40]	X [32]	None identified	X [2]	3
Service Delivery	Staff	X [14, 28]	X [32, 42]	X [9]	X [27]	6

Table 3 Barriers of access for Indigenous populations at the end-of-life

Issues		Australia	Canada	NZ	USA	No of articles
Accessibility to services	Challenges in Rural and Remote Areas	X [14, 28, 31, 40]	X [32, 42, 66]	X [26, 65]	X [2, 23, 25, 29, 39]	14
	Affordability	X [14]	X [66]	X [11, 24]	X [2, 29, 39]	6
	Lack of Awareness and Knowledge	X [14, 28]	X [66]	X [11, 24, 36, 65]	X [2, 25, 29, 39]	11
Service Delivery	Lack of Funding and Resources	None Identified	X [22, 32, 42]	X [65]	X [2, 6, 23, 25, 39]	9
	Health Service Provider Perceptions	X [28]	None Identified	X [24]	X [43]	3
	Policy	None Identified	None Identified	None Identified	X [2, 6, 23, 25]	4
	Services not Culturally Appropriate	X [14, 40]	X [32, 35]	X [24, 30]	X [29]	7
	Built Environment	X [40]	X [35]	X [26, 65]	None Identified	4
	Staffing Issues	X [14, 28, 40, 67]	X [32, 42, 66]	None Identified	X [2, 23, 25, 29, 39]	12
	Communication	X [14, 28, 31, 67]	X [35, 42, 66]	X [24]	X [6, 25]	11
Cultural Influences	Indigenous Perceptions of Palliative Care	X [14, 40]	X [32]	X [11, 24, 26, 36, 41]	X [25]	10
	Family Conflicts	X [28]	X [32, 33]	X [11, 30]	None Identified	5
	Death Issues	X [28]	None Identified	X [30]	X [29, 39]	4
	Historical, Cultural and Social Context	X [14, 28, 67]	X [22, 42]	X [24, 26]	X [6]	8

intercultural space, both worldviews should be respected. Being able to make these connections with families, kin, communities, and land was reported as helping people gain energy and in turn facilitating a strong spirit and peace of mind.

Open and honest communication from physicians, physicians respecting patients' choices [32], 'compassion with kindness' in attitudes [35] and having access to Indigenous staff [42, 44] were expressed as preferences. It was reported in one Canadian study that 'offering foods that bring comfort to the dying person may be more spiritually and emotionally healing than restrictive diets' (p.11) [35].

Barriers
As expected, distance and affordability of services (along with other indirect expenses related to treatment such as leaving families behind to travel) were identified as key barriers to access palliative care services [6, 14, 22, 24, 26, 42, 45]. Other important service delivery issues included staffing, lack of funding and resources in the sector, and poor availability of culturally appropriate services [6, 14, 22, 24, 26, 42, 45].

Differences between Western medical models and Indigenous cultures in understandings of and priorities for EOL care pose a major issue within the health care setting. Disrespectful and racist treatment by HSPs, and difficulty in regards to communicating EOL care issues to Indigenous patients and families, were also identified as barriers [35, 46, 47]. Hospital policies restricting extended family members from gathering around a dying Indigenous person, or practicing prayers and ceremonies at EOL were highlighted [35]. More training and education for HSPs in

order for them to work effectively with Indigenous people who are dying [35], and the employment of more Indigenous staff in the health sector, were seen as possible solutions to these service delivery issues. Misinformation and misunderstandings regarding palliative care and hospice services were also documented among Indigenous people [14, 24, 26], with providing an adequate and continuing health literacy program in the community seen as a requirement for making progress in better EOL care.

Innovations and models of care
A range of models and innovative service delivery strategies, for delivering EOL care for Indigenous communities across the four countries, were identified from the literature (Table 4). The most comprehensive conceptual model was developed in Australia by McGrath and colleagues [12]. They outlined seven key principles for Indigenous palliative care service delivery: equity (equal access); autonomy/empowerment (respecting patients' choices); trust (acknowledgement and consideration of the historical context of colonisation and its impact on the lives of Indigenous people and empathy while providing care); humane (non-judgemental care with a focus on quality of life and choice for patients and their families); seamless care (collaboration of a multidisciplinary team of health professionals and community-based organisations, working together across the continuum of care); emphasis on living (rather than on dying), and cultural respect (respect towards cultural practices and beliefs, culturally-based lifestyle) [12].

Hands-on, practical, and innovative service delivery models were identified as having adopted diverse strategies to deliver palliative care into communities. The

Table 4 Summary of the Key Articles that describe the Models of Care

Author(s), Year, Country, Location	Types of Services	Study Population	Methodology	Models	Critical Elements	Outcomes/ Indicators of Success	Daly's Hierarchy of Evidence
Braun et al. (2012), USA (mainly rural)	Multiple settings but mainly linking communities and hospitals	Poor and underserved communities including American Indians and Alaska Natives (AI/ANs)	Program analysis using the 'continuum of cancer care' and the 'five A's of quality care' frameworks	Patient Navigation (PN) Model	• Early introduction to PC • Focus on the whole cancer continuum • Personal features of patient navigators, such as, capacity to learn about cancer, track cancer services, communicate with professionals, know when and where to refer clients for help, cultural brokers or interpreters for their clients. • Training and orientation to navigators • Continuing education • Flexible approach	Cancer patients have a better quality of life and longer survival when they receive PC concurrently with treatment Cancer PN programs should collect data to track key PN outcomes	Level III
Byock et al. (2006), USA (urban and rural)	Multiple settings, including nursing homes, dialysis clinics, inner city public health and safety net systems and prisons	AI/AN African Americans Medically underserved populations in the city Paediatric patients Mental health patients	Mixed methods evaluation of 22 different projects	Integrated Health Service Delivery (IHSD)	• Community needs assessmentStable institution • Clinician endorsement • Peer-to-peer teaching. • Partnership between the funding bodies and administrators • Successful partnerships, co-ownership and collaboration among academic medical centre, local providers and the community [rural] • Successful projects established working partnerships with local city, country or federal programs [city settings] • Patients and families accepted the delivery model • Established Quality Improvement • Techniques and Routine data collection • PC embedded in cancer care • Creative, careful realignment of existing health system resources • Availability of outpatient PC • Community outreach to raise awareness • On-the-job training • Formal psycho-social and spiritual care QoL assessment tools used to uncover domains of patient or family-reported QoL	Evaluation results are positive: Practicality: Feasibility and Acceptability - 20 of 22 projects were sustained beyond the conclusion of the Grant project - Acceptable to clinicians, administrations, payers, patients and families Access: Availability and use of services - Days for palliative care patients enhanced than national average- Developed partnership with local hospices and with local public health systems to reach to 'hard-to-reach' people - Advance Care Planning - Over half of the projects provided education to patients and families Quality: standards, protocols and quality of care - Symptom protocols measured - Regular data collection proved difficult - Good outpatient PC prevented or managed crises that would otherwise require hospitalisation Financial impact: Health care utilization and costs - Costs did not increase - Total health care costs were moderately reduced - Creative, careful realignment of existing health system resources can improve service delivery Ongoing evaluations	Level III

Table 4 Summary of the Key Articles that describe the Models of Care *(Continued)*

Author(s), Year, Country, Location	Types of Services	Study Population	Methodology	Models	Critical Elements	Outcomes/ Indicators of Success	Daly's Hierarchy of Evidence
						Project led culture change within the organisations Interest increased in pain management and the social needs of all patients	
DeCourtney et al. (2003), USA (remote)	Decentralised home visiting service	Alaskan Native Villages	Qual Focus groups	Decentralised model	• Community input and engagement • Education and training for Community Health Aides/Practitioners • Multiple referral pathways onto program • Home Health Nurse visits patient • Volunteer coordinator determines support needed • Doctor visits during scheduled village visits 4/5 times/year • Hospital provides out of hours telephone support • Volunteer village youths receive training, help with chores, record traditional knowledge in journal • Integrate all health care and social service resources • Flexible, innovative, patient	• More successful than expected • More patients than anticipated • Patients thrived in home environment and lived longer than expected • Formal evaluation: • - Percentage of home deaths increased from 33% in 1997 to 77% in 2001. - Big increase in number of patients with DNR orders - Caregivers were glad as family member remained in village - AN Health Consortium and "investigating possibility of expanding program to other parts of Alaska"	Level III
Fernandes et al. (2010), USA (mixed)	Kokua Kalihi Valley, a Federally qualified health centre. Offering home based palliative care.	91 HBPC clients enrolled, 46 adult patients	Mixed A prospective design. Data collected upon admission then every month afterwards. Different measures included. A caregiver satisfaction survey & telephone interviews.	Home Based Palliative Care Service Model	• Multidisciplinary team delivers medical care, assesses caregivers for stress & burnout, provides patient & family education • Community partnerships • Routine home visits scheduled every 2–3 months • Bilingual case managers were key to building trust • Local partnerships with universities, churches • Counselling provided • Monthly caregiver support groups • Medical insurance was provided by the physician and psychologist • Family based decision-making • The health centre also serves as a PC clinical rotation for nursing, medical and law schools	• This model has been evaluated • Significant reduction in acute care admissions. • The most utilised support service was case management • High caregiver satisfaction rates • Patients reported significant improvements in wellbeing • The program demonstrated the ability to stabilize the care of seriously and terminally ill patients at home, minimize the pain and anxiety for most clients, improve advance care planning, reduce hospitalisations, and increase appropriate use of community resources	Level I
Finke et al. (2004), USA (rural)		AI/AN	Qual Focus group discussions Interviews	Integrated Health Service Delivery Model	• Collaboration among local health services, communities and university Culturally appropriate materials developed • PC training for clinical staff	• Development of stakeholder support • Self sustainable	Level III

Table 4 Summary of the Key Articles that describe the Models of Care *(Continued)*

Author(s), Year, Country, Location	Types of Services	Study Population	Methodology	Models	Critical Elements	Outcomes/ Indicators of Success	Daly's Hierarchy of Evidence
					• Respect and consistency regarding cultural beliefs on death • Strong administrative and management support • Community consultation and needs identified • Local tribal leadership led program • Tribal cultural and spiritual consultation • Distinct PC home health chart • Interdisciplinary team meetings • Coordination with the Zuni EMS • Skilled nursing care • Telephone consultation • Home visits • Adopted policies and procedures		
Kitzes et al. (2004), USA (rural/ remote)	AI/AN Health Care System (IHS facilities)	Secondary data analysis/ 114 Medical Record Review	Mixed methods Medical Record Review and Semi-structured interview	Integrated Service Model in health service settings	• The first IHS Area policy on Palliative Care and Pain Management • Space for traditional ceremonies; • Hospital had an "open door policy" regarding traditional healing; • Spiritual care and cultural practices; • Accommodated families' desires; • Individualise care; • Not make assumptions about preferences; • Pain Management was developed; • A new version of the IHS patient contact form developed • Policies made available to IHS Elder • Innovative PC programs established involving multiple agencies	This itself was an evaluation paper of one Indian Health Service	Level IV
Kitzes et al. (2003), USA (rural/ remote)	AI/AN Health Care System	Case Studies	Description of multiple initiatives	Service Model	• Cross-trained Home Health Agency employees provided EOL care services, rather than a separate hospice staff. • Medical oncologist provides physician support • "High touch, low tech" program designed • Before start of the program, great effort was ensured to make the services culturally appropriate (medical anthropologist worked with the development team; FGDs conducted to enhance understanding) • Home-based PC and staffed by family and village members. • Nurse's availability on "on-call"	• Evaluation was conducted in some health services • There has been a 500% growth in chronic care patients and a 350% growth in the HHA patients	Level III

Table 4 Summary of the Key Articles that describe the Models of Care *(Continued)*

Author(s), Year, Country, Location	Types of Services	Study Population	Methodology	Models	Critical Elements	Outcomes/ Indicators of Success	Daly's Hierarchy of Evidence
					basisInterdisciplinary team discussion		
Mann et al. (2004), NZ (urban)	Mixed medical/ surgical Intensive Care Unit (ICU)	17 ICU patients (14 NZ Maori, 2 Cook Is Maori, 1 Samoan)	Mixed methods Medical Record Review and discussions with family and health professionals		• Maori patients led • Nurses are experienced, confident, close relationship with family • Palliation plan in place • Multidisciplinary approach • Support from GPs, district nurses, • Hospice Service • Bereavement team – available 24/7 • Approach families of all Maori and Samoan ICU patients facing death • Transport patient home to die • Explain families the process • Patient transported home by 2 ICU nurses, all treatment ceases, pain medication provided • If death is not imminent, PC provided by district nurses, GPs and Hospice	All families reported this as a positive experience	Level III
Slater, et al., (2015), NZ (urban)	Hospice	17 participants	Maori-centered, qualitative research 17 semi-structured, face-to-face interviews with patients, and family members and service providers were undertaken	Hospice-based care	• Importance of building relationships with families, communities and primary health care providers • Building networks with Maori providers, traditional healers • Maori staff partnered with hospice nurse (collaborative model) • Work with volunteer services • Helpful staff • 24 h service • Worked as respite care • Working with family • Accommodating and supportive for large family gathering • Spiritual support provided	• Positive experiences reported • Patients and family members felt more confident with regard to communication • Further needs for improvements explored and documented	Level III
Cottle et al. (2013), NZ (urban)	Hospice	1 woman of Maori and Samoan heritage	Qualitative Single person case study	Whare Tapa Wha Model of Maori health	• Organisational changes occurred to ensure collectivist approach to care • Community engagement and ownership • Support from Maori elders • Coordination between multiple-agencies to deal with the complex case • Multi-systemic and wraparound care • Partnership between cultural community and health care professionals • Clear and regular communication between all parties • A "one size fits all" MOC does not work	• Hui created conditions for significant change to hospice services: • Nursing clinic held during hui meetings • Hui volunteers attended initial assessment • Hui volunteers raised awareness in community • Increased use of hospice by Maori and Pacific people • Availability of and access to palliative care for patients can improve QOL	Level IV

Table 4 Summary of the Key Articles that describe the Models of Care *(Continued)*

Author(s), Year, Country, Location	Types of Services	Study Population	Methodology	Models	Critical Elements	Outcomes/ Indicators of Success	Daly's Hierarchy of Evidence
					• Support from hospice – staff time, physical space, management support, nursing clinic • Hui (weekly local gathering) created conditions for significant change to services		
Fruch, et al., (2016), Canada (urban)	Community-based palliative care	Canadian Aboriginal people	Process described	Palliative Shared Care Outreach Team	• Haudenosaunee traditional teachings • Community-based Project Advisory Committee led • Local and regional palliative care partners led implementation; partnership with researchers • Vision was to deliver compassionate, coordinated and comprehensive EOL • Community capacity development • Locally initiated and driven • Dedication, leadership and commitment from key community members and local healthcare providers • Bottom up approach • Built on existing resources and infrastructure • Community had required infrastructure, i.e., health services and providers • Shared vision for change • Effective collaboration among community healthcare providers and members • Community members feeling empowered • 24/7 Palliative Shared Care Outreach Team providing medical, spiritual and cultural support	• Palliative care guidelines and client care pathways are in effect • Increased home deaths as opposed to hospital or hospice deaths • Number of referrals increased • Increased access to palliative care education • Mentorship opportunity for local healthcare providers • Incorporation of traditional teachings to support clients and staff dealing with death and dying	Level III
Kelly et al. (2009), Canada (rural)	Hospital, Palliative Care Service	10 bereaved Aboriginal family members	Qual Semi structured interviews	Service model in hospital setting	• Services extended to visiting family • Interpreter service • Empower patient to decide place of death • Infrastructure • Involvement of all hospital staff • Spiritual care • Participant experiences considered to make changes in services, cultural practices and physical surroundings	Yes – ongoing qualitative evaluation	Level III
St Pierre-Hansen et al. (2010), Canada	Rural Health Centre	3 different baseline studies:	Qual Patient survey, Group discussion	Service Model	• Leadership and governance based on the cultural values and beliefs	• Some form of evaluationMore planned - telephone follow-up of	Level III

Table 4 Summary of the Key Articles that describe the Models of Care *(Continued)*

Author(s), Year, Country, Location	Types of Services	Study Population	Methodology	Models	Critical Elements	Outcomes/ Indicators of Success	Daly's Hierarchy of Evidence
(rural/ remote)		Community Consultation: 50 elders FN PC Study: Qualitative study: 10 participants whose family members received PC	In-depth interviews		• Active community engagement in decision-making and planning stage • Minimise communication barriers and provide support services • Cultural training to staff • Infrastructural/ environmental transformation occurred • Traditional healing and cultural needs incorporated • Elders provided patient support • Interpreters trained as certified medical interpreters • Planned telephone follow-up of bereaved families • Two-day cultural orientation and conflict-resolution training program	bereaved families • Interpreter availability increased from 50 h/month to 250 h/month - patient satisfaction increased	
McGrath (2010), AUS (remote)		72 participants – patients (10), carers (19), AHWs (11), health professionals (30), interpreters (2)	Qualitative Open-ended qualitative interviews	The Living Model for Aboriginal Palliative Care Service Delivery – Conceptual Model	• Considered patients within the context of the extended family • Cultural safety, Community participation, Personal advocacy, Choice, Empowerment • Understand/support/ respect cultural grief practices • Focus on staying at home • Education – consumer and professional • Facilitate family meetings • Service availability in the communities • Address psychosocial and practical problems • Effective communication • Use of Indigenous workers • Provision of respite • Carer and escort support • Advocacy for resources and infrastructure	Not evaluated	Level I
McGrath et al. (2006), AUS (remote)		72 participants	Qualitative Open-ended qualitative interviews	Indigenous Palliative Care Service Delivery Conceptual Model	1) Equity 2) Autonomy and Empowerment 3) The Importance of Trust 4) Humane, Non-judgmental Care 5) Seamless Care 6) Emphasis on Living 7) Cultural Respect	Not evaluated	Level I

Table 4 Summary of the Key Articles that describe the Models of Care (Continued)

Author(s), Year, Country, Location	Types of Services	Study Population	Methodology	Models	Critical Elements	Outcomes/ Indicators of Success	Daly's Hierarchy of Evidence
McGrath et al. (2009), AUS (remote)		72 participants	Qualitative Open-ended qualitative interviews	Service model	• Generic features of palliative care: - 24 h access to palliative care - Focus on living - Respect for choice and autonomy - Patient advocacy - Support to patients, families - Patience and compassion - Multidisciplinary skill - Expert advice - Interagency cooperation - Seamless care - Dedicated professionalism - Carer upskilling - Provision of respite care • Rural and remote specific factors: - Practical assistance (support [oxygen] and organisational [Meals on Wheels]) - Flexible and creative approach to solve some practical issues - Health professionals visit communities • Cultural respect - Relationship and trust-building - Family and community network - Respect for grieving practices - Physical environment - Use of traditional healer and respect for spiritual practices	Not clear	Level I
Carey, et al., (2016), AUS (remote)	Alice Spring Palliative Care Service, NT	Patients accessing the services	Cross-sectional qualitative study/ evaluation study	Day Respite Facility	• Respite care available in the locality • Flexibility of the staff; Staff attitudes • Relationship and friendship with staff • Provision for caring for complex patients, and looking after their clinical, personal needs • Transportation provided • Service was flexible and accommodating	• Qualitative evaluation • Impact has been strongly positive • Therapeutic needs ensured • Client satisfaction • Symptom management, medication compliance, QoL and service coordination – all improved • Act as a 'safe place' for isolated and marginalised community members • ED attendances and hospital admissions dropped	Level II

service models included: Patient Navigators Model [48], Outreach Care [11] and Palliative Shared Care Outreach Model [49] and Home-based service [4], Hospice based care [9, 11], and Integrated Health Service Delivery (IHSD) Model [7, 23, 50]. Eleven of the 17 articles that discussed service models were based on rural/remote locations, two covered mixed locations and four were based in an urban context [mostly within health services settings except for Fruch et al. [49].

In most cases, evaluations of these service models have been included in the published literature, with the following positive short-term outcomes reported (Table

4): symptom management, medication adherence and patients' QoL improved [4, 7, 11, 48, 51, 52]; total health care costs moderately decreased [7]; emergency department (ED) attendances and hospital admissions diminished [52]; service use and patient satisfaction increased [34, 52]; number of deaths at home increased [2, 49]; and families and caregivers reporting positive experiences with the services [4, 9, 51]. Kelly et al., [33] reported there would be ongoing qualitative evaluation. Two remote communities in Australia's Northern Territory (NT) developed their palliative care services according to McGrath's 'Living Model' (Table 4) [14] although it was unclear whether the model had been evaluated in these settings.

The contexts for implementing these innovations varied: some were in-patient hospital or hospice settings whereas others were in community-based care settings. Common themes and critical elements that have facilitated EOL service delivery to Indigenous populations are discussed below (Table 5).

Community engagement

Effective service models implemented in rural or remote settings demonstrated strong community connection and involvement from the outset [2, 7, 11, 33, 49]. Some had built partnerships with local services, some had involved Elders from the communities in the program design and materials development, others reported that they had explored community palliative care needs before designing the projects [2, 7, 23], while some promoted services that were already well-established in the local communities. One study reported that an eight person Elders' Council had influenced strategic planning and operations, and that this Council had shaped the program in the locality [34]. Elders also provided patient support by visiting patients in their residences and as interpreters. Kitzes et al. [6] included tribal and community values in planning, and considered the diversified community and their rich history, sacred culture and traditions [6]. Fruch and colleagues [49] also reported traditional philosophies guiding the project development. Cottle et al. [11], in their case analysis in one urban-based hospice service, explained how they adopted the Whare Tapa Wha Model of Maori health (consisting of four dimensions: spiritual, mental, physical, extended family) into their service delivery [11]. They worked with a Hui (weekly local gathering) to make significant changes to that hospice service, including reallocating staff time, rearranging the physical space, and re-orienting the management format. They made efforts to ensure clear and regular communication between all parties. These initiatives increased use of that particular hospice service by Māori and Pacific peoples.

Education and training

Providing continuing education and training to upskill HSPs and community stakeholders and family members is an integral part of all community-based program models [2, 7, 11, 23, 48]. Byock and colleagues [7] highlighted the significance of peer-to-peer teaching within their program. The palliative care and primary health care (PHC) partnership model described by DeCourtney et al. [2] provided training to village-based workers to develop a cadre of trained workers and volunteers in each Alaskan Native Village. Specific culturally sensitive program materials were developed and used to educate and train patients, families, staff, and volunteers. Training for navigators is an integral part of the Patient Navigators' model [48]. McGrath et al. [14] also highlighted the importance of consumers and professionals' education in their conceptual model. The service models that were implemented in the hospital or health service settings adopted other strategies, such as cultural orientation and conflict-resolution training programs for staff.

Culturally safe service delivery strategy

Various service delivery strategies have been identified. Attributes of individual staff were identified as particularly crucial for service delivery models like the Navigator Model, whereas the IHSD Model [7] adopted a whole-of-service approach (team-based palliative care) in which all staff within the service were informed and involved in delivering palliative care to clients. Where palliative care was integrated within the existing services, funds and resources were generally more sustainably shared and allocated [7, 11, 23, 33], and strong support was usually received from administrative and management staff [23]. Clinicians' endorsement was identified as particularly important to ensuring implementation and continuing delivery of palliative care in health services settings. DeCourtney et al. [2] reported that they did not want to introduce new strategies to deliver palliative care, but instead utilised an existing rural health care delivery model in the Alaskan Native Villages to expand the continuum of care to the EOL setting. They described it as a decentralised model that combined trained volunteers and health care workers in villages, with medical direction from a central urban location and home visits by nurses. They allowed for multiple referral pathways into the program, including by family members. Three studies described decentralised home-based outreach palliative care service models [2, 4, 49] with a large multidisciplinary team including outreach workers, delivering clinical care by making regular home visits every 2–3 months. Bilingual case managers, monthly caregiver support groups and a family-based decision-making process were also part of the service model. DeCourtney et al. [2] stated that doctors visited remote villages 4–5 times per year whereas

Table 5 Critical elements of models of care in an Indigenous setting identified from the published, peer-reviewed literature

Community Engagement	• Community/ local needs identified • Strong community connection and engagement in decision-making, planning, designing the program/ project • Community leadership
Education & Training: Providers, Support Workers & Carers	• Upskilling staff through training • Providing training and education to community members (peer-to-peer teaching) • Culturally-appropriate resources and materials
Culturally Safe Service Delivery Strategy	• Palliative Care integrated with cancer care (palliative care is not separated rather included within the cancer treatment continuum, Link to an established Program) • A team-based whole-of-service approach (Support from all staff) • Creative, careful realignment of existing health system resource utilisation • Clinician endorsement is critical
Flexible Organisation/ Program Structure	• Sufficient flexible funding • Stable institution • Infrastructure (physical environment, Built Environment, accessibility and availability of services) • Organisational policy • Partnership with local agencies, hospitals, academic institutions, etc.
Patient-centered Care	• Culturally safe care (respect for traditional practices and medicine, respectful of traditional beliefs, providing cultural and spiritual care) • Delivery of Care (Inter-disciplinary care, multidisciplinary team, coordination of care, outreach services/ home visit, interpreter services) • Family involvement in care and decision-making, place of death, home visit, outreach services, provide various forms of support, patient empowerment, compassionate care)
Quality Service Delivery	• Ongoing evaluation • Systematic record-keeping to capture progressive data

Fruch et al. [49] described a Palliative Shared Care Outreach team that offered medical, spiritual and cultural care 24/7 to the communities. Carey et al. [52] described a 'Day Respite Facility' in the Alice Spring EOL service in the Northern Territory in Australia which had helped reduce emergency attendances and hospital admissions at the end stages of life while addressing therapeutic needs and client satisfaction.

Flexible organisation/ program structure
A report on innovative palliative care programs noted that they tended to be more successful when implemented in stable institutions, i.e., those not experiencing severe financial stress or undergoing structural changes [7]. Successful programs were flexible in nature and embraced co-ownership and collaborative partnerships. In rural settings, partnerships occurred between academic medical centres, local providers and the community [23]. In urban settings, established working partnerships operated with local city, county or federal programs. These programs mostly worked with established support services, such as volunteer programs [7].

Organisational level changes were reported in Outreach Care, a non-residential, community-based hospice organisation in New Zealand, when the organisation was required "to move beyond Eurocentric individualism to a more collectivist approach to care" [11]. Outreach Care ensured holistic assessment of patients' physical, emotional, psychosocial and economic needs; invited local community members to tell the service about their unmet needs; involved multiple agencies to deal with individual

cases; and maintained clear and regular communication between all parties [11].

Palliative care service providers sometimes underwent infrastructure refurbishments to make their service more comfortable and accessible to Indigenous patients and their families [14, 33, 34, 53, 54]. Examples included: the construction of a new building with a smudge room (in which the smoke of sacred herbs is used for ceremonial purification), enlarging a common area in order to accommodate large family groups, and ensuring the availability of large patient rooms [11, 52].

Patient-centred care
Patient-centred care that is "respectful of and responsive to the preferences, needs and values of patients and consumers" was prioritised in all these service models. The dimensions of patient-centred care are "respect, emotional support, physical comfort, information and communication, continuity and transition, care coordination, involvement of family and carers, and access to care" [55] p.13.

The availability of navigators' support during EOL phases was successful in ensuring that patients found cancer care understandable, available, accessible, affordable, appropriate, and accountable. Navigators work as cultural brokers and interpreters for their clients, and ensure that the clients are participating fully and actively in care [48]. One navigator noted,

"when a client is terminal, we work hard to take a neutral position relative to cancer treatment. We

provide information and allow them to make their own decisions about continuing chemotherapy and other treatments. If a client starts saying he/she is 'tired of treatment and pain' and 'it's time to return to God,' we discuss what the client and family want of the future, and provide information about advance directives, palliative care, and hospice." [48]

As part of the IHSD Model, implemented through the Promoting Excellence in EOL Care program in the USA, different communities adopted different locally suitable strategies to promote EOL care. The IHSD model introduced new standards and protocols to ensure delivery of core palliative care services: pain and symptom management, psychosocial care, spiritual counselling and support, QoL improvement and continuity of care, value-based care, and life-review [7]. Twenty of the 22 projects were sustained in some form by their home institutions beyond the conclusion of the program funding. DeCourtney et al. [39] described how, as part of the IHSD program, they established a village-focused, culturally sensitive, regionally based physician- and home health nurse-led multidisciplinary palliative care program in rural Alaska Native communities. The Helping Hands Program provided training to village-based health care providers on palliative care, and these trained health care providers provided at-home care during EOL. This model allowed for multiple referral pathways while helping to decentralise services, by ensuring central technical support from a local health service. When patients were admitted into the program, four steps were followed: 1) individual needs-based assessment; 2) identification of differences in goals between patient and service providers; 3) individual care plan development concordant with community values; and 4) establishment of trust. Patients and family members were pleased with the option to remain at home in familiar surroundings as they neared the EOL. The frequency of nurses' visits to patients' homes was increased if the patient's condition worsened and bereavement support to family members after a patient's death was also provided.

Quality improvement in service delivery

Most of the projects, especially those under the Promoting Excellence in Palliative Care program in the USA [7], used established quality improvement techniques for systematic record-keeping and to monitor and observe program impacts on patient outcomes. Byock et al. [7] described how various projects refined their palliative care service delivery strategies based on feedback from clients and observed changes in outcomes. Clinical data were used in care planning, including the use of QoL assessment tools to highlight domains of patient or family-reported needs and helped to focus therapeutic attention.

Discussion

This comprehensive review of the literature has identified a variety of key innovative strategies for delivering palliative care to Indigenous communities in Australia, NZ, Canada, and the USA. Preferences, barriers and needs that can influence quality of palliative care for Indigenous patients and their families have also been examined. Despite diversity amongst the included Indigenous communities, similarities in terms of the needs and preferences were observed in the literature. Many of the issues identified are not likely to be very different from those of other people at the EOL; however, HSPs drawing on those that were more unique to Indigenous people might make a big difference to the care for Indigenous people globally. Overwhelmingly the included publications focused on community-based palliative care services. There were very few examples in the literature of culturally safe palliative care delivery within hospital inpatient settings or specifically designed 'stand-alone' inpatient palliative care facilities (for example, hospices). This could be because of the preference of Indigenous people to be cared for at home [56] (as identified in this review) or because many Indigenous people do not feel safe in hospitals [57]. Clearly, admission to a specialised palliative care inpatient facility may be required for brief episodes of care (i.e. respite, acute symptom stabilisation).

Key preferences identified are: family and community involvement; dying at home; provision for cultural and spiritual ceremonies within service settings; open and honest communication from health professionals; respectful treatment by HSPs, and availability of Indigenous staff. Indigenous people expressed a strong preference to spend time with families and communities at EOL. Families are pivotal to the wellbeing of dying Indigenous patients [11, 24, 41]. In congruence with that need, service models have been developed to ensure that families are included in clinical decision-making. Efforts have been made to build relationships with family members and carers, to promote respect for family caregivers' roles, and to facilitate death at home when appropriate. Reconnection with the land before death is frequently highlighted as a strong preference for Indigenous people across the four countries. It was observed that some innovative services endeavour to bring people back to their 'homeland' to die. However, additional staffing of personal support workers, outreach community workers, nurses and case managers are required to facilitate the choice of dying on the homeland, and for some people, at home. When quality palliative care enables people to die at home, community members are more willing to engage in the care process [49]. Hospices in New Zealand have tailored their services to meet the needs of Māori patients by increasing flexibility, partnering Māori hospice staff with both non-Indigenous staff and primary health care providers, working closely with families, creating physical space for large families to visit, and regular communication between multiple agencies [11]. Community leadership of EOL program development in rural and remote Indigenous communities facilitates education and training of support workers, in turn creating employment opportunities.

The major barriers that restrict access to culturally appropriate palliative care services include: distance from and cost of services; a paucity of culturally safe service environments; disrespectful treatment by HSPs, poor communication, and differences in understanding of and priorities at the EOL between HSPs and Indigenous people. We have identified six critical elements within the identified models that attempted to deliver culturally sensitive palliative care services to Indigenous populations and address the above-mentioned preferences and needs: community engagement, education and training, culturally safe service delivery strategy, flexible organisation/ program structure, patient-centred care, and quality service delivery.

Key models and innovative service strategies for improving Indigenous access to palliative care services must ensure a culturally safe environment for Indigenous families by employing appropriate Indigenous health workers within the services, providing compulsory cultural awareness programs for all staff, and creating opportunities for community awareness-raising [57]. Where these preferences were addressed adequately, improved quality of care was achieved in terms of access to services, client satisfaction, symptom management, and corresponding declining ED and hospital admissions. Engagement and partnership of palliative care programs with existing local health services has been a key to success, especially in rural and remote settings. Likewise, within the urban context and for inpatient settings, strong relationships and regular communication with primary health care providers can play a pivotal role in expediting referrals to palliative care services, and in endorsing the value of palliative care facilities to patients, families and other health services [49]. Such actions can facilitate the trust-building process between patients, family members and service providers, and alleviate fears around palliative care services. However, further research is required to explore the palliative care needs and experiences of Indigenous people living in urban areas.

Health partnerships at national, provincial and regional levels are important in promoting culturally safe palliative care service delivery for Indigenous populations. Despite 'palliative care' being identified as a 'priority area' at all levels of care and to the whole population in international policy documents, major barriers such as, lack of public and professional awareness of the benefits of palliative care, workforce shortages, lack of infrastructure and care delivery models and an inadequate evidence base have made EOL care inaccessible to many people [58]. Moreover, in the developed world, palliative care has become synonymous with service provision, rather than with its original purpose, as an ethos and approach to care. Under this ethos, palliative care begins at the time of the diagnosis, however in practice, care has tended to be provided only the last months and weeks of life, due to limited resources. Therefore, many population and disease groups lack access to specialist palliative care. From the studies synthesised in this comprehensive review, Indigenous peoples seem to be supported during the terminal illness and end of life in ways that fit with the key principles of a palliative approach to care. A palliative approach to caring emphasises patient- and family-centred care that focuses on the person and not just the disease, the importance of therapeutic relationships between care providers and the patient and family and clear communication throughout the illness trajectory about goals of care, comfort measures, and needs and wishes [59, 60]. Therefore, the way forward, is to upskill primary care professionals in indigenous communities in the principles and practice of a palliative approach to care for a more sustainable model of care. Although not Indigenous-specific, one such upskilling program has been successful in the field of Motor Neurone Disease [61].

More recently, in the wealthy nations, including Australia, NZ and Canada, government funding is being allocated strategically [58]. In Australia, increasing government interest in all aspects of reducing disparities in Indigenous health and closing service gaps has been evident in Close the Gap campaigns and other programs. Government contracts for a broad spectrum of health and education services now contain a clause specifically requiring providers to address Indigenous issues. There have also been many Indigenous-specific EOL initiatives developed by non-governmental organisations, i.e., Palliative Care Australia (Program of Experience in the Palliative Approach [PEPA] [62]), the Palliative Care Outcomes Collaboration [PCOC]) [63] and Cancer Australia.

In this context, it is hoped that evidence of practical, context-specific frameworks or models of care will contribute to enhancing the understanding of particular needs of different population groups, which in turn will ensure universal coverage of appropriate delivery of palliative care to all population groups.

Conclusion

Health equity is an important goal and includes efforts to ensure equitable access to quality treatment, resources and appropriate support. However, Indigenous people have been underrepresented in palliative care services and this is an important issue for attention. This review has highlighted the key features of culturally safe service delivery that have been reported to be working well in the Indigenous palliative care context. "'Good care' is defined by those receiving the care, and not those who provide it" [64]. A flexible approach, adaptability to the context and 'buy-in' from local communities are reported to be some of the essential features of successful service models to deliver palliative care services to Indigenous populations and the literature emphasises that a 'one size fits all' approach is not appropriate [11]. This flexibility must incorporate family involvement in decision-making [4] and extend to the referral process, such that family members are able to refer patients to specialist palliative care services [2, 23]. McGrath et al. [14], reiterated that, "a static model … [should not] be imposed on services or communities but rather a living, flexible model is required to assist with service delivery and health policy" [p59]. Flexibility in these settings also augments Indigenous representation and retention within the health workforce [9].

Abbreviations
AI/ANs: American Indians and Alaska Natives; ED: Emergency Department; EoL: End-of-Life; FGDs: Focus Group Discussion; GP: General Practitioners; IHS: Indian Health Service; HSPs: Health Service Providers; ICU: Intensive Care Unit; IHSD: Integrated Health Service Delivery; MOL: Model of Care; NT: Northern Territory; NZ: New Zealand; PC: Palliative Care; PCOC: The Palliative Care Outcomes Collaboration; PEPA: Program of Experience in the Palliative Approach; PHC: Primary Health Care; PN: Patient Navigation; PRISMA: Preferred Reporting Items for Systematic Review and Meta-Analysis; QoL: Quality of Life; USA: The United States of America

Funding
The review was undertaken under the auspices of the Centre of Research Excellence in Discovering Indigenous Strategies to improve Cancer Outcomes Via Engagement, Research Translation and Training (DISCOVER-TT CRE, funded by the Australian National Health and Medical Research Council #1041111), and the Strategic Research Partnership to improve Cancer control for Indigenous Australians [STREP Ca-CIndA, funded through Cancer Council NSW (SRP 13–01)], with supplementary funding from Cancer Council WA. We also acknowledge the ongoing support of the Lowitja Institute, Australia's National Institute for Aboriginal and Torres Strait Islander Health Research. Shaouli Shahid was supported by an NHMRC Early Career Fellowship (#1037386). JW is supported by NHMRC Postgraduate Research Scholarship (#1133793) and a University of Western Australia Athelstan and Amy Saw Top-Up Scholarship.

Authors' contributions
SS and SCT conceived the study. SS coordinated the whole process, contributed to the reference screening, analysed data and drafted the manuscript; EVT and JAW undertook the literature search. EVT and SC contributed substantially to reference screening and data analysis. All authors made considerable contributions to writing the manuscript and approved the final draft.

Competing interests
The authors declare that they have no competing interests.

Author details
[1]Centre for Aboriginal Studies (CAS), Curtin University, Kent Street, Bentley, WA 6102, Australia. [2]Western Australian Centre for Rural Health (WACRH), School of Population and Global Health, The University of Western Australia, Geraldton, WA 6530, Australia. [3]School of Nursing, Midwifery and Paramedicine, Curtin University, Kent Street, Perth, WA 6102, Australia. [4]Palliative Care Unit, School of Psychology and Public Health, La Trobe University, Melbourne 3086, Australia. [5]Institute for Health Research, Notre Dame University, Fremantle, WA 6160, Australia.

References
1. World Health Organisation. Palliative Care. Fact sheet N°402. WHO. 2015. http://www.who.int/mediacentre/factsheets/fs402/en/. Accessed 04 Apr 2018.
2. DeCourtney CA, Jones K, Merriman MP, Heavener N, Branch PK. Establishing a culturally sensitive palliative care program in rural Alaska Native American communities. J Palliat Med. 2003;6:501–10.
3. Meier D. Increased access to palliative care and hospice services. Opportunities to improve value in health care. Milbank Q. 2011;89:343–80.
4. Fernandes R, Braun KL, Ozawa J, Compton M, Guzman C, Somogyi-Zalud E. Home-based palliative care services for underserved populations. J Palliat Med. 2010;13:413–9.
5. National Hospice and Palliative Care Organisation. Ground-breaking palliative care resolution is adopted at World Health Assembly in Geneva. Media release. 2014. http://www.globalpartnersincare.org/news/ground-breaking-palliative-care-resolution-adopted-world-health-assembly-geneva. Accessed 03 Apr 2018.
6. Kitzes J, Berger L. End-of-life issues for American Indians/Alaska Natives: insights from one Indian Health Service area. J Palliat Med. 2004;7:830–8.
7. Byock I, Twohig J, Merriman M, Collins K. Promoting excellence in end-of-life care: a report on innovative models of palliative care. J Palliat Med. 2006;9:137–51.
8. Hampton M, Baydala A, Drost C, McKay-McNabb K. Bridging conventional Western health care practices with traditional Aboriginal approaches to end of life care: a dialogue between Aboriginal families and health care professionals. Can J Nurs Inform. 2009;4:22–66.
9. Slater T, Matheson A, Ellison-Loschmann L, Davies C, Earp R, Gellatly K, Holdaway M. Exploring Maori cancer patients', their families', community and hospice views of hospice care. Int J Palliat Nurs. 2015;21:439–45.
10. Australian Institute of Health and Welfare. Australia's health 2014. Australia's health series no. 14. Cat. no. AUS 178. Canberra: AIHW; 2014.
11. Cottle M, Hughes C, Gremillion H. A community approach to palliative care: embracing Indigenous concepts and practices in a hospice setting. J Syst Ther. 2013;32:56–69.
12. McGrath P, Holewa H. Seven principles for Indigenous palliative care service delivery: research findings from Australia. Austral-Asian J Cancer. 2006;5:179–86.
13. McMichael C, Kirk M, Manderson L, Hoban E, Potts H. Indigenous women's perceptions of breast cancer diagnosis and treatment in Queensland. Aust N Z J Public Health. 2000;24:515–9.
14. McGrath P. The living model: an Australian model for Aboriginal palliative care service delivery with international implications. J Palliat Care. 2010;26:59–64.
15. Agency for Clinical Innovation. Understanding the process to develop a Model of Care–An ACI Framework. Version 1.0. Chatswood: Agency for Clinical Innovation; 2013.

16. Greenhalgh T, Robert G, MacFarlane F, Bate P, Kyriakidou O. Diffusion of innovations in service organizations: systematic review and recommendations. Milbank Q. 2004;82:581–629.

17. Liberati A, Altman DG, Tetzlaff J, Mulrow C, Gøtzsche PC, Ioannidis JP, et al. The PRISMA statement for reporting systematic reviews and meta-analyses of studies that evaluate healthcare interventions: explanation and elaboration. BMJ. 2009;339:b2700.

18. Dixon-Woods M, Cavers D, Agarwal S, Annandale E, Arthur A, Harvey J, et al. Conducting a critical interpretive synthesis of the literature on access to healthcare by vulnerable groups. BMC Med Res Methodol. 2006;6:35.

19. Daly J, Willis K, Small R, Green J, Welch N, Kealy M, Hughes E. A hierchachy of evidence for assessing qualitative health research. J Clin Epidemiol. 2007;60:43–9.

20. Aoun S, Kristjanson L. Evidence in palliative care research: how should it be gathered? Med J Aust. 2005;183:264–6.

21. Nicholson E, Murphy T, Larkin P, Normand C, Guerin S. Protocol for a thematic synthesis to identify key themes and messages from a palliative care research network. BMC Res Notes. 2016;9:1.

22. Castleden H, Crooks VA, Hanlon N, Schuurman N. Providers' perceptions of Aboriginal palliative care in British Columbia's rural interior. Health Soc Care Community. 2010;18:483–91.

23. Finke B, Bowannie T, Kitzes J. Palliative care in the Pueblo of Zuni. J Palliat Med. 2004;7:135–43.

24. Frey R, Gott M, Raphael D, Black S, Teleo-Hope L, Lee H, Wang Z. 'Where do I go from here'? A cultural perspective on challenges to the use of hospice services. Health Soc Care Community. 2013;21:519–29.

25. Isaacson M, Karel B, Varilek BM, Steenstra WJ, Tanis-Heyenga JP, Wagner A. Insights from health care professionals regarding palliative care options on South Dakota reservations. J Transcult Nurs. 2014;26:473–9.

26. Taylor JE, Simmonds S, Earp R, Dip PT. Māori perspectives on hospice care. Divers Equal Health Care. 2014;11:61–70.

27. Schrader S, Nelson M, Eidsness L. Reflections on end of life. Comparison of American Indian and non-Indian peoples in South Dakota. Am Indian Culture Res J. 2009;33:67–87.

28. Shahid S, Bessarab D, Van Schaik KD, Aoun SM, Thompson SC. Improving palliative care outcomes for Aboriginal Australians: service providers' perspectives. BMC Palliat Care. 2013;12:26.

29. Colclough YY, Brown GM. American Indians experiences of life-threatening illness and end of life. J Hosp Palliat Nurs. 2014;16:404–13.

30. Frey R, Raphael D, Bellamy G, Gott M. Advance care planning for Maori, Pacific and Asian people: the views of New Zealand healthcare professionals. Health Soc Care Community. 2014;22:290–9.

31. Fried O. Palliative care for patients with end-stage renal failure: reflections from Central Australia. Palliat Med. 2003;7:514–9.

32. Hotson KE, Macdonald SM, Martin BD. Understanding death and dying in select First Nations communities in Northern Manitoba: issues of culture and remote service delivery in palliative care. Int J Circumpol Health. 2004;63:25–38.

33. Kelly L, Linkewich B, Cromarty H, St Pierre-Hansen N, Antone I, Giles C. Palliative care of First Nations people: a qualitative study of bereaved family members. Can Fam Physician. 2009;55:394–5. e397.

34. St Pierre-Hansen N, Kelly L, Linkewich B, Cromarty H, Walker R. Translating research into practice: developing cross-cultural First Nations palliative care. J Palliat Care. 2010;26:41–6.

35. Hampton M, Baydala A, Bourassa C, McKay-McNabb K, Placsko C, Goodwill K, et al. Completing the circle: elders speak about end-of-life care with Aboriginal families in Canada. J Palliat Care. 2010;26:6–14.

36. Bray Y, Goodyear-Smith F. Patient and family perceptions of hospice services: 'I knew they weren't like hospitals'. J Prim Health Care. 2013;5:206–13.

37. Brooke NJ. Needs of Aboriginal and Torres Strait Islander clients residing in Australian residential aged-care facilities. Aust J Rural Health. 2011;19:166–70.

38. Colqhoun S, Dockery A. The link between Indigenous culture and wellbeing: qualitative evidence for Australian Aboriginal peoples. CLMR Discussion Paper Series 2012/01. Perth: Curtin University; 2012.

39. Decourtney CA, Branch PK, Morgan KM. Gathering information to develop palliative care programs for Alaska's Aboriginal peoples. J Palliat Care. 2010; 26:22–31.

40. Dembinsky M. Exploring Yamatji perceptions and use of palliative care: an ethnographic study. Int J Palliat Nurs. 2014;20:387–93.

41. Bellamy G, Gott M. What are the priorities for developing culturally appropriate palliative and end-of-life care for older people? The views of healthcare staff working in New Zealand. Health Soc Care Community. 2013;21:26–34.

42. Kelly L, Minty A. End-of-life issues for Aboriginal patients: a literature review. Can Fam Physician. 2007;53:1459–65.

43. Marr L, Neale D, Wolfe V, Kitzes J. Confronting myths: the Native American experience in an academic inpatient palliative care consultation program. J Palliat Med. 2012;15:71–6.

44. Davidson PM, Jiwa M, DiGiacomo ML, McGrath SJ, Newton PJ, Durey AJ, et al. The experience of lung cancer in Aboriginal and Torres Strait Islander peoples and what it means for policy, service planning and delivery. Aust Health Rev. 2013;37:70–8.

45. Shahid S, Finn L, Bessarab D, Thompson S. 'Nowhere to room ... nobody told them': logistical and cultural impediments to Aboriginal peoples' participation in cancer treatment. Aust Health Rev. 2011;35:235–41.

46. Oetzel J, Simpson M, Berryman K, Iti T, Reddy R. Managing communication tensions and challenges during the end-of-life journey: perspectives of Maori kaumatua and their whanau. Health Commun. 2015;30:350–60.

47. Oetzel JG, Simpson M, Berryman K, Reddy R. Differences in ideal communication behaviours during end-of-life care for Maori carers/patients and palliative care workers. Palliat Med. 2015;29:764–6.

48. Braun KL, Kagawa-Singer M, Holden AEC, Burhansstipanov L, Tran JH, Seals BF, et al. Cancer patient navigator tasks across the cancer care continuum. J Health Care Poor Underserved. 2012;23:398–413.

49. Fruch V, Monture L, Prince H, Kelley ML. Coming home to die: six nations of the Grand River Territory develops community-based palliative care. Int J Indig Health. 2016;11:50–74.

50. Kitzes JA, Domer T. Palliative care: an emerging issue for American Indians and Alaskan Natives. J Pain Palliat Care Pharmacother. 2003;17:201–10.

51. Mann S, Galler D, Williams P, Frost P. Caring for patients and families at the end of life: withdrawal of intensive care in the patient's home. N Z Med J. 2004;117:U935.

52. Carey TA, Schouten K, Wakerman J, Humphreys JS, Miegel F, Murphy S, Arundell M. Improving the quality of life of palliative and chronic disease patients and carers in remote Australia with the establishment of a day respite facility. BMC Palliat Care. 2016;15:62.

53. McGrath P. Exploring Aboriginal peoples' experience of relocation for treatment during end-of-life care. Int J Palliat Nurs. 2006;12:102–8.

54. McGrath PD, Phillips EL. Insights from the Northern Territory on factors that facilitate effective palliative care for Aboriginal peoples. Aust Health Rev. 2009;33:636–44.

55. Australian Commission on Safety and Quality in Healthcare. Patient-centred Care: Improving quality and safety by focusing care on patients and consumers. Discussion Paper. Sydney: ACSQHC; 2010.

56. McGrath P, Holewa H, Kail-Buckley S. "They should come out here ...": research findings on lack of local palliative care services for Australian Aboriginal people. Am J Hosp Palliat Care. 2007;24:105–13.

57. Australian Commission on Safety and Quality in Healthcare (ACSQHC). Consumer health information needs and preferences: Perspectives of culturally and linguistically diverse and Aboriginal and Torres Strait Islander people. Sydney: Cultural & Indigenous Research Centre Australia; 2017.

58. Morrison RS. A National Palliative Care Strategy for Canada. J Palliat Med. 2017;20(Suppl 1):S63–75.

59. Kristjanson LJ, Toye C, Dawson S: New dimensions in palliative care: a palliative approach to neurodegenerative diseases and final illness in older people. Med J Aust. 2003; 179(Suppl 6):S41-3.

60. Stajduhar KI, Tayler C: Taking an "upstream" approach in the care of dying cancer patients: the case for a palliative approach. Can Oncol Nurs J. 2014;24:144-53.

61. McConigley R, Aoun S, Kristjanson L, Colyer S, Deas K, O'Connor M, et al. Implementation and evaluation of an education program to guide palliative care for people with motor neurone disease. Palliat Med. 2012;26:994–1000.

62. Shahid S, Ekberg S, Holloway M, Jacka C, Yates P, Garvey G, Thompson SC. Experiential learning to increase palliative care competence among the Indigenous workforce: an Australian experience. BMJ Support Palliat Care. 2018. https://doi.org/10.1136/bmjspcare-2016-001296.

63. Eager K, Watters P, Currow DC, Aoun SM, Yates P. The Australian palliative care outcomes collaboration (PCOC) – measuring the quality and outcomes of palliative care on a routine basis. Aust Health Rev. 2010;34:186–92.

64. Ramsden IM. Cultural safety and nursing education in Aotearoa and Te Waipounamu (PhD Thesis). Wellington: Victoria: University of Wellington; 2002.

65. Lawrenson R, Smyth D, Kara E, Thomson R. Rural general practitioner
     perspectives of the needs of Maori patients requiring palliative care. N Z
     Med J. 2010;123:30–6.
66. Prince H, Kelley M. An integrative framework for conducting palliative care
     research with First Nations communities. J Palliat Care. 2010;26:47–53.
67. McGrath PD, Patton MA, Ogilvie KF, Rayner RD, McGrath ZM, Holewa HA.
     The case for Aboriginal Health Workers in palliative care. Aust Health Rev.
     2007;31:430–9.

11

Redefining diagnosis-related groups (DRGs) for palliative care

Matthias Vogl[1,2†], Eva Schildmann[3*†] ⓘ, Reiner Leidl[1,2], Farina Hodiamont[3], Helen Kalies[3], Bernd Oliver Maier[4], Marcus Schlemmer[5], Susanne Roller[5] and Claudia Bausewein[3]

Abstract

Background: Hospital costs and cost drivers in palliative care are poorly analysed. It remains unknown whether current German Diagnosis-Related Groups, mainly relying on main diagnosis or procedure, reproduce costs adequately. The aim of this study was therefore to analyse costs and reimbursement for inpatient palliative care and to identify relevant cost drivers.

Methods: Two-center, standardised micro-costing approach with patient-level cost calculations and analysis of the reimbursement situation for patients receiving palliative care at two German hospitals (7/2012–12/2013). Data were analysed for the total group receiving hospital care covering, but not exclusively, palliative care (group A) and the subgroup receiving palliative care only (group B). Patient and care characteristics predictive of inpatient costs of palliative care were derived by generalised linear models and investigated by classification and regression tree analysis.

Results: Between 7/2012 and 12/2013, 2151 patients received care in the two hospitals including, but not exclusively, on the PCUs (group A). In 2013, 784 patients received care on the two PCUs only (group B). Mean total costs per case were € 7392 (SD 7897) (group A) and € 5763 (SD 3664) (group B), mean total reimbursement per case € 5155 (SD 6347) (group A) and € 4278 (SD 2194) (group B). For group A/B on the ward, 58%/67% of the overall costs and 48%/53%, 65%/82% and 64%/72% of costs for nursing, physicians and infrastructure were reimbursed, respectively. Main diagnosis did not significantly influence costs. However, duration of palliative care and total length of stay were (related to the cost calculation method) identified as significant cost drivers.

Conclusions: Related to the cost calculation method, total length of stay and duration of palliative care were identified as significant cost drivers. In contrast, main diagnosis did not reflect costs. In addition, results show that reimbursement within the German Diagnosis-Related Groups system does not reproduce the costs adequately, but causes a financing gap for inpatient palliative care.

Keywords: Diagnosis related groups, DRG, Costs and cost analysis, Reimbursement, Palliative care, Palliative care funding

* Correspondence: eva.schildmann@med.uni-muenchen.de
†Equal contributors
[3]Munich University Hospital, Department of Palliative Medicine,
Ludwig-Maiximilians-Universitaet Munich, Marchioninistr. 15, 81377 Munich,
Germany
Full list of author information is available at the end of the article

Background

Patients in palliative care (PC) usually suffer from cancer or advanced neurological, cardiac, pulmonary or renal disease, with a highly individual care utilization [1]. Needs of patients and their family members are diverse. They include relief of symptoms, psychosocial and spiritual as well as practical support [2, 3] – care taking dimensions which need to be reflected by reimbursement calculation. After its introduction in 2003, it has continuously been discussed whether the German Diagnosis-Related Groups (G-DRG) system is an appropriate payment scheme for hospital palliative care units (PCUs) [4, 5]. PC focuses on specific patient and family needs regardless of the underlying diagnosis. In contrast, patient classification by the DRG system mainly relies on main diagnosis or procedures.

In Australia, where the G-DRG system is derived from, [6] "acute care" (treatment driven primarily by patient's diagnosis) is distinguished from "subacute care" (treatment driven primarily by patient's functional status and quality of life) [7–9]. It is acknowledged that "sub-acute care" episodes - including PC - are not adequately classified by DRGs and require a different classification approach [10, 11]. A large Australian study demonstrated that the complexity of the patients' situation, reflected by factors such as phase of illness (stable, unstable, deteriorating, terminal), functional status, severity of symptoms and age, best predicts the resource use and cost in PC, together with the model of PC in the ambulatory setting (multidisciplinary or nursing or medical therapy only) [1, 9]. Consequently, Australia has implemented a special PC reimbursement system outside the DRG-system, based on these factors [7].

Hospital treatment costs and related cost drivers in PC are poorly analysed [12]. It remains unknown whether current G-DRGs, merely accounting for main diagnosis or procedure and developed for acute inpatient care episodes, reproduce costs in PC in Germany adequately. Specifically, it is unknown to which extent, in which direction and in which categories PC costs deviate from the DRG reimbursement.

The aim of this study therefore was to analyse inpatient PC costs and reimbursement, and to identify patient and care characteristics predictive of case costs.

Methods

Study design, setting and costing

PC costs were analysed in a cross-sectional, two-center approach. Data were acquired from two German hospitals for all patients who received care on their PCUs from July 2012 to December 2013 ("group A"): a university hospital providing 10 PCU beds, and a non-university hospital providing PCU 30 beds. Data for group A, including length of stay (LOS) data, refer to the complete stay of the patients in the hospital, not only encompassing the stay on the PCU, but also possible days on a normal ward or the intensive care unit. A subgroup of cases with a PCU stay only in 2013 (group B) was also analysed. For 2012, data were unavailable to identify this subgroup.

Clinical and socio-demographic data were acquired from hospital medical records, inpatient costs on patient level from the hospitals' costing systems. Costs had been calculated using the InEK costing scheme (Institute for the Hospital Remuneration System) [13, 14]. Investment costs for PC were not calculated [15]. The InEK costing scheme is an activity-based full cost approach which has become a generally accepted national costing standard [13]. Each cost center and cost category in a hospital is represented in a cost-matrix, where a cost classifier is defined for each cost module (combination of cost center and cost category). For example, costs of physicians (cost category) on the PCU are allocated to patients based on their LOS (cost classifier). PC is part of the normal ward cost center within this calculation, and is not specifically reflected by any subgrouping. For most cost categories on the ward, LOS is used as the cost classifier to allocate costs to patients. For diagnostic or procedural cost centers such as operating room, radiology or laboratory tests, point systems, actual duration or surgery time are used as cost classifiers. This kind of activity-based micro costing is used in several countries alike and allows comparison of costs between health care systems [16–18].

In the G-DRG-system, a procedure code for specialist palliative care (SPC) was introduced, defined by criteria for SPC acknowledgement and the duration of SPC provision (< 7 days, 7–13 days, 14 to 20 days or > 20 days). A supplementary fee is provided for SPC > 7 days, increasing with the duration of SPC. We used the actual reimbursement of each case, including supplementary fees (e.g. for duration of SPC and for time-consuming nursing care), and distributed it based on the national average cost matrix for the respective DRG, to analyse differences between costs and reimbursement (profit) at the cost-module level of the cost-matrix. We set profit distribution in relation to LOS.

Statistical analysis

Cost and reimbursement data are given as mean and standard deviation (SD). Spearman's rank correlation was used to test the relationship of current cost classifiers and costs. The relationship of LOS and costs is visualized by a scatterplot with a linear and LOESS fit line (locally weighted scatterplot smoothing). LOESS was chosen to give an intuitive, optical view on trends in the scatterplot. Therefore, the best fitting models on localized subsets of points in the plot are used instead of a global function, to generate an overall fit line [19].

To analyse the effects of key cost drivers, such as clinical and socio-demographic factors, on case costs, we used a generalized linear model (GLM) with gamma distribution and log link function. A simple ordinary least squares (OLS) model would have required Gaussian distribution, and was thus not able to process the right skewed (*Kolmogorov-Smirnov-Test*, $p < 0.000$) case cost data (Fig. 1) [20]. The GLM suits best for the integration of high cost cases to a single model and can reduce heteroscedasticity of OLS residuals [21, 22]. The GLM model provides relative cost differences for each key cost driver via exponentiated coefficients. For the nearly normal distributed case costs per day, we used OLS regression. Covariates included in regression analyses (independent of being significant in bivariate analysis) were location, age, gender, discharge reason, kind of supplementary fees for SPC, other supplementary fees (e.g. for very costly drugs), LOS, Major diagnostic category (MDC), number of side diagnoses and number of operation and procedure codes. Main diagnosis and DRG were not considered in regression analysis due to too many values (degrees of freedom) to be reported.

To test in multivariate analyses whether the current DRG differentiation by main diagnosis is discriminative for costs, MDC was used as a proxy for main diagnosis and DRG. A p-value of < 0.05 was considered significant. Statistical analyses were performed with SPSS 22.

To test a DRG-grouping based on current cost classifiers and determine cut-off values, we used classification and regression tree (CART) analysis. CART is a decision tool that has been used in defining the Australian casemix classification for PC [9] and is able to maximise homogeneity within DRGs by defining cut-off values for the strongest predictors of costs, which serve as the splitting variables [23].

The study was approved by the ethics committee of Ludwig-Maximilians-Universität Munich (reference number: 24–15).

Results

Sample characteristics

Between July 2012 and December 2013, 2151 patients received care in the two hospitals including, but not exclusively, on the PCUs (group A). In 2013, 784 patients received care on the two PCUs only (group B). Both groups were similar regarding age, gender, and proportions of malignant disease. Proportions of patients who died on the unit, of patients who received SPC for at least 7 days and the mean number of secondary diagnoses were also similar between groups. Mean LOS was 12 ± 10 days for group A and 10 ± 6 days for group B (Table 1).

Costs and reimbursement

For group A, mean total costs per case were €7392 (SD 7897, range 134–132769). Mean total reimbursement per case, including supplementary fees, was €5155 (SD 6347), creating a total financing gap of €2237 per case. Mean case costs per day were €578 (SD 143). 84% of the costs per case occurred on the ward, 10% were related to diagnostics and therapy and 4% to intensive care. However, only 70% of reimbursement was distributed to the cost centre "ward" (i.e. all wards, including the PCU). 62% of the overall financing gap was related to nursing, 15% to physicians, and 35% to medical and non-medical infrastructure on the cost centre "ward", respectively. For laboratory tests, reimbursement was more than double the costs (270%). The financing gap on the cost centre "ward" (all wards including the PCU) was €2599. For this cost centre, 58% of the overall costs, and 48%, 65% and 64% of costs for nursing, physicians and (medical and non-medical) infrastructure were reimbursed, respectively (Table 2). For group B, i.e. the subgroup of patients with a stay on a PCU only, mean total costs per case were €5763 (SD 3664), mean total reimbursement per case €4278 (SD 2194), creating a total financing gap of €1485. On the PCU, the financing gap was €1767. 67% of overall costs, and 53%, 82%, 72% of costs for nursing, physicians

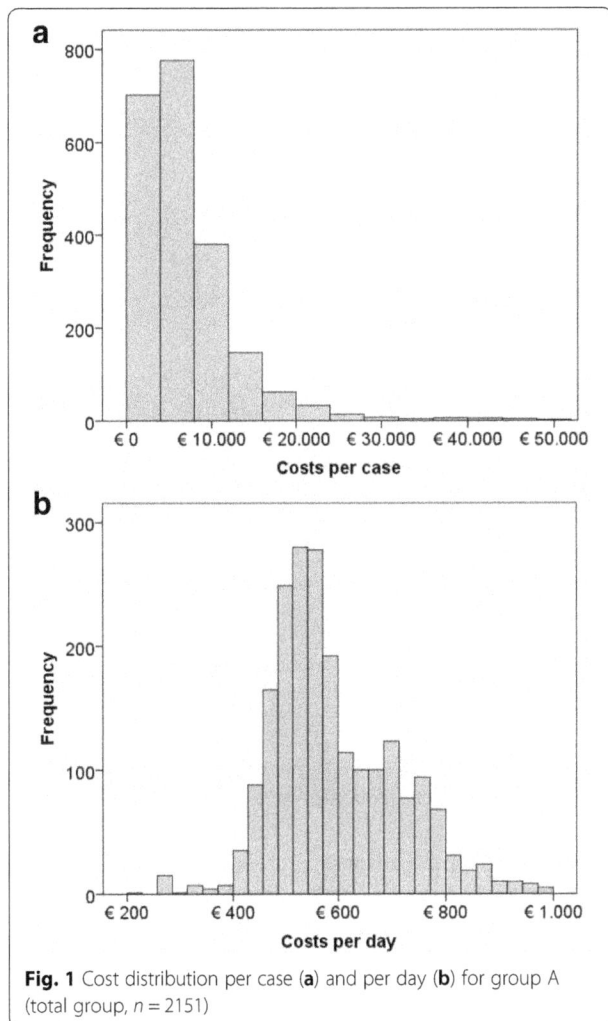

Fig. 1 Cost distribution per case (**a**) and per day (**b**) for group A (total group, $n = 2151$)

Table 1 Sample characteristics

Group		A = total group		B = "pall. Care only" group	
Number of patients		n = 2151		n = 784	
Variable		n; mean	%; SD	n; mean	%; SD
Location	BBM	1555	72.3%	659	84.1%
	LMU	596	27.7%	125	15.9%
Year	2012	1070	49.7%		
	2013	1081	50.3%	784	100%
Gender	male	1031	47.9%	350	44.6%
	female	1120	52.1%	434	55.9%
MDC	respiratory system	331	15.4%	99	12.6%
	hepatobiliary system and pancreas	309	14.4%	123	15.7%
	digestive system	296	13.8%	127	12.2%
	nervous system	288	13.4%	91	11.6%
	other	262	12.2%	116	14.8%
	skin, subcutaneous tissue & breast	191	8.9%	60	7.7%
	kidney and urinary tract	126	5.9%	42	5.4%
	female reproductive system	120	5.6%	35	4.5%
	poorly differentiated neoplasms	119	5.5%	43	5.5%
	male reproductive system	109	5.1%	48	6.1%
Discharge	death	1299	60.4%	455	58%
	home	590	27.4%	237	30.2%
	hospice	159	7.4%	55	7.0%
	nursing home	55	2.6%	25	3.2%
	other hospital	30	1.4%	6	0.8%
	other	18	0.8%	6	0.8%
Cancer	yes	1497	69.6%	549	70%
	no	654	30.4%	235	30%
Kind of suppl. Fee for SPC	palliative care ≤6 days (=no fee)	732	34.0%	240	30.6%
	palliative care 7–13 days	797	37.1%	313	39.9%
	palliative care 14–20 days	466	21.7%	181	23.1%
	palliative care ≥21 days	156	7.3%	50	6.4%
age (years)		69.8	12.37	70.7	11.8
length of stay (days)		12.2	10.10	9.8	6.3
number of secondary diagnoses		14.3	6.50	14.3	5.8
number of operation/ procedure codes		4.7	5.28	3.3	1.7

BBM (Hospital Barmherzige Brüder München), LMU (University Hospital Munich), MDC (main Diagnostic Category)

and (medical and non-medical) infrastructure on the PCU were reimbursed, respectively (Table 3). For laboratory tests, more than 7-fold (730%) of the costs were reimbursed.

Including both standard G-DRG reimbursement and supplementary fees, the benefit distribution of cases with highest profit to highest loss shows that about 21% of all cases generated a profit of on average €1078, while 79% of all cases generated a loss of on average €3086 Euros (Fig. 2a). The benefit distribution according to total LOS shows that for the average case, the break-even point was around 6–9 days, while longer stays caused losses in most cases (Fig. 2b).

Bi- and multivariate analysis

Spearman's correlation with costs identified total LOS, the kind of supplementary fee for SPC (generally reflecting duration of SPC) and the number of operation and procedure codes (German classification used to encode surgical and medical procedures) as the most relevant factors

Table 2 Mean costs and reimbursement per case in Euros, separated by cost categories and cost centers for group A (total group, $n = 2151$)

	Physicians	Nursing	Medical/ technical staff	Drugs	Implants/ grafts	Material	[b]Medical infrastructure	[b]Non-medical infrastructure	Sum	%
Cost matrix of palliative care cases										
Ward (including palliative care ward)	982	2658	45	208	0	140	500	1659	6193	83.8%
Intensive care	47	114	1	46	0	27	22	55	312	4.2%
Dialysis	2	7	0	0	0	7	1	2	18	0.2%
Operating room	21	0	23	2	18	22	11	15	112	1.5%
Anesthesia	21	0	14	2	0	5	3	6	51	0.7%
Cardiac diagnostics/ therapy	1	0	0	0	1	2	0	0	5	0.1%
Endoscopic diagnostics/ therapy	6	0	7	1	2	11	5	5	36	0.5%
Radiology	29	0	36	0	3	21	16	19	125	1.7%
Laboratory tests	4	0	22	47	0	48	4	7	133	1.8%
Further diagnostics/ therapy	87	0	170	5	0	16	42	86	406	5.5%
sum	1200	2778	318	313	25	299	604	1855	7392	
%	16.2%	37.6%	4.3%	4.2%	0.3%	4.0%	8.2%	25.1%		
Matrix used for reimbursement[a]										
Ward (including palliative care ward)	638	1276	26	160	0	121	337	1035	3594	69.7%
Intensive care	55	116	2	21	0	23	19	49	286	5.5%
Dialysis	4	11	0	1	0	11	1	3	31	0.6%
Operating room	34	0	27	2	20	28	14	21	146	2.8%
Anesthesia	23	0	14	2	0	5	3	6	53	1.0%
Cardiac diagnostics/ therapy	0	0	0	0	1	1	0	0	3	0.1%
Endoscopic diagnostics/ therapy	6	0	7	0	0	6	3	5	27	0.5%
Radiology	55	0	65	1	0	19	30	47	218	4.2%
Laboratory tests	32	0	124	18	0	109	18	59	359	7.0%
Further diagnostics/ therapy	99	0	183	3	0	20	27	105	437	8.5%
sum	945	1403	450	208	22	343	453	1331	5155	
%	18.3%	27.2%	8.7%	4.0%	0.4%	6.7%	8.8%	25.8%		

[a]overall absolute value represents actual reimbursement, distribution of absolute value represents hypothetical InEK calculation based on study patients
[b]medical infrastructure: e.g. pharmacy, hygiene; non-medical infrastructure: e.g. management, energy, laundry

influencing costs. The number of secondary diagnoses, main diagnosis, DRGs, and MDCs were also significantly associated with costs, but did not correlate highly (see Additional file 1). LOESS fit line analysis confirms total LOS as a good cost driver in the current costing scheme (Fig. 3).

Multivariate analysis showed that total LOS, the kind of supplementary fee for SPC (reflecting the duration of SPC), number of side diagnoses and location influenced costs per case for the total group of patients (group A) and for the patients with purely SPC (group B) (Table 4).

Each additional day increased case costs by 5.6% (group A) and 11.3% (group B), and each additional side diagnosis increased costs by 1.5% (group A) and 1.1% (group B). Compared to the shortest duration of SPC, costs increased between 62% and 79% (group A) and between 39% and 91% (group B) dependent on the duration of SPC – with highest costs for 14–20 days SPC. Costs were higher in the university hospital than in the non-university hospital. MDC did not significantly influence costs.

Linear regression on costs per day showed that location and the number of procedure codes significantly

Table 3 Mean costs and reimbursement per case in Euros, separated by cost categories and cost centers for group B ("palliative care only" 2013; n = 784)

	Physicians	Nursing	Medical/ technical staff	Drugs	Implants/ grafts	Material	[b]Medical infrastructure	[b]Non-medical infrastructure	Sum	%
Cost matrix of palliative care cases										
Ward	782	2465	35	87	0	100	464	1450	5382	93.4%
Intensive care	0	0	0	0	0	0	0	0	0	0.0%
Dialysis	0	0	0	0	0	0	0	0	0	0.0%
Operating room	3	0	4	0	3	3	2	2	17	0.3%
Anesthesia	3	0	2	0	0	1	0	1	7	0.1%
Cardiac diagnostics/ therapy	0	0	0	0	0	0	0	0	0	0.0%
Endoscopic diagnostics/ therapy	3	0	4	0	0	2	3	2	15	0.3%
Radiology	4	0	5	0	0	2	2	3	15	0.3%
Laboratory tests	1	0	6	8	0	11	1	2	29	0.5%
Further diagnostics/ therapy	27	0	148	4	0	12	36	71	298	5.2%
Sum	823	2465	204	100	4	130	507	1531	5763	
%	14.3%	42.8%	3.5%	1.7%	0.1%	2.3%	8.8%	26.6%		
Matrix used for reimbursement[a]										
Ward	643	1295	12	158	0	63	340	1044	3615	84.5%
Intensive care	0	0	0	0	0	0	0	0	0	0.0%
Dialysis	0	0	0	0	0	0	0	0	0	0.0%
Operating room	3	0	2	0	6	1	1	2	18	0.4%
Anesthesia	2	0	1	0	0	0	0	1	5	0.1%
Cardiac diagnostics/ therapy	0	0	0	0	0	0	0	0	0	0.0%
Endoscopic diagnostics/ therapy	4	0	5	0	0	1	2	3	16	0.4%
Radiology	19	0	20	0	0	3	9	15	69	1.6%
Laboratory tests	18	0	77	4	0	34	11	36	212	5.0%
Further diagnostics/ therapy	90	0	142	3	0	8	20	72	343	8.0%
Sum	780	1295	259	166	6	111	383	1172	4278	
%	18.3%	27.2%	8.7%	4.0%	0.4%	6.7%	8.8%	25.8%		

[a]overall absolute value represents actual reimbursement, distribution of absolute value represents hypothetical InEK calculation based on study patients
[b]medical infrastructure: e.g. pharmacy, hygiene; non-medical infrastructure: e.g. management, energy, laundry

influenced costs per day for group A and B. LOS only influenced costs per day for group A (see Additional file 2).

CART also identified total LOS as the most important cost driver, followed by the kind of supplementary fee for SPC which reflects duration of SPC (only for group A). All other regression variables were no good classifiers in CART (see Additional file 3).

Discussion
Cost and reimbursement situation
To our knowledge, this is the first study analysing costs and reimbursement for individual SPC cases. Results show that the current reimbursement system in Germany does

not reflect the costs for SPC cases in the hospital. Given the growing evidence that certain interventions or treatments, e.g. laboratory tests or imaging, are less likely after involvement of SPC, over-reimbursement for SPC in a diagnosis-based reimbursement system would also have been conceivable [24, 25]. On the contrary, both absolute and relative differences between overall costs and overall reimbursement in the study sample as well as between costs and reimbursement of cost modules (ward vs. other cost centers, and e.g. nurses versus other cost categories) were large. This applies both for group A (all patients on the PCU, including those treated on other hospital wards before referral to the PCU) and for group B (patients

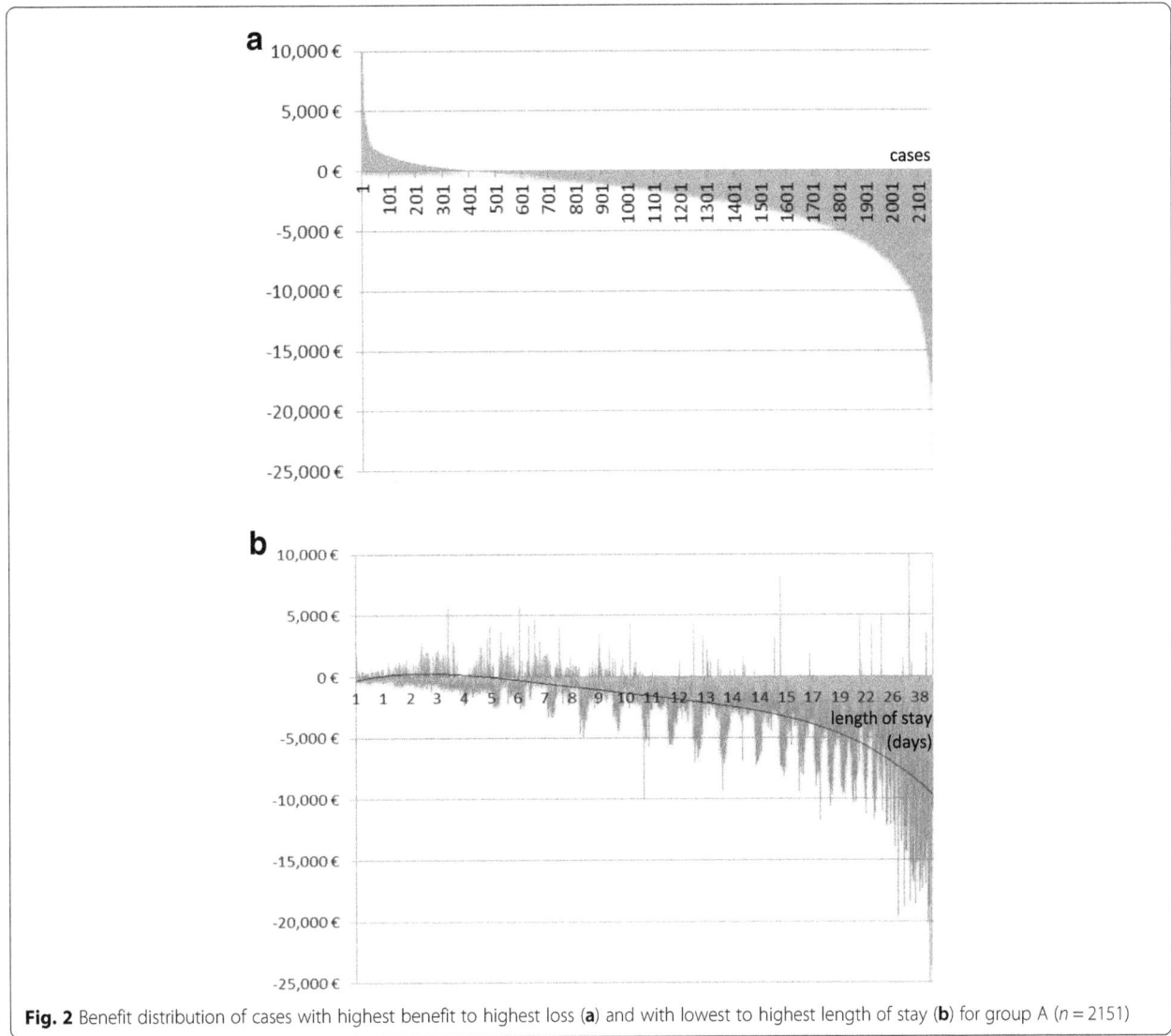

Fig. 2 Benefit distribution of cases with highest benefit to highest loss (**a**) and with lowest to highest length of stay (**b**) for group A (n = 2151)

treated on the PCU only). The patients of group B were externally referred, had a shorter LOS, lower costs and smaller differences between costs and reimbursement. The main reason for the smaller financing gap for group B is probably the shorter LOS and the fact, that most costs in PC are attributed to cases via LOS, whereas reimbursement in the DRG system is not mainly influenced by LOS. Thus, our data show that G-DRGs do not reproduce costs for patients treated on the PCU, whether they had a phase of "acute care" on a non-PC ward before referral to the PCU or were treated on the PCU only. As costs or reimbursement for group A could not be differentiated by "acute care phase" or PCU phase, it is not possible to draw any conclusions regarding acute care alone.

Most of the financing gap between costs and reimbursement appeared for nursing costs on the cost centre "ward", while for laboratory tests, reimbursement was up to 7-fold higher (group B) than the costs. Within

reimbursement calculation in the DRG-system, PC patients and non-PC cases are mixed up in a single DRG. As ordinary cases are much more frequent, the more complex and costly PC cases barely influence DRG reimbursement [4]. Within this costing system, the PCU is thus treated like an ordinary ward, and use of resources such as professionals' time is poorly reflected. Nursing and physician costs, however, are the biggest cost pool for PC, and the ward makes up 84% of overall case costs for group A and 93% for group B, while laboratory costs play a marginal role. The situation is mitigated by supplementary fees for the duration of SPC, otherwise the discrepancy between costs and reimbursement would be even higher.

Most studies on costs or cost-effectiveness in PC focus on specific diseases, [26–28] few report on general inpatient and outpatient PC costs [29–32]. Most work on cost drivers and reimbursement is on the development

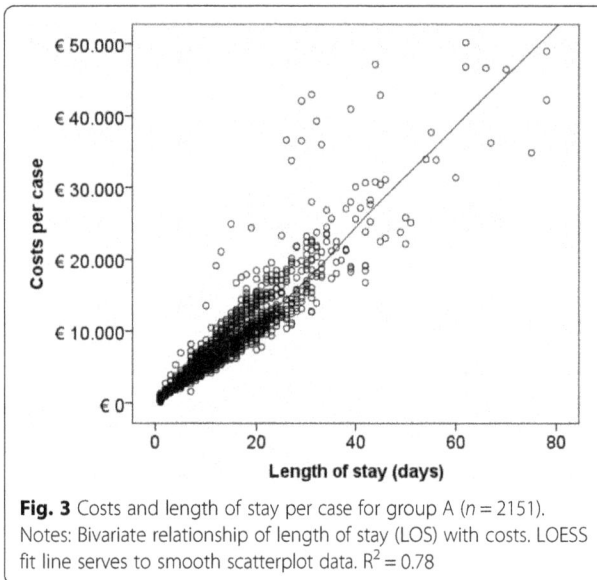

Fig. 3 Costs and length of stay per case for group A (n = 2151). Notes: Bivariate relationship of length of stay (LOS) with costs. LOESS fit line serves to smooth scatterplot data. $R^2 = 0.78$

of the Australian PC reimbursement system outside the DRG-system.[7, 9, 33]. Within the UK, a special reimbursement system for PC patients is currently evolving [34]. This study shows that the German reimbursement system needs changes, too, in order to meet the costs of inpatient PC – for patients treated on non-PC wards and then referred to the PCU as well as for those treated on the PCU only. The current loss-making system may disincentivise hospital palliative care. This is especially problematic, as incentives for SPC at home are lacking, too, and SPC at home is still not available all over the country [35]. For an adequate, needs-oriented care for PC patients, changes to the current reimbursement system in order to achieve adequate reimbursement are essential. In heavily ageing populations, the challenge to adapt the DRG system to more complex needs in a multimorbid, multiply restricted patient population may even extend beyond the scope of PC.

Redefining DRGs for palliative care
One of our most important findings is that main diagnosis, by which current DRGs are mainly generated, is not an adequate parameter to define costs for PC patients. Significant cost drivers were the kind of supplementary fee for SPC, which reflects the duration of SPC, and total LOS. Both might only be sensitive cost drivers because the current costing system allocates most relevant costs to cases dependent on their LOS. Cost drivers identified in Australia like the complexity of the patient's situation - which is reflected in the time nurses and physicians spend for the patient – are not assessed in the current system. Actual time spent is used increasingly as a cost classifier in healthcare, and detailed costing

systems, so-called time-driven activity-based costing (TDABC), exist to measure costs incurred [13, 36, 37].

There is an ongoing debate on G-DRG's in PC. The new hospice and palliative care law introduced in Germany in 2015 allows hospitals to leave the DRG system and negotiate day-related fees for PCUs with the sickness funds. From 2017 onwards, individual supplementary fees for SPC hospital advisory teams can be negotiated, which will be standardised for Germany in 2019. To adequately link reimbursement to the complexity of the patients' situation, we see a need to include the variables used in Australia such as phase of illness, functional status and problem severity [9, 33]. This could be introduced on different levels: 1) Revising the supplementary fee for SPC by inclusion of factors reflecting complexity, 2) Introducing new "DRGs" for PC patients, as already proposed by other authors, [4] separating cases based on complexity of the patients' situation, and 3) development of an entirely new reimbursement system for PC outside the DRG system. Guided by the Australian and UK experiences, pilot studies are currently underway to develop a casemix classification for German PC, based on complexity of the patients' situation. On the cost side, elements of TDABC will be used in accordance with the Australian study [9, 13, 36, 37].

Palliative care has been found to be cost-saving compared to usual care, [24, 25, 31, 38–43] and the aging of societies will considerably increase the need of palliative care [44, 45]. An adequate financing system for inpatient palliative care is thus key to a cost-conscious health care system. Hospitals will benefit from adequate reimbursement for PC patients that is calculated from actual PC patients and not mainly from patients in similar DRGs on normal wards. From a long-term policy perspective, this will turn PCUs from loss-making units that have to be cross-subsidised to economically viable units.

Strengths and limitations and a future perspective
A strength of this study is that we used actual reimbursement of our cases and distributed it on the matrix according to the national calculation dataset, to make cost and reimbursement calculation comparable. A limitation is that we analysed only cases from two centres. These may not be representative of all German PCUs. If they were less efficient than other units, this could have increased the financing gap [13]. In fact, costs were higher in the university hospital than in the non-university hospital, but this may well be explained by the more complex conditions and needs of the patients cared for. To reach a more representative case-mix for PC in Germany, a multi-centre study is necessary. However, in the present study, a large number of cases was analysed, and study patients were treated at a university

Table 4 GLM log link regression on costs per case

Group		A = total group			B = "palliative care only" group		
Number of patients		*n* = 2151			*n* = 784		
Variable		exp(b)	(95% CI)	*p*-value	exp(b)	(95% CI)	*p*-value
Location	BBM	−36.3%	(−39.2%; −33.3%)	**0.000**	−38,0%	(−42,0%; − 33,8%)	**0.000**
	LMU	ref.			ref.		
Gender	male	−4.2%	(−7.3%; −1.0%)	**0.011**	0,9%	(−3,0%; 4,9%)	0.646
	female	ref.			ref.		
Kind of suppl. Fee for SPC	SPC for 7–13 days	62.1%	(55.7%; 68.8%)	**0.000**	39,4%	(17,1%; 66,0%)	**0.000**
	SPC for 14–20 days	79.3%	(69.7%; 89.5%)	**0.000**	90,9%	(66,7%; 118,5%)	**0.000**
	SPC for ≥21 days	69.2%	(55.3%; 84.5%)	**0.000**	60,9%	(45,3%; 78,1%)	**0.000**
	SPC for 0–6 days (=no fee)	ref.			ref.		
Other suppl. Fee	no	−38.4%	(−45.3%; − 30.8%)	**0.000**	−5,8%	(−27,7%; 22,8%)	0.659
	yes	ref.			ref.		
Discharge	home	6.8%	(2.8%; 10.8%)	**0.001**	5,7%	(1,0%; 10,7%)	**0.018**
	to other hospital	3.6%	(−9.0%; 17.8%)	0.595	30,7%	(5,9%; 61,4%)	**0.013**
	to hospice	7.5%	(1.1%; 14.4%)	**0.022**	−0,3%	(−7,7%; 7,6%)	0.935
	to nursing home	8.5%	(−1.6%; 19.7%)	0.101	6,3%	(−4,4%; 18,2%)	0.259
	other	−5.7%	(−20.0%; 11.2%)	0.485	−27,5%	(− 41,0%; −10,8%)	**0.002**
	death	ref.			ref.		
MDC	other	4.6%	(−3.1%; 13.0%)	0.251	−0,2%	(−8,6%; 9,0%)	0.973
	nervous system	9.4%	(1.3%; 18.1%)	**0.022**	7,9%	(−1,1%; 17,7%)	0.086
	respiratory system	2.6%	(−4.8%; 10.5%)	0.499	4,6%	(−3,8%; 13,9%)	0.292
	digestive system	−0.1%	(−7.4%; 7.7%)	0.973	4,7%	(−4,3%; 14,4%)	0.316
	hepatobiliary system & pancreas	3.1%	(−4.4%; 11.1%)	0.431	4,2%	(−4,3%; 13,4%)	0.348
	skin, subcutaneous tissue & breast	−0.8%	(−8.6%; 7.7%)	0.848	0,7%	(−8,6%; 11,1%)	0.882
	kidney and urinary tract	1.3%	(−7.3%; 10.7%)	0.777	0,9%	(−9,1%; 12,1%)	0.861
	male reproductive system	4.4%	(−4.9%; 14.7%)	0.367	−3,7%	(−14,0%; 7,7%)	0.509
	female reproductive system	−0.4%	(−9.1%; 9.1%)	0.924	4,2%	(−6,3%; 15,8%)	0.452
	poorly differentiated neoplasms	ref.			ref.		
Age		0.1%	(0.0%; 0.2%)	0.169	0,0%	(−0,1%; 0,2%)	0.887
Length of stay		5.6%	(5.3%; 6.0%)	**0.000**	11,3%	(10,4%; 12,2%)	**0.000**
No. of side diagnoses		1.5%	(1.1%; 1.8%)	**0.000**	1,1%	(0,6%; 1,5%)	**0.000**
No. of procedure codes		0.0%	(−0.4%; 0.5%)	0.982	1,8%	(0,5%; 3,1%)	**0.008**

BBM (Hospital Barmherzige Brüder München), LMU (University Hospital Munich), MDC (main Diagnostic Category)
Bold numbers: significant results (α-level 0.05)

hospital and a general hospital PCU, well reflecting the German PC situation.

A further limitation is a time gap in the data used, as InEK cost calculations refer to the preceding year. In 2012, a new procedure code was introduced in the G-DRG system, reflecting the duration of SPC on PCUs. The supplementary fee for this was introduced in 2014. Therefore, the reimbursement data used here do not yet entail this new supplementary fee, which may contribute to a reduction of the financing gap in the future. Besides, the G-DRG system is updated annually, which means that every year slightly different base rates and DRG weights are applied. However, as we compare costs and reimbursement on case level, this difference between 2012 and 2013 does not affect the total financing gap. These aspects reflect a general challenge of evaluations of international health care systems, which are continuously changing. Evaluations are only possible with a time lag due to the reasons mentioned above. If the system has changed before the analysis is finished, the question is open once again, whether the current reimbursement system is reflecting the costs.

A general limitation of this study is that all reported costs were calculated based on cost classifiers predefined by the InEK costing scheme such as LOS, and that the data do not include the variables identified as significant cost drivers in Australia [9]. However, this cost calculation method is the current national standard in Germany, and thus provides a relevant starting point for analysing the current situation. To better reflect the costs accrued by the care for the individual patients, the resources used by the patients, especially the time spent with the patients by SPC team members, has to be recorded, i.e. a TDABC approach, as done in the Australian study, the ongoing UK study and planned in future studies in Germany [9, 46].

Conclusions

Main diagnosis, by which current DRGs are mainly generated, is not an adequate parameter to define costs for PC patients. Besides, G-DRGs do not reproduce costs for inpatient PC episodes adequately. Possible reasons for this are 1) the fact that PC patients differ from acute patients on normal wards regarding the complexity of their situation and the care they need, and 2) that the cost classifiers currently used for DRG grouping poorly reflect resource use – especially the use of professionals' time, which accounts for the biggest cost pool in PC. Studies collecting resource-use based cost data as well as data on the cost drivers identified in Australia are needed as a basis for further development of our costing and reimbursement system for PC. Changes to the current system are crucial to make PCUs economically viable and enable them to provide adequate care to the increasing number of patients in need of PC in the future.

Additional files

Additional file 1: Spearman's correlation coefficient on costs per case for group A ($n = 2151$). (DOCX 18 kb)

Additional file 2: Multiple linear regression on costs per day. (DOCX 19 kb)

Additional file 3: Results of the Classification and regression tree analysis (CART) for group A and B. (DOCX 17 kb)

Abbreviations

BBM: Hospital Barmherzige Brüder München; CART analysis: Classification and regression tree analysis; G-DRG: German Diagnosis-Related groups; GLM: Generalized linear model; InEK: Institute for the Hospital Remuneration System (Institut für das Entgeltsystem im Krankenhaus); LMU: University Hospital Munich; LOS: Length of stay; MDC: Major diagnostic category; OLS model: Ordinary least squares model; PC: Palliative care; PCU: Palliative care unit; SD: Standard deviation; SPC: Specialist palliative care

Acknowledgements
We thank the data providers for this study: the costing systems of Munich university hospital and Krankenhaus Barmherzige Brüder München.

Funding
This article represents independent research funded by a private charity. The organisation that provided funding does not wish to have its name published. This organisation had no role in the design of the study, the collection, analysis and interpretation of data and the writing of the manuscript.

Authors' contributions
MV, ES, RL, BOM and CB obtained the funding. The authors made the following contributions: conception and design of the study: MV, ES, RL, BOM and CB. Organisation of study and acquisition of study data: MV, ES, RL, MS, SR and CB. Development of analysis plan: MV and RL, with input from ES, FH, BOM and CB. Data analysis: MV supervised by RL. Interpretation of study results, with additional statistical support by HK: all authors. MV wrote the first draft of the paper with significant input from ES and input from FH, RL and CB. All authors critically commented on, contributed to the first draft and agreed with the manuscript results and conclusions. ES significantly revised the first draft of the paper based on the comments of all authors. All authors meet the ICMJE criteria for authorship, CB is the guarantor. MV and ES contributed equally to this manuscript and therefore claim shared first authorship. All authors read and approved the final version of the manuscript.

Competing interests
The authors declare that they have no competing interests.

Author details
[1]Helmholtz Zentrum Munich, German Research Center for Environmental Health, Institute of Health Economics and Health Care Management, Munich, Germany. [2]Ludwig-Maximilians-Universitaet Munich, Munich School of Management, Institute of Health Economics and Health Care Management & Munich Centre of Health Sciences, Munich, Germany. [3]Munich University Hospital, Department of Palliative Medicine, Ludwig-Maiximilians-Universitaet Munich, Marchioninistr. 15, 81377 Munich, Germany. [4]St. Josephs-Hospital, Department of Palliative Medicine and Interdisciplinary Oncology, Wiesbaden, Germany. [5]Krankenhaus Barmherzige Brüder Munich, Department of Palliative Medicine, Munich, Germany.

References
1. Eagar K, Gordon R, Green J, Smith M. An Australian casemix classification for palliative care: lessons and policy implications of a national study. Palliat Med. 2004;18:227–33.
2. Docherty A, Owens A, Asadi-Lari M, Petchey R, Williams J, Carter YH. Knowledge and information needs of informal caregivers in palliative care: a qualitative systematic review. Palliat Med. 2008;22:153–71.
3. Steinhauser KE, Christakis NA, Clipp EC, McNeilly M, McIntyre L, Tulsky JA. Factors considered important at the end of life by patients, family, physicians, and other care providers. JAMA. 2000;284:2476–82.
4. Roeder N, Klaschik E, Cremer M, Lindena G, Juhra C. DRGs in der Palliativmedizin: Ist die palliativmedizinische Begleitung Schwerstkranker pauschalierbar? das Krankenhaus. 2002;12:1000–4.
5. Weber M. Fallpauschalen: Sterbenden Patienten nicht angemessen. Dtsch Aerztebl. 2013;110:A-2272–C-1934.

165

6. Vogl M. Assessing DRG cost accounting with respect to resource allocation and tariff calculation: the case of Germany. Heal Econ Rev. 2012;2(1):15.
7. Gordon R, Eagar K, Currow D, Green J. Current funding and financing issues in the Australian hospice and palliative care sector. J Pain Symptom Manag. 2009;38:68–74.
8. The Australian National Sub-Acute and Non-Acute Patient (AN-SNAP) Casemix Classification: report of the National Sub-Acute and Non-Acute Casemix Classification Study [http://ro.uow.edu.au/chsd/7/].
9. Eagar K, Green J, Gordon R. An Australian casemix classification for palliative care: technical development and results. Palliat Med. 2004;18:217–26.
10. Eagar K, Cromwell D, Kennedy C, Lee L. Classifying sub-acute and non-acute patients: results of the new South Wales Casemix area network study. Aust Health Rev. 1997;20:26–42.
11. Eagar K, Innes K. Creating a common language: the production and use of patient data in Australia. Canberra: Department of Health, Housing and Community Services; 1992.
12. Murtagh F, Groeneveld I, Kaloki Y, Calanzani N, Bausewein C, Higginson IJ. Capturing activity, costs, and outcomes: the challenges to be overcome for successful economic evaluation in palliative care. Progress in Palliative Care. 2013;21:232–5.
13. Vogl M. Improving patient-level costing in the English and the German 'DRG' system. Health Policy. 2013;109:290–300.
14. Institut für das Entgeltsystem im Krankenhaus (InEK). Handbuch zur Kalkulation von Fallkosten Version 3.0. Düsseldorf: Deutsche Krankenhaus Verlagsgesellschaft mbH; 2007.
15. Vogl M. Hospital financing: calculating inpatient capital costs in Germany with a comparative view on operating costs and the English costing scheme. Health Policy. 2014;115:141–51.
16. Busse R, Geissler A, Quentin W, Wiley MW. Diagnosis-related groups in Europe: moving towards transparency, efficiency and quality in hospitals. New York: McGraw-Hill, Open University Press; 2011.
17. Kimberly JR, de Pouvourville G, D'Aunno T. The globalization of managerial innovation in health care. Cambridge: Cambridge University Press; 2009.
18. Porter ME. What is value in health care? N Engl J Med. 2010;363:2477–81.
19. Cleveland W, Devlin SJ. Locally-weighted regression: an approach to regression analysis by local fitting. J Am Stat Assoc. 1988;83:596–610.
20. Blough D, Ramsey S. Using generalized linear models to assess medical care costs. Health Serv Outcomes Res Methodol. 2000;1:185–202.
21. Kilian R, Matschinger H, Loeffler W, Roick C, Angermeyer MC. A comparison of methods to handle skew distributed cost variables in the analysis of the resource consumption in schizophrenia treatment. J Ment Health Policy Econ. 2002;5:21–31.
22. Haas L, Stargardt T, Schreyoegg J, Schlosser R, Hofmann T, Danzer G, Klapp BF. Introduction of DRG-based reimbursement in inpatient psychosomatics– an examination of cost homogeneity and cost predictors in the treatment of patients with eating disorders. J Psychosom Res. 2012;73:383–90.
23. Fonarow GC, Adams KF Jr, Abraham WT, Yancy CW, Boscardin WJ. Risk stratification for in-hospital mortality in acutely decompensated heart failure: classification and regression tree analysis. JAMA. 2005;293:572–80.
24. May P, Garrido MM, Cassel JB, Kelley AS, Meier DE, Normand C, Smith TJ, Morrison RS. Cost analysis of a prospective multi-site cohort study of palliative care consultation teams for adults with advanced cancer: where do cost-savings come from? Palliat Med. 2017;31:378–86.
25. May P, Garrido MM, Cassel JB, Kelley AS, Meier DE, Normand C, Smith TJ, Stefanis L, Morrison RS. Prospective cohort study of hospital palliative care teams for inpatients with advanced cancer: earlier consultation is associated with larger cost-saving effect. J Clin Oncol. 2015;33:2745–52.
26. Pace A, Di Lorenzo C, Capon A, Villani V, Benincasa D, Guariglia L, Salvati M, Brogna C, Mantini V, Mastromattei A, Pompili A. Quality of care and rehospitalization rate in the last stage of disease in brain tumor patients assisted at home: a cost effectiveness study. J Palliat Med. 2012;15:225–7.
27. Higginson IJ, McCrone P, Hart SR, Burman R, Silber E, Edmonds PM. Is short-term palliative care cost-effective in multiple sclerosis? A randomized phase II trial. J Pain Symptom Manag. 2009;38:816–26.
28. Iskedjian M, Iyer S, Librach SL, Wang M, Farah B, Berbari J. Methylnaltrexone in the treatment of opioid-induced constipation in cancer patients receiving palliative care: willingness-to-pay and cost-benefit analysis. J Pain Symptom Manag. 2011;41:104–15.
29. Dumont S, Jacobs P, Turcotte V, Anderson D, Harel F. The trajectory of palliative care costs over the last 5 months of life: a Canadian longitudinal study. Palliat Med. 2010;24:630–40.
30. Gomes B, McCrone P, Hall S, Koffman J, Higginson IJ. Variations in the quality and costs of end-of-life care, preferences and palliative outcomes for cancer patients by place of death: the QUALYCARE study. BMC Cancer. 2010;10:400.
31. Morrison RS, Penrod JD, Cassel JB, Caust-Ellenbogen M, Litke A, Spragens L, Meier DE. Cost savings associated with US hospital palliative care consultation programs. Arch Intern Med. 2008;168:1783–90.
32. Mercadante S, Intravaia G, Villari P, Ferrera P, David F, Casuccio A, Mangione S. Clinical and financial analysis of an acute palliative care unit in an oncological department. Palliat Med. 2008;22:760–7.
33. Green J, Gordon R. The development of version 2 of the AN-SNAP casemix classification system. Aust Health Rev. 2007;31(Suppl 1):S68–78.
34. Developing a new approach to palliative care funding: A first draft for discussion [https://www.england.nhs.uk/wp-content/uploads/2014/10/pall-care-fund-new-appr-fin.pdf].
35. Stellungnahme der Deutschen Gesellschaft für Palliativmedizin: SAPV: Die spezialisierte Ambulante Palliativversorgung ist kein Wettbewerbsfeld! [https://www.dgpalliativmedizin.de/stellungnahmen/stellungnahme-der-deutschen-gesellschaft-fuer-palliativmedizin-sapv-die-spezialisierte-ambulante-palliativversorgung-ist-kein-wettbewerbsfeld.html].
36. Kaplan RS, Anderson SR. Time-driven activity-based costing: a simpler and more powerful path to higher profits. Boston: Harvard Business Press; 2007.
37. Kaplan RS, Porter ME. How to solve the cost crisis in health care. Harv Bus Rev. 2011;89:46–52, 54, 56–61 passim.
38. Smith TJ, Cassel JB. Cost and non-clinical outcomes of palliative care. J Pain Symptom Manag. 2009;38:32–44.
39. Penrod JD, Deb P, Dellenbaugh C, Burgess JF Jr, Zhu CW, Christiansen CL, Luhrs CA, Cortez T, Livote E, Allen V, Morrison RS. Hospital-based palliative care consultation: effects on hospital cost. J Palliat Med. 2010;13:973–9.
40. McGrath LS, Foote DG, Frith KH, Hall WM. Cost effectiveness of a palliative care program in a rural community hospital. Nurs Econ. 2013;31:176–83.
41. Bendaly EA, Groves J, Juliar B, Gramelspacher GP. Financial impact of palliative care consultation in a public hospital. J Palliat Med. 2008;11:1304–8.
42. Smith S, Brick A, O'Hara S, Normand C. Evidence on the cost and cost-effectiveness of palliative care: a literature review. Palliat Med. 2014;28:130–50.
43. May P, Garrido MM, Del Fabbro E, Noreika D, Normand C, Skoro N, Cassel JB. Does modality matter? Palliative care unit associated with more cost-avoidance than consultations. J Pain Symptom Manag. 2017;55:766–774.e4.
44. Simon ST, Gomes B, Koeskeroglu P, Higginson IJ, Bausewein C. Population, mortality and place of death in Germany (1950-2050) - implications for end-of-life care in the future. Public Health. 2012;126:937–46.
45. DiBello K, Coyne N. Palliative care hits a triple win: access, quality, and cost. Home Healthc Nurse. 2014;32:183–90. quiz 191-182
46. C-Change [http://www.kcl.ac.uk/lsm/research/divisions/cicelysaunders/research/studies/c-change/c-change.aspx].

12

Perceptions of trained laypersons in end-of-life or advance care planning conversations

Elizabeth Somes[1†], Joanna Dukes[2†], Adreanne Brungardt[4], Sarah Jordan[4], Kristen DeSanto[5], Christine D. Jones[6], Urvi Jhaveri Sanghvi[7], Khadijah Breathett[8], Jacqueline Jones[7] and Hillary D. Lum[3,4*]

Abstract

Background: Laypersons including volunteers, community health navigators, or peer educators provide important support to individuals with serious illnesses in community or healthcare settings. The experiences of laypersons in communication with seriously ill peers is unknown.

Methods: We performed an ENTREQ-guided qualitative meta-synthesis. We conducted a systematic search of MEDLINE, PsycINFO, CINAHL, Cochrane Library, and AMED to include qualitative studies with data regarding communication and laypersons in advance care planning, palliative care, or end-of-life settings. Study quality was appraised using a standardized tool. The analysis identified key domains and associated themes relating specifically to laypersons' perspectives on communication.

Results: Of 877 articles, nine studies provided layperson quotations related to layperson-to-peer communication associated with advance care planning ($n = 4$) or end-of-life conversations ($n = 5$). The studies were conducted in United Kingdom (n = 4) or United States settings (n = 5). The synthesis of layperson perspectives yielded five main domains: 1) layperson-to-peer communication, focusing on the experience of talking with peers, 2) layperson-to-peer interpersonal interactions, focusing on the entire interaction between the layperson and peers, excluding communication-related issues, 3) personal impact on the layperson, 4) layperson contributions, and 5) layperson training. Laypersons described using specific communication skills including the ability to build rapport, discuss sensitive issues, listen and allow silence, and respond to emotions.

Conclusions: Published studies described experiences of trained laypersons in conversations with peers related to advance care planning or end-of-life situations. Based on these layperson perspectives related to communication, programs should next evaluate the potential impact of laypersons in meaningful conversations.

Keywords: Volunteers, Communication, Hospice care, Palliative care, Terminal care, Lay health navigators, Advance care planning, Peer educators

* Correspondence: Hillary.lum@ucdenver.edu
†Elizabeth Somes and Joanna Dukes contributed equally to this work.
[3]VA Eastern Colorado Geriatric Research Education and Clinical Center, Denver, CO, USA
[4]Division of Geriatric Medicine, University of Colorado School of Medicine, University of Colorado Anschutz Medical Campus, 12631 E. 17th Ave, Mail Stop B179, Aurora, CO 80045, USA
Full list of author information is available at the end of the article

Background

Advance care planning is a process that supports adults at any age or stage of health in understanding and sharing their values, goals, and preferences regarding future medical care [1]. Advance care planning is associated with increased hospice use, decreased hospital admissions, reduced medical care costs, and increased patient satisfaction [2, 3]. To increase participation in advance care planning, national recommendations suggest raising public awareness of advance care planning and enabling people to think about future medical care planning in their own life situations [4–6]. One strategy to increase community engagement and promote advance care planning is through non-medical laypersons such as volunteers, community health navigators, and peer educators [7, 8].

Trained laypersons have been involved in supporting advance care planning among general older adult populations and specific populations such as ethnic minorities with multiple comorbidities, patients with end-stage renal disease, and patients with cancer [9–11]. These layperson-based programs suggest that individuals value the opportunity to exchange stories with peers who belong to their community group, are a similar age, or share similar experiences [12]. The involvement of volunteers in advance care planning conversations is a natural extension of the long-standing role volunteers have played in interdisciplinary hospice and palliative care teams [13–15].

Laypersons in hospice and palliative care settings serve in multiple capacities, including providing physical, spiritual, and emotional comfort to patients and family caregivers; assisting with information exchange and referral support (e.g., acting as a "bridge to the hospice"); socialization; and companionship [16–19]. Layperson-to-peer communication related to living with serious illness occurs in multiple settings including hospitals and clinics, palliative care programs, hospice programs, and community settings [7, 11, 20–22]. Given the formal and informal involvement of laypersons in communicating with individuals with serious illness, the specific experiences that non-medical laypersons have related to end-of-life communication, including advance care planning conversations, warrants close examination.

Systematic reviews that summarize layperson perspectives on communication related to end-of-life situations are lacking. To address this gap, we performed a meta-synthesis of qualitative studies to address the study question: "What are the perspectives of laypersons on communication with individuals with serious illness or advance care planning?" The intention of this study is to provide a rich description of how trained non-medical laypersons engage in layperson-to-peer conversations related to advance care planning or end of life situations, including palliative care and hospice care.

Methods

Design

This study is an interpretive thematic synthesis which uses a structured team-based meta-synthesis approach consistent with the ENTREQ standards. Specifically, we extracted salient information about each study, developed descriptive data-driven themes, and then synthesized themes through a process called reciprocal translation [23, 24]. We conducted a comprehensive search to identify articles on non-medical laypersons (i.e., volunteers, patient navigators, peer educators) in communication related to serious illness or advance care planning. We use the term "layperson" to streamline presentation of the results, while acknowledging differences in how various non-medical trained laypersons may be compensated, trained, and integrated into community or healthcare-based programs. We use the term "peer" in recognition that some of individuals that laypersons interacted with were in community-based settings and could be considered a peer, even if they did not personally know them. We also use the term "patient" in recognition that some individuals were in a healthcare context. We chose to perform a meta-synthesis because it provides a mechanism for exploring layperson-to-peer communication across a variety of settings from multiple studies. As a rigorous systematic interpretive study of a defined body of qualitative research, this process produces new knowledge beyond the individual studies and does not include quantitative studies. The analysis involves an integrative synthesis with the following assumptions: 1) the whole published study, not just participant quotations, is treated as qualitative data for interpretation; 2) a multidisciplinary analytic team adds context variation to study interpretation, and 3) when qualitative studies include similar findings, they can be amassed to draw larger and different interpretative meaning [23, 24].

Search strategy and study selection

A comprehensive search was performed by a medical librarian (K.D.) on March 20, 2017. Table 1 summarizes the key search terms used. Relevant publications were identified by searching the following databases: MEDLINE, PsycINFO, CINAHL, Cochrane Library, and AMED. No limiters were used for language or publication date. Publication/source types were limited in PsycINFO and CINAHL to exclude dissertations, theses, and book chapters to improve efficiency of searching and to ensure all included studies had been peer-reviewed and were easily discoverable. Appendix 1 describes the comprehensive search strategies for each database. Reference lists of included studies were hand-searched for additional relevant studies.

The inclusion and exclusion criteria are presented in Table 1. One author (H.L./J.D./A.B.) examined titles for general relevance to the study question of layperson perspectives on communication with individuals with serious

Table 1 Search strategy and study selection

Search terms	1. Volunteers OR lay navigators OR peer groups 2. Advance care planning OR advance directives OR palliative care OR hospice 3. Education OR experience OR sharing OR encouraging 4. Qualitative methods OR phenomenological study OR focus groups OR grounded theory OR observation
Inclusion criteria	1. Qualitative methods 2. Participants are non-medical peers (i.e., volunteer, patient navigator, peer educator) 3. Setting related to advance care planning, palliative care, hospice, or end-of-life
Exclusion criteria	1. Non-English language 2. Not full papers (i.e., abstracts, posters) 3. No extractable data from peers 4. No data relating to communication

illness or advance care planning. One author (J.D./A.B.) examined study abstracts for relevance, and then two authors (H.L. and J.D.) independently reviewed full studies based on the inclusion and exclusion criteria. The final inclusion of nine studies in the meta-synthesis was confirmed by the study team.

Quality appraisal

The quality appraisal is an important first step in a meta-synthesis and is a process of immersion into the data. It provides a deeper understanding of each article and helps the team determine the relevance and value of each study toward understanding key findings of the meta-synthesis. To assess study quality (Appendix 2), all articles were independently reviewed using the McMaster University tool [25] by at least two members of an multidisciplinary team including a nurse researcher (U.S.), a palliative care-trained geriatrician (H.L.), and two hospital-based physician researchers (C.J. and K.B.). The tool assesses for the presence or absence of 17 quality domains, including additional subdomains, for a total of 22 items that together address study rigor and other qualitative methodological issues. Any appraisal differences were resolved by consensus and input from another team member (S.J.) who has expertise in qualitative methods. To aid in comparing study quality, each domain received 0 points for No, 1 point for Yes. Not applicable (N/A) ratings were excluded from the total possible score. Scores for each domain were summed and divided by the total possible score (22 minus number of "N/A") multiplied by 100 to provide an overall quality score with a possible range of 0 to 100%. The appraisal was not used to exclude articles.

Meta-synthesis

Using a meta-synthesis approach based on Thomas and Harden, [24] we extracted study aim, design, methods, type of layperson participants, and main findings of the original studies. Three authors (H.L., J.D., A.B.) reviewed all articles, extracted layperson quotations, and coded meaningful ideas within and across studies. We used an inductive approach for thematic analysis to identify themes and analyze similarities and differences across the studies [24]. In studies with mixed methods, the analysis focused on the qualitative portion of the study. The process was iterative, building consensus through visual mapping of broader domains, themes, and subthemes; naming and renaming; and contextualizing themes through team discussion and re-immersion into the articles to determine whether the emerging results resonated with the original data. Congruent with a meta-synthesis approach, we then used a reciprocal translation approach to create a reciprocal theme table that displayed the synthesized domains and themes alongside themes from the original studies [24]. We maintained an audit trail of decisions and presented and received feedback from multidisciplinary palliative care researchers and clinicians on the derived themes and primary data to contextualize our findings and maintain a high degree of rigor.

Results

Among 1566 titles identified with the initial search strategy, 690 were duplicates. One additional study was found by hand searching. Of 877 titles screened for general relevance to the study question, 694 titles were removed. Next, 183 abstracts were screened based on the inclusion criteria, and an additional 98 were removed. The full text of 85 articles were assessed, and 76 were excluded (two were not in English, seven were not full studies, 26 did not have discrete qualitative layperson data, and 41 did not address communication). Nine studies remained eligible for inclusion in the meta-synthesis as shown in the PRISMA diagram (Fig. 1) [26].

Table 2 shows study characteristics. Studies were conducted in the United Kingdom (UK) or the United States (US) and published between 2002 and 2017. Most studies used a qualitative descriptive approach with interviews, focus groups, or a combination. Two studies included a participatory action approach and one study used ethnography. Four studies specifically focused on communication related to advance care planning; whereas, five studies addressed the role of laypersons in communicating with

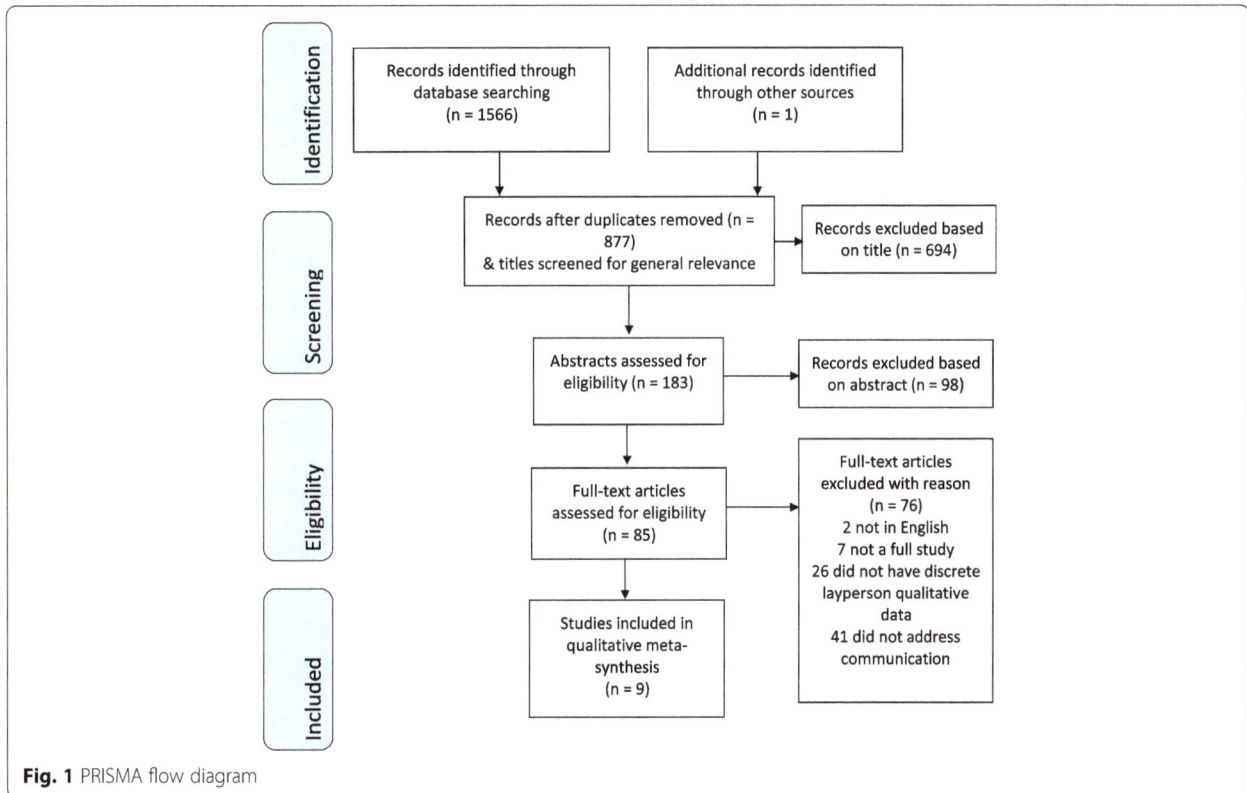

Fig. 1 PRISMA flow diagram

patients who were hospitalized at the end-of-life, had palliative care needs, or were receiving hospice care. Studies included laypersons as volunteers, peer educators, or lay health navigators. Sample sizes ranged from 8 to 351 participants. The combined qualitative data from the nine studies represent a total of 692 laypersons.

In the initial immersion into the data and assessment of study quality, study quality varied with overall quality scores ranging from 50 to 95% (Appendix 2). Across the nine studies, areas of poor quality were description of sampling methods; description of study site; identification of researchers' biases; and confirmability of data to minimize bias.

Meta-synthesis of themes

Across nine studies, five major domains with themes and subthemes emerged related to laypersons' involvement in communication related to end-of-life or advance care planning conversations. The major domains were 1) *layperson-to-peer communication*, focusing on the experience of talking with peers, 2) *layperson-to-peer interpersonal interactions*, focusing on the entire interaction between the layperson and peers, excluding communication-related issues, 3) *personal impact on the layperson*, 4) *layperson contributions*, and 5) *layperson training*. Figure 2 provides a graphical representation of the domains and associated themes. Table 3 presents each domain, related themes, and subthemes, as well as themes from the original studies to provide additional context.

I. Layperson-to-peer communication

The domain of layperson-to-peer communication includes six key themes: a) *building rapport*, b) *talking about sensitive issues*, c) *listening and allowing silence*, d) *responding to patient and family emotions*, e) *communication facilitators*, and f) *communication barriers*. These themes describe the layperson's process of engaging in conversations with a seriously ill peer or initiating advance care planning conversations.

Laypersons focused on *building rapport*, which included building trust and developing relationships over time. They noted that longitudinal relationships over multiple encounters allowed for time and space to have unhurried discussions about sensitive subject matter. One volunteer described the process as follows,

"You just … need to hit the ball back over the net when you're talking to someone… who has that disorder. You're not seeking things, you're not negotiating a peace treaty here, and you're not making a business deal here… All you need to do is just hit the ball back over the net. They're gonna hit it right back to you, you just hit it back" [27].

Moreover, laypersons noted that being perceived as a "peer" enhanced trust; "I think she sees me as a friend, also someone to maybe pass on some of her wisdom" [28]. Laypersons often felt most comfortable focusing on life-related subject matter through "life review" conversations.

Layperson-to-peer communication involved *talking about sensitive issues*, such as advance care planning,

Table 2 Studies of layperson perspectives on layperson-to-peer communication related to serious illness or advance care planning

Study	Study aim	Design and method	Participants and setting	Results from primary study	Overall score from critical appraisal of study quality
1 Berry and Planalp, USA, 2009 [30]	To explore ethical issues hospice volunteers confront in their work	Thematic analysis of interviews	39 hospice volunteers in urban and rural areas in Southwestern US. Mean age 64, 76% female, 100% White	Four themes of ethical issues: 1) dilemmas about gifts, 2) patient care and family concerns, 3) issues related to volunteer roles and boundaries, and 4) suicide/ hastening death.	60%
2 Brighton et al., UK, 2017 [20]	To explore hospital volunteers' end-of-life care training needs and learning preferences, and the acceptability of training evaluation methods	Thematic analysis of focus groups	25 hospital volunteers with at least 3 months experience. Mean age 50 (range 19–80 years), 76% female, highly ethnically diverse sample	Four themes emerged: 1) preparation for volunteering role; 2) end-of-life care training needs, including a) communication skills, b) understanding grief and bereavement, c) understanding spiritual diversity, d) understanding symptoms at end-of-life, and e) volunteers' self-care; 3) learning preferences, including a) teaching methods, b) teachers, c) optional vs mandatory training, d) consolidating learning; and 4) evaluation preferences.	95%
3 Clarke et al., UK, 2009 [36]	To evaluate whether researchers successfully worked with peer educators to develop and pilot an education program for advance care planning	Participatory action research; analysis of questionnaires, field notes, interviews	5 "older adult" peer educators from community organizations, who were research advisors and volunteer peer educators	Peer educator findings from the program development process included: 1) enjoying project meetings, 2) involvement in reviewing material, 3) enhanced awareness of advance care planning, 4) training encouraging action, and 5) training enabling action.	61%
4 Foster, USA 2002 [28]	To describe volunteer-patient relationships and communication at the end-of-life	Narrative ethnography using interviews, observations, small groups	9 hospice volunteers and researcher over 12-months in 1 hospice	Three themes related to volunteer-patient relationships emerged: 1) focus on the life of the patient – "The patient is alive", 2) volunteer prioritizes the patient – "It's not about me", and 3) importance of presence – "Being there".	60%
5 Jones et al., UK, 2015 [29]	To evaluate volunteers' experiences of advance care planning in a hospice	Mixed-method descriptive case studies, data from open-ended questions	10 advance care planning -trained hospice volunteers completed questionnaires, providing 23 statements for analysis	The first theme was benefits of being an advance care planning volunteer, including a) positive interactions, b) gratitude shown by peers, and c) personal impact. The second theme was challenges of being an advance care planning volunteer, including: a) no engagement by peer, b) negative attitude of caregiver, c) being asked for inappropriate advice, and d) denial by peers.	50%
6 Planalp and Trost, USA, 2008 [22]	To understand difficult communication issues or dilemmas experienced by hospice volunteers, patients, and their families	Qualitative analysis of data from 3 open-ended questions	351 hospice volunteers from urban and rural areas in Southwestern US. Mean age 55 (range 15–88 years), 75% female.	Three themes of communication issues were identified: 1) denial between the dying person and their caregiver/family; 2) dealing with many negative feelings experienced by the patient and their caregiver/family; 3) family issues, including a) within-family conflicts, b) conflicts about patient care/treatment, c) financial/estate issues, d) unresolved relationship issues. Sources of communication difficulties were physical and/ or mental impairments that made it difficult to	68%

Table 2 Studies of layperson perspectives on layperson-to-peer communication related to serious illness or advance care planning (*Continued*)

Study	Study aim	Design and method	Participants and setting	Results from primary study	Overall score from critical appraisal of study quality
				talk with the dying person.	
7 Planalp et al., USA, 2011 [27]	To describe conversations volunteers had with patients that they considered meaningful	Qualitative analysis of data from open-ended questions and in-depth interviews	350 hospice volunteers from 32 hospices in Southwestern US completed questionnaires, 31 volunteers interviewed	Prominent themes about meaningful conversations were: 1) meaning of life, experiences and life stories, 2) talk about death and spirituality, 3) families and relationships, 4) shared interests with volunteers, 5) unfinished business, and 6) loss of capacities. Volunteers appreciated gaining life lessons.	60%
8 Rocque et al., USA, 2017 [11]	To evaluate implementation of lay navigator-led advance care planning	Mixed-methods design, including thematic content analysis of lay navigator interviews	26 lay navigators in Respecting Choices advance care planning Facilitator training in Southeastern US. Mean age 45, 81% female; 39% Black, 58% White.	Navigators identified key facilitators and barriers of implementation of advance care planning. Facilitators included physician buy-in, patient readiness, and prior advance care planning experience. Barriers included space limitations, identifying the "right" time to start conversations, and personal discomfort discussing end-of-life.	95%
9 Seymour et al., UK, 2013 [37]	To report volunteers' perspectives on a advance care planning peer education program and feelings on role of volunteer peer educator	Participatory action research; mixed methods including interviews and focus groups	24 older adult volunteers and 8 care staff. 25% below 55 years, 9% over 75 years; 81% white, 6% black	At 6 and 12 months after training, the volunteers' perspectives related to 1) personal and emotional implications of being a peer educator, and 2) report of community engagement activities in the year after peer education training.	84%

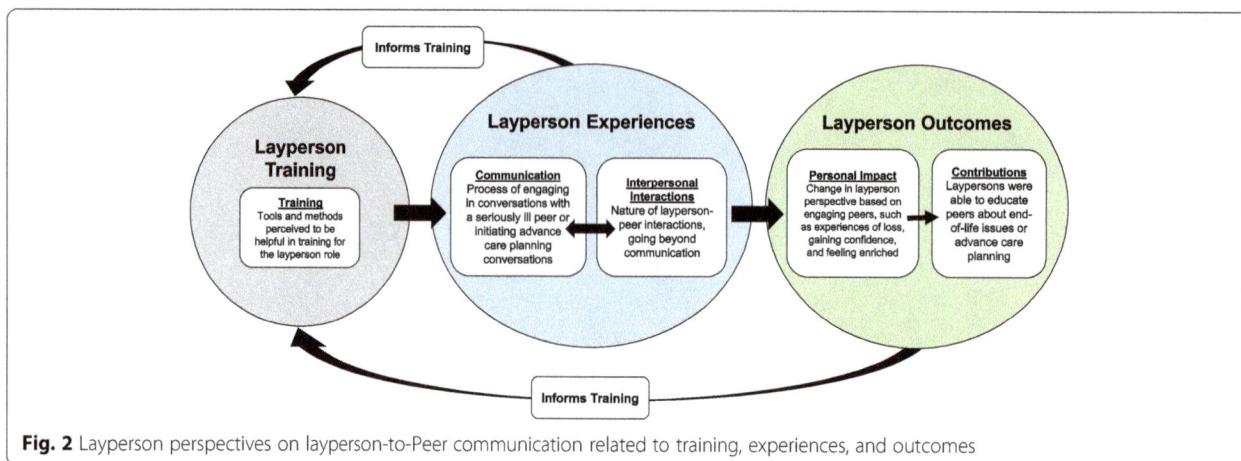

Fig. 2 Layperson perspectives on layperson-to-Peer communication related to training, experiences, and outcomes

prognosis, death, family and caregiver issues, bereavement, and suicide. Laypersons were able to engage in these diverse conversation topics because of their training and by overcoming their own obstacles, such as initial avoidance of death-related subjects and lacking sufficient knowledge of a peer's medical or social situation. When laypersons did initiate difficult conversations with a peer, it was ultimately met with a sense of relief. Through discussions with laypersons, hospice patients and loved ones often overcame denial of death and were able to address end-of-life practicalities, such as funeral planning and care of pets.

Listening and allowing silence was another theme of layperson communication. Some laypersons indicated that silence was anxiety-provoking because initially they worried about their contribution to the conversation and how the patient would perceive them. They reported that over time, they relinquished their self-concern and focused on the patient. They learned that listening, and being present or "in the moment," were the greatest gifts they could give because patients often needed someone to listen without judgement.

Responding to patient and family emotions was another theme of layperson-to-peer communication. Laypersons perceived several negative emotions experienced by patients including fear, anger, regret, guilt, loss of dignity, and feeling like a burden to their families. Laypersons also described that families appeared to experience grief, fatigue, discouragement, feeling trapped, and feeling guilty for wanting the process to be over. Families were fearful of losing their loved one, fearful of not being present at the time of death, and concerned about the loved one's pain and not being able to alleviate it. Laypersons wanted to learn how to sensitively and appropriately respond to these emotions.

Laypersons identified *communication facilitators* of layperson-to-peer communication, including physician endorsement and healthcare team involvement. For example,

they felt that physician endorsement of layperson-led advance care planning conversations would help to reinforce its importance. They also felt that the support and involvement of healthcare team members helped when a patient's questions surpassed the layperson's role. One volunteer noted,

"If they start askin' questions that I'm not sure of, then I'll get a nurse. I'll ask her questions, and I'll come back to 'em. I've had one that would ask about, well, how long would they keep feeding me before they would turn me off or whatever...I wasn't sure, so I went and got an MD to answer the question for me" [11].

Laypersons also identified several *communication barriers*. Laypersons noted peer-related obstacles to conversations, including denial of death, lack of readiness, limited health literacy, and family conflicts. Specific barriers included physical or cognitive impairments, such as Parkinson's disease or dementia, or the active dying process. In these situations, non-verbal communication became even more important when a patient's disease made verbal communication difficult. Patients seemed to be reassured by the layperson's presence. Specific to advance care planning conversations, laypersons noted health literacy limitations, including how the peers they were supporting seemed overwhelmed by medical information and jargon provided by the healthcare teams. At the broader community or healthcare system-level, a lack of time and space for advance care planning conversations, lack of widespread healthcare provider support, and cultural suspicion about talking about death and dying were the primary communication barriers. A volunteer in an advance care planning program stated, "I found it stressful with the pressure of completing an advance care planning quickly. It was like hitting a target" [29].

II. Layperson-to-peer interpersonal interactions

The second domain describes the nature of the layperson-to-peer interactions, going beyond communication. The themes included: a) *discomfort with the peer's situation,*

Table 3 Domains and themes exploring layperson perspectives about communication in serious illness or advance care planning

Derived domains, themes and subthemes	Theme from primary study (# refers to Table 2)	Exemplar layperson quotations for each subtheme (# refers to Table 2)
Domain 1. Layperson-to-peer communication		
Building rapport (Subthemes: Building trust; Developing relationships over time)	Benefits as an advance care planning: Positive interactions (5); Difficult communication: Volunteer's role (6); Navigator-level facilitators to advance care planning (8)	Of course, all of these patients have a relationship with me. Have rapport with me. I have seen them several times previously before I bring it up, so they know who I am and what I look like. They trust me. (8) I'll explain the type of services I can offer. The first time I may just mention it and tell them that one of the things that we can offer is advance care planning and we can talk about that another time if you're more interested. (8)
Talking about sensitive issues (Subthemes: Advance care planning; Prognosis; Death; Family/caregiver issues; Bereavement; Suicide)	Patient care and family concerns (1); Suicide and Hastening Death (1); End-of-Life Care Training Needs: Symptoms; Communication skills (2); Training encouraging action (3); The Patient is Alive (4); Personal Impact (5); Difficult communication: Denial; Dealing with pain/discomfort; Negative feelings of caregiver/family (6); Meaningful conversations: Life stories; death and spirituality; families and relationships; unfinished business (7); Patient-level barriers to advance care planning (8); Increased confidence in the topic (9)	Before [advance care planning] always felt like a major topic, you know 'Oh how am I going to raise this?' … [the training has] made it seem like something more natural to talk about, not to feel so awkward about discussing end-of-life matters and decisions … so that was really helpful. (9) It was just…had I known how serious the prognosis was, I would have handled the situation much differently. So, you know, it is very difficult going in cold sometimes because you can end up really putting your foot in your mouth. (2) It means that you have the opportunity to say to a family member who is quite distressed, 'Actually, it is okay. This is all that's happening', and that can be the most powerful thing you can possibly say, to know that actually that's okay. It is not anything out of the ordinary. (2, discussing dying) The most meaningful conversation was with the mother and the young kids. The topic was her concerns and fears about her family. (7) The most difficult thing seems to be business-type problems that need to be dealt with prior to or after the death. Families seem to find it an insensitive topic but usually recognize the necessity. (6) She was so miserable, she wanted me to contact this Dr. Kevorkian, and so trying to talk her out of it without disparaging her wishes, or you know, disappointing her…she wanted to be right with God, but she was talking about having, you know, ending her own life. It was her discussion, and I didn't promote it or anything. It was just a discussion to talk about, so I guess talking about that with somebody would be considered…kind of like I shouldn't be doing it, but it interested me to talk to her about it, and she was a very open person. (1)
Listening and allowing silence	End-of-Life Care Training Needs: Communication skills (2); Being There (4); Shared interests (5); Difficult communication: Physical/mental impairment (6); Meaningful conversations: Life Stories (7)	Most striking was how much he needed somebody to listen and not judge. (7)
Responding to patient and family emotions	End-of-Life Care Training Needs: Communication skills (2); Difficult communication: Negative feelings (6)	[The patient] was in one of the rooms where you have to wear extra protective clothing as well, and I remember his children there. And they were really upset, and obviously me and him

Table 3 Domains and themes exploring layperson perspectives about communication in serious illness or advance care planning (*Continued*)

Derived domains, themes and subthemes	Theme from primary study (# refers to Table 2)	Exemplar layperson quotations for each subtheme (# refers to Table 2)
		were having…He is telling me about times he went to Jamaica, and we're talking, but I could see that his children were visibly upset. So I asked them if they wanted me to leave, and they were like no, no, no. To them, they are seeing their dad, someone who has looked after them, in an ill position, but I didn't really know what to say to them. (2)
Communication facilitators (Subthemes: Physician endorsement; Healthcare team involvement)	System-level facilitators to advance care planning (8)	I want to get into the clinics and I want to have the doctor say to the patient, 'Your navigator is gonna come in, and they're gonna cover all of this, including advance directive, and I think that everybody should get it done.' (8)
Communication barriers (Subthemes: Physical or cognitive limitations; Health literacy limitations; Limited time for advance care planning conversations; Cultural norms)	End-of-Life Care Training Needs: Communication Skills (2); It's Not About Me (4); Personal Impact (5); Difficult communication: Physical/ mental impairment; Religious differences (6); Patient-level barriers to advance care planning (8); System-level barriers and facilitators to advance care planning (8)	I think the hardest issue for me was when my lady couldn't think of the word she wanted to say. She would get very frustrated and would cry. The best way I could get through this was to try to understand the concept of what she was talking about, then redirect the conversations. Sometimes I would use humor or we would listen to her favorite music. (6) Sure, they're anxious about whether or not they want to be on what they deem to be life-supportive equipment or whether they want a CPR. It kinda gets into the medical jargon. (8) I found it stressful with the pressure of completing an advance care planning quickly. It was like hitting a target. (5) It's just hard to deliver given our time with the patient and actually space to actually have a private conversation with them. (8) There's a cultural suspicion about it…. they call people who would discuss these things like death panels…I don't know if that's just our region or whatever…the difficulty is, I think, getting people to understand this is for their benefit. (8)
Domain 2: Layperson-to-peer interpersonal interactions		
Discomfort with peer's situation (Subthemes: Witnessing symptoms; Witnessing family distress)	Patient care and family concerns (1); End-of-Life Care Training Needs: Symptoms; communication skills (2); Being There (4); Difficult communication: Denial; Dealing with pain and discomfort; Family issues (6)	I actually thought he was dead because he didn't say anything for a while, and I was like 'Oh no, what am I going to do'. Because he had really heaving breathing, I don't know what was actually wrong with him. Air would get caught in him and it seemed like he was choking, so I told the nurse straight away. And she was like, 'No, don't worry'. (2) The family wouldn't mention that the patient is dying in front of him and refused to discuss it. They were really in denial. I told them that he knows he is dying - they were shocked that I knew because the patient told me. This opened up dialogue between them. We all felt some relief. (6)
Uncertainty of layperson role (Subtheme: Responding to patient/family requests; Gifts; Responding to symptoms)	Patient care and family concerns (1); Dilemmas about Gifts (1); Volunteer roles and boundaries (1); Difficult communication: Conflicts about patient care (6)	The person asked me if I would…If I would stay 8 h - for the day, and I told 'em, "Now, that's really not my job." I said, "It's a four-hour shift and I'll be glad to do that, but 8 h… that's really a lot." (1) …and I said, "I really can't accept that." She says, "You will hurt me if you don't accept that." So I thought, "What do I do? What do I do? It's almost like a gift." And I know it didn't cost

Table 3 Domains and themes exploring layperson perspectives about communication in serious illness or advance care planning (Continued)

Derived domains, themes and subthemes	Theme from primary study (# refers to Table 2)	Exemplar layperson quotations for each subtheme (# refers to Table 2)
		her anything, but that's not the principle, and I said, "Do I give it away?" And she was very adamant that I accept it, and so I didn't want to hurt her feelings, so I took it, right or wrong or indifferent… (1)
Interpersonal differences between layperson and peer (Subthemes: Cultural/religious differences; Socioeconomic differences)	End-of-Life Care Training Needs: Understanding spiritual diversity (2); The Patient is Alive (4); Difficult communication: Religious differences (6)	The one that stood out for me the most is understanding spiritual, cultural, and environmental aspects of dying because nowadays we are living in a society where people are very religious. And even though there may be some patients that aren't religious, you just have to respect what somebody believes. (2)
Domain 3: Personal impact on the layperson		
Building meaningful relationships (Subthemes: Learning from the peer; Receiving gratitude; Experiencing loss)	End-of-Life Care Training Needs: Self-care (2); The patient is alive; Being There (4); Benefits as an advance care planning volunteer: positive interactions; gratitude shown by peers; personal impact (5); Peer loss (6); Meaningful conversations; Shared interests; Gaining life lessons (7); Implications of being a peer educator (9)	Some things I don't understand and he explains to me. He wants to be informed about the future. He's not - he doesn't stop living here in the present. He makes me understand that, too, the way he talks about politics. He's all into that. I'm ashamed sometimes, I think, "Gosh, you know, I'm 23 and I don't know that a bomb exploded here or there." I think he keeps his life, very simple, day-to-day, to live in the moment. Maybe that's a lesson I'm supposed to learn. (4) The benefits are the gratitude for engaging with people to discuss such delicate issues at this very sensitive time in their lives. (5)
Gaining awareness of end-of-life (Subthemes: Personal reflection; Personal application; Personal difficulty with mortality)	Training encouraging action; training enhancing awareness (3); It's Not About Me (4); Difficult communication: Denial (6); Navigator-level barriers to advance care planning (8); Implications of being a peer educator (9)	The subject of dying and death is very delicate and how it is presented makes a difference. Over the months, the training we received has helped me become comfortable with the subject and, to a certain extent, more knowledgeable. (3) It certainly brought home to me that I myself might find this situation occurring in my life and yet I'd not done anything about it. So it made me think a lot and it made me talk to my family about it. (3) The difficulty is just dealing with somewhat your own - not issues, but your own reserves about this. (8)
Domain 4: Layperson contributions		
Educating others	Training encouraging action (3); Training enabling action (3);	I certainly didn't feel fazed by any of the questions that we were asked and, fortunately, other people participating in the group also answered questions, it wasn't just left to us as the leaders. (3) Older people have always been good educators for younger people but with support we can educate each other on more serious issues like these. (3)
Engaging in community outreach	Community engagement activities (9)	I'll be quite frank, I certainly wouldn't have got as involved as I am if I hadn't done it (the training). After the last training day we had a meeting [and] said well okay, we'll go and meet these people and see what they're doing … one thing we found was who knows what is out there as far as care provision. So we went and saw the hospice. We went and saw the PCT [Primary Health Care Trust]. We went and saw the Council… We literally pressed our PCT to get an (end-of-life) care strategy together because we went and saw them and we said okay we're going to hold an information day and we

Table 3 Domains and themes exploring layperson perspectives about communication in serious illness or advance care planning (*Continued*)

Derived domains, themes and subthemes	Theme from primary study (# refers to Table 2)	Exemplar layperson quotations for each subtheme (# refers to Table 2)
		will invite them to come and talk. So it pressurized them into having something ready. (9)
Domain 5: Layperson training		
Strategies (Subthemes: Experiential learning; Meetings over time; Supervision; Group-based learning)	Learning preferences (2); Program development process; Training encouraging action (3); Helpful additional supervision (5); Personal and emotional implications of being a peer educator (9)	If I know that it actually happens and this was the scenario that someone actually faced, it makes it seem more than just an exercise [sounds of agreement]. (2) I think role play is probably one of the best ways. So do I, because it puts you on the spot. (2) We've had a chance to take things in and think about it and then come to another meeting and that's been helpful, I think. (3) Actual structured supervision with feedback. (5)
Instructional personnel	Learning preferences (2); Training encouraging action (3)	I think both [staff and volunteers], because you will get the professional experience or the professional knowledge of the situation and they might have been dealing with it for years, so their training, and then a bit from the volunteers because they are hands on also. So I think both is important. (2) There were three groups. In each, there were 6–8 people from various backgrounds, and then two peer educators supported by a researcher. We rotated roles within the group, taking turns to be a facilitator, co-facilitator and observer. (3)
Materials	Learning preferences (2); Reviewing training materials (3); Suggestions for programme improvement (5)	The material is too detailed for use in a peer education guide. Most people, myself included, would find it most daunting to prepare an advance directive after reading the book. The subject presentation is too complicated for a peer guide where simplicity should be of the essence. (3) General information about what is available locally so we can signpost more effectively. (5)

b) *uncertainty of the layperson role*, and c) *interpersonal differences between layperson and peer. Discomfort with the peer's situation* encompassed witnessing symptoms and witnessing family distress. Laypersons described feeling helpless when observing patients' symptoms and not knowing what to do. Some were upset when witnessing a patient's distress over not being able to communicate, and felt unsure of how to help a patient with dementia. Witnessing a patient's or family's denial about death, hurtful family interactions, or emotional distress also caused discomfort. Laypersons identified these circumstances as opportunities for further training and desired clear preparation for encounters with distress, the dying process, and death.

A second theme that characterized interpersonal interactions was laypersons' *uncertainty of their role*. This theme included uncertainty regarding responding to patient/family requests, gifts, and responding to symptoms. A commonly cited reason for this uncertainty was the position of being neither friend nor provider. Laypersons felt that they were in a nebulous in-between role. One volunteer described:

"[The patient] was in pain, and made it very clear that he wanted his morphine, which is an absolute…you know, no-no. I'm not supposed to be dispensing medication. It was, for me, a very uncomfortable and difficult situation to be in, 'cause on the one hand, you don't want to watch a human being suffer. On the other hand, it was made very clear to me that, you know, 'this is something you don't do!'" [30].

Laypersons recounted requests from patients and families that were inappropriate for this in-between role, such as dispensing pain medications, staying at the facility beyond their volunteer shift, or performing conspiratorial favors, such as throwing away an item that the patient didn't want his family to see. This nebulous role also meant receiving gifts put them in an awkward position. If the layperson was a personal friend, they would have no problem receiving gifts. If they were a healthcare team member, they would have clear boundaries for declining gifts. Laypersons' uncertainty also related to responding to symptoms or the peer's self-care needs. They were uncertain about their role when advocating for the patient when concerns about a patient's care or needs were raised. Laypersons often needed to navigate their role with the peer, family members, and healthcare team members, each of whom may have had different expectations of the layperson's role and appropriate level of involvement.

Interpersonal differences between layperson and peer was a third theme and included the subthemes of cultural or religious differences and socioeconomic differences. Some laypersons perceived that religious differences could be a barrier. For example, some laypersons described feeling disconnected from a peer whose beliefs contradicted their own, while others admitted it was difficult to refrain from sharing their own beliefs. Awareness of these differences, however, did not necessarily cause a rift between the layperson and peer. One layperson recalled a patient with whom she connected despite their very different socioeconomic backgrounds:

"We instantly connected because we left out all the bullshit and just connected on a human level. And there's a lot of female connection that we have, too. We connect as two women. We can talk about men, our husbands, what society expects of us as women, and what we want out of life. So she, I realized, shares the dreams and desires and aspirations that I have. We're sisters under the skin" [28].

III. Personal impact on the layperson

The third domain is the personal impact on the layperson as they engaged in training, meeting peers with serious illness, or initiating advance care planning conversations. A key theme of this domain was *building meaningful relationships*, including learning from the peer, receiving gratitude, and experiencing loss. Laypersons describe "enriching" and "rewarding" experiences, gleaning wisdom from their patient as a "living history." They felt rewarded by gratitude from the patient, which they felt accounted for the challenges of discussing death and dying. By forming strong connections with patients, however, they also experienced loss. Laypersons commented on the difficulty of letting go of friendships that had formed, stating:

"It does affect you at times when you know someone, you may be seeing them… [and] during two or three weeks you get to know them, and then they are gone" [20].

Personal impact on the layperson also included *gaining awareness of end-of-life*. Laypersons elaborated on this awareness in subthemes of personal reflection, personal application, and personal difficulty with mortality. Several laypersons commented that death became less daunting as a result of their experiences, especially when seen through the eyes of a peer with a positive outlook. They gained a better appreciation of how others approach end-of-life issues, and a deeper understanding of loss. They applied these lessons to their own lives, feeling better prepared to support those who had lost someone and how to advocate for their own wishes. One layperson commented that his experience had been a "re-education," and he had become more compassionate as a result. Not all experiences were positive. Some laypersons discussed their own anxieties about mortality limited their ability to help patients.

IV. Layperson contributions

The fourth domain is layperson contributions and includes the themes of *educating others* and *engaging in community outreach*. Through effective training programs, laypersons discovered that they were able to educate their peers about end-of-life issues or advance care planning. They felt satisfaction when seeing the results of their hard work, such as completing a workbook for advance care planning with a peer. Some felt emboldened to engage their own families in end-of-life care discussions and even expanded their work into the wider community. For example, some trained peer educators hosted information sessions and meetings with local community stakeholders. They became further involved in local and national organizations aimed at increasing awareness of death and advance care planning.

V. Layperson training

The final domain is layperson training. Several studies described the processes of preparing laypersons to be peer navigators, educators, or hospice or hospital-based volunteers to support individuals with serious illnesses or to initiate advance care planning conversations. Layperson training focused on communication skills and provided laypersons with knowledge, experience, and confidence to address specific communication issues, as well as the broader role of supporting a peer. In addition to the content-focused suggestions that laypersons had related to the aforementioned domains, layperson input specific to training included *strategies, instructional personnel,* and *materials.* Suggestions for training strategies included experiential learning, meetings over time, supervision, and group-based learning. Laypersons preferred experiential learning, using real case examples and role playing, over computer-based "e-learning" or virtual classrooms. In terms of timing, they valued attending trainings that continued after starting the layperson role because they were able to learn from their real-life experiences, reflect between sessions, and receive on-going support from other laypersons. Structured supervision with feedback was another training need. Lastly, laypersons felt co-leading a group discussion related to advance care planning, rather than independently leading groups, helped peer education to go more smoothly.

A second theme related to layperson training was *instructional personnel.* Laypersons found that the most effective training was provided by experienced lay volunteers and healthcare professionals (e.g., palliative care providers), in addition to the program coordinators. The third training suggestion related to *materials.* Laypersons felt that simpler, more layperson-friendly materials were more effective than advance care planning printed materials that used complicated jargon. They also suggested that advance care planning materials for peers be based on stories or examples to make the concepts more understandable.

Discussion
Main findings of the study
This meta-synthesis addresses the study question: "What are the perspectives of laypersons on communication with individuals with serious illness or advance care planning?" We provide an integrated synthesis of the thoughts and experiences of non-medical laypersons as they communicate with peers experiencing serious illnesses, end-of-life care, or related to advance care planning conversations. In focusing on layperson-to-peer communication, this analysis describes commonalities in how trained laypersons approached and experienced conversations. It also highlights the variety of interactions, social or clinical context, benefits, and challenges of those conversations. The findings provide additional support to the role of laypersons in having meaningful conversations, though healthcare provider or physician endorsement of the layperson role may improve their effectiveness [8, 14]. Together with specific input from laypersons on their training needs, these findings can inform best practices for training and ongoing support systems for community or healthcare system-based programs that involve lay individuals. The synthesized results provide a foundation for the design and adaptation of peer-based programs that focus on communication skills and training.

This study offers insight into the benefits and challenges of laypersons' engagement in advance care planning conversations. While other research studies focus on advance directive documentation, this study describes how engaging with seriously ill patients or peers in advance care planning conversations can be a challenging yet rewarding experience from the layperson's perspective [31]. A future analysis should also include perspectives of the peer/patient and family caregivers [32]. Laypersons also shared similar sentiments regarding end-of-life communication: being with the patient and his/her loved ones and talking about death could be anxiety-provoking or uncomfortable, especially with inadequate training. Many laypersons and patients still found the experience to be positive. Laypersons specifically described increased awareness of end-of-life issues for themselves and, in turn, initiated conversations with families, friends, and sometimes their broader community. Thus, the investment of training a layperson for involvement in palliative care, hospice, or other programs to support seriously ill individuals may yield community-level benefits related to discussions about death and dying. Additionally, for programs that utilize older adult volunteers, this analysis aligns with a theoretical benefit between volunteering and successful aging through opportunities for communication [33, 34].

As a meta-synthesis, this study included individual studies that involved laypersons in highly varied settings, including hospices, hospitals, and community-based outreach programs to enhance advance care planning conversations. There were diverse types of non-health laypersons, including hospital volunteers, hospice volunteers, lay health navigators, and peer educators. The laypersons may have been part of a specific communication-based program or may have had opportunities for communication as part of their broader role. Although this meta-synthesis provides access to context variation within and across studies, the application of the key findings must be re-contextualized to the particular type of layperson, type of peer/patient, and program implementation setting. The laypersons' suggestions on training, planning for program sustainability, and legal and ethical aspects of the involvement of laypersons in communication-based roles need to be adapted to regional or national policy considerations. The unique position of laypersons may require training measures specific to them because laypersons experienced uncertainty in their role, being neither a caregiver nor a health care professional. However, laypersons reported building and using communication skills such as building rapport, responding to patient and family emotions, and talking about sensitive issues which are skills also used by health care professionals. Because these skills are commonly used by health and social care professionals, there may be opportunities to adapt existing training models for use in layperson programs. Additionally, further study could evaluate the potential benefit and challenges of shared training, at least in part, for health care providers and laypersons in communication skills for a particular program. Given the significant difference in the role of a healthcare provider and a trained layperson, skills which may seem transferable between the two may still require different training methods and would require further evaluation.

Further research on the impact of laypersons in advance care planning or end-of-life conversations is warranted. This meta-synthesis focuses on the perspectives of laypersons, but future work should focus on the perspectives of patients, family members, and members of the healthcare team regarding the role and impact of laypersons. Prior to widespread adoption of laypersons in this role, specific evaluation of the safety and potential effectiveness of trained laypersons on communication and other meaningful person-centered outcomes is needed.

Limitations of the study

This study has several limitations. As a meta-synthesis, we did not have access to the original data sets, including complete transcripts or field notes, and were limited in our ability to interpret the linguistic and cultural context of the published quotations. Additionally, the focus on qualitative studies, inclusion criteria, and exclusion criteria resulted in unintentionally limiting the geographical location of the studies to the US and the UK. For example, in choosing to exclude grey literature such as dissertations, theses, and book chapters, we may have

biased the findings toward established programs that had desire and ability to publish in peer-reviewed journals. The literature search yielded studies involving laypersons in palliative care or end-of-life settings conducted elsewhere, such as Canada and Uganda, but those studies did not specifically examine communication or use qualitative methods [18, 35]. Still, the majority of studies relating to volunteer or other layperson experiences are based in the US, Canada, or UK, making it difficult to broadly apply the findings of this meta-synthesis beyond these regions. Future work should include grey literature as this literature may have insights from additional settings, making the results of a meta-synthesis more broadly applicable. Additionally, the scope of this study did not include quantitative outcomes related to advance care planning programs involving trained laypersons [31]. An additional limitation to the study is that there was no layperson on the research team contributing to the analysis of themes.

Conclusions

The findings from layperson perspectives on communication with peers experiencing serious illness or related to advance care planning have practical implications. Since volunteers are more likely to commit to an activity that is personally satisfying, volunteer laypersons may constitute a reliable and cost-effective way to enhance advance care planning efforts and support individuals with palliative care needs, especially in community-based settings [35]. Training, and even paying, laypersons could be a viable alternative to training existing healthcare providers in specific advance care planning communication skills, especially in resource-limited settings. Moreover, because laypersons may have more time or common life factors on which to establish rapport, laypersons are uniquely positioned to engage in end-of-life conversations with peers experiencing serious illnesses.

In conclusion, we synthesized the perspectives of a diverse group of laypersons who were involved in communicating with individuals with serious illnesses or as part of advance care planning programs. Together the studies described the involvement of laypersons in meaningful conversations with their peers and outlined interpersonal interactions, personal impact, contributions, and training that laypersons experienced. Laypersons may complement and potentially enhance the work of healthcare providers in meeting the educational and psychosocial needs of individuals and their family caregivers in palliative care settings. Programs that involve laypersons should include training specifically for layperson-to-peer conversations related to the end-of-life period, as well as a mechanism for

Appendix 1

Table 4 Search strategies. Comprehensive search strategies used to identify articles for each database

MEDLINE, including Ovid MEDLINE Epub Ahead of Print, In-Process & Other Non-Indexed Citations, and Ovid MEDLINE Daily (1946-present)	(exp Peer Group/ or exp. Volunteers/ or exp. Mentors/ or exp. Patient Navigation/ or (voluntary or peer* or volunteer* or mentor* or navigator* or lay*).tw,kf.) and (exp Advance Care Planning/ or exp. Hospices/ or exp. Hospice and Palliative Care Nursing/ or exp. Palliative Medicine/ or exp. Palliative Care/ or exp. Terminal Care/ or (Living Will* or Medical Power* Attorney or Health Care Power* Attorney or Healthcare Power* Attorney or advance* care plan* or advance* directive* or advance* health care plan* or advance* healthcare plan* or advance* medical plan* or hospice* or palliative or terminal care or end-of-life).tw,kf.) and (exp Patient Education as Topic/ or exp. Counseling/or exp. Information Dissemination/ or exp. Teaching/ or exp. Consumer Health Information/ or (discussion* or coaching or navigation* or navigating or learning or awareness or training or conversation* or engag* or promotion* or story or stories or experienc* or sharing or educator* or education* or educating or encourag* or teaching or counseling or information or knowledge or communicat*).tw,kf.) and (exp Qualitative Research/ or exp. Grounded Theory/ or exp. Interviews as Topic/ or exp. Focus Groups/ or exp. Nursing Methodology Research/ or exp. anecdotes as topic/ or exp. narration/ or exp. "surveys and questionnaires"/ or exp. personal narratives as topic/ or exp. Observational Studies as Topic/ or exp. interview/ or exp. personal narratives/ or exp. observational study/ or (qualitative or ethnograph* or phenomenol* or grounded theor* or purposive sampl* or hermeneutic* or heuristic* or semiotics or lived experience* or narrat* or life experience* or cluster sample* or action research or observational method* or content analys* or thematic analys* or constant comparative method* or field stud* or theoretical sampl* or discourse analys* or focus group* or ethnological research or ethnomethodolog* or interview* or mixed method* or mixed model* or mixed design* or survey* or questionnaire* or anecdote*).tw,kf.)	Results = 745
PsycINFO via Ovid (1806 to March Week 2 2017)	(exp peers/ or exp. volunteers/ or mentor/ or (voluntary or peer* or volunteer* or mentor* or navigator* or lay*).ab,ti.) and (exp advance directives/ or exp. Palliative Care/ or exp. hospice/ or (Living Will* or Medical Power* Attorney or Health Care Power* Attorney or Healthcare Power* Attorney or advance* care plan* or advance* directive* or advance* health care plan* or advance* healthcare plan* or advance* medical plan* or hospice* or palliative or terminal care or end-of-life).ab,ti.) and (exp peer education/ or exp. Community Counseling/ or exp. Educational Counseling/ or exp. Peer Counseling/ or exp. information dissemination/ or exp. teaching/ or exp. consumer education/ or exp. death education/ or (discussion* or coaching or navigation* or navigating or learning or awareness or training or conversation* or engag* or promotion* or story or stories or experienc* or sharing or educator* or education* or educating or encourag* or teaching or counseling or information or knowledge or communicat*).ab,ti.) and (exp qualitative research/ or exp. grounded theory/ or exp. Interviews/ or exp. Narratives/ or exp. surveys/ or exp. questionnaires/ or exp. narratives/ or (qualitative or ethnograph* or phenomenol* or grounded theor* or purposive sampl* or hermeneutic* or heuristic* or semiotics or lived experience* or narrat* or life experience* or cluster sample* or action research or observational method* or content analys* or thematic analys* or constant comparative method* or field stud* or theoretical sampl* or discourse analys* or focus group* or ethnological research or ethnomethodolog* or interview* or mixed method* or mixed model* or mixed design* or survey* or questionnaire* or anecdote*).ab,ti.) *Publication types were limited to ("0100 journal" or "0110 peer-reviewed journal" or "0120 non-peer-reviewed journal" or "0130 peer-reviewed status unknown").*	Results = 277
CINAHL Cumulative Index to Nursing and Allied Health Literature (CINAHL) via EBSCOhost	(MH "Peer Group" OR MH "Volunteer Workers" OR MH "Volunteer Experiences" OR TI (voluntary or peer* or volunteer* or mentor* or navigator* or lay*) OR AB (voluntary or peer* or volunteer* or mentor* or navigator* or lay*)) AND (MH "Advance Care Planning" OR MH "Advance Directives+" OR MH "Hospice Patients" OR MH "Hospice and Palliative Nursing" OR MH "Hospices" OR MH "Terminal Care+" OR MH "Palliative Care" OR TI (Living Will* or Medical Power* Attorney or Health Care Power* Attorney or Healthcare Power* Attorney or advance* care plan* or advance* directive* or advance* health care plan* or advance* healthcare plan* or advance* medical plan* or hospice* or palliative or terminal care or end-of-life) OR AB (Living Will* or Medical Power* Attorney or Health Care Power* Attorney or Healthcare Power* Attorney or advance* care plan* or advance* directive* or advance* health care plan* or advance* healthcare plan* or advance* medical plan* or hospice* or palliative or terminal care or end-of-life)) AND (MH "Patient Education+" OR MH "Counseling+" OR MH "Teaching" OR MH "Death Education" OR MH "Consumer Health Information+"	Results = 359

Table 4 Search strategies. Comprehensive search strategies used to identify articles for each database *(Continued)*

	OR TI (discussion* or coaching or navigation* or navigating or learning or awareness or training or conversation* or engag* or promotion* or story or stories or experienc* or sharing or educator* or education* or educating or encourag* or teaching or counseling or information or knowledge or communicat*) OR AB (discussion* or coaching or navigation* or navigating or learning or awareness or training or conversation* or engag* or promotion* or story or stories or experienc* or sharing or educator* or education* or educating or encourag* or teaching or counseling or information or knowledge or communicat*)) AND (MH "Qualitative Studies+" OR MH "Ethnological Research" OR MH "Action Research" OR MH "Phenomenological Research" OR MH "Ethnographic Research" OR MH "Field Studies" OR MH "Grounded Theory" OR MH "Multimethod Studies" OR MH "Survey Research" OR MH "Phenomenology" OR MH "Focus Groups" OR MH "Interviews+" OR MH "Narratives" OR MH "Surveys+" OR MH "Observational Methods+" OR MH "Discourse Analysis" OR MH "Thematic Analysis" OR MH "Content Analysis" OR MH "Qualitative Validity+" OR TI (qualitative or ethnograph* or phenomenol* or grounded theor* or purposive sampl* or hermeneutic* or heuristic* or semiotics or lived experience* or narrat* or life experience* or cluster sample* or action research or observational method* or content analys* or thematic analys* or constant comparative method* or field stud* or theoretical sampl* or discourse analys* or focus group* or ethnological research or ethnomethodolog* or interview* or mixed method* or mixed model* or mixed design* or survey* or questionnaire* or anecdote*) OR AB (qualitative or ethnograph* or phenomenol* or grounded theor* or purposive sampl* or hermeneutic* or heuristic* or semiotics or lived experience* or narrat* or life experience* or cluster sample* or action research or observational method* or content analys* or thematic analys* or constant comparative method* or field stud* or theoretical sampl* or discourse analys* or focus group* or ethnological research or ethnomethodolog* or interview* or mixed method* or mixed model* or mixed design* or survey* or questionnaire* or anecdote*)) *Dissertation/thesis was excluded as a source type.*	
Cochrane Library (via Wiley, including Cochrane Database of Systematic Reviews, Database of Abstracts of Reviews of Effect, Cochrane Central Register of Controlled Trials, Cochrane Methodology Register, Health Technology Assessment Database, and NHS Economic Evaluation Database)	#1 → MeSH descriptor: [Peer Group] explode all trees #2 → MeSH descriptor: [Volunteers] explode all trees #3 → MeSH descriptor: [Mentors] explode all trees #4 → MeSH descriptor: [Patient Navigation] explode all trees #5 → voluntary or peer or volunteer or mentor or navigator or lay:ti orab orkw (Word variations have been searched) #6 → MeSH descriptor: [Advance Care Planning] explode all trees #7 → MeSH descriptor: [Hospices] explode all trees #8 → MeSH descriptor: [Hospice and Palliative Care Nursing] explode all trees #9 → MeSH descriptor: [Palliative Medicine] explode all trees #10 → MeSH descriptor: [Palliative Care] explode all trees #11 → MeSH descriptor: [Terminal Care] explode all trees #12 → "Living Will" or "Medical Power of Attorney" or "Health Care Power Attorney" or "Healthcare Power of Attorney" or "advance care planning" or "advance directive" or "advance health care plan" or "advance healthcare plan" or "advance medical plan" or hospice or palliative or "terminal care" or "end of life":ti orab orkw (Word variations have been searched) #13 → MeSH descriptor: [Patient Education as Topic] explode all trees #14 → MeSH descriptor: [Counseling] explode all trees #15 → MeSH descriptor: [Information Dissemination] explode all trees #16 → MeSH descriptor: [Teaching] explode all trees #17 → MeSH descriptor: [Consumer Health Information] explode all trees #18 → discussion or coaching or navigation or navigating or learning or awareness or training or conversation or engagement or promotion or story or stories or experience or sharing or educator or education or educating or encouragement or teaching or counseling or information or knowledge or communication:ti orab orkw (Word variations have been searched) #19 → MeSH descriptor: [Qualitative Research] explode all trees #20 → MeSH descriptor: [Grounded Theory] explode all trees #21 → MeSH descriptor: [Interviews as Topic] explode all trees #22 → MeSH descriptor: [Focus Groups] explode all trees #23 → MeSH descriptor: [Nursing Methodology Research] explode all trees #24 → MeSH descriptor: [Anecdotes as Topic] explode all trees #25 → MeSH descriptor: [Narration] explode all trees #26 → MeSH descriptor: [Surveys and Questionnaires] explode all trees #27 → MeSH descriptor: [Personal Narratives as Topic] explode all trees #28 → MeSH descriptor: [Observational Studies as Topic] explode all trees #29 → MeSH descriptor: [Interview] explode all trees #30 → MeSH descriptor: [Personal Narratives] explode all trees	Results = 37

Table 4 Search strategies. Comprehensive search strategies used to identify articles for each database *(Continued)*

	#31 → MeSH descriptor: [Observational Study] explode all trees
	#32 → qualitative or ethnography or phenomenoly or "grounded theory" or "purposive sample" or hermeneutics or heuristics or semiotics or "lived experience" or narrative or "life experience" or "cluster sample" or "action research" or "observational method" or "content analysis" or "thematic analysis" or "constant comparative method" or "field study" or "theoretical sample" or "discourse analysis" or "focus group" or "ethnological research" or ethnomethodology or interview or "mixed method" or "mixed model" or "mixed design" or survey or questionnaire or anecdote:ti,ab,kw (Word variations have been searched)
	#33 → (#1 or #2 or #3 or #4 or #5) and (#6 or #7 or #8 or #9 or #10 or #11 or #12) and (#13 or #14 or #15 or #16 or #17 or #18) and (#19 or #20 or #21 or #22 or #23 or #24 or #25 or #26 or #27 or #28 or #29 or #30 or #31 or #32)
Allied and Complementary Medicine (AMED) via Ovid (1985 to March 2017)	(exp Peer group/ or exp. Voluntary workers/ or exp. Mentors/ or (voluntary or peer* or volunteer* or mentor* or navigator* or lay*).ab,ti.) AND (exp advance directives/ or exp. hospices/ or exp. palliative care/ or exp. terminal care/ or (Living Will* or Medical Power* Attorney or Health Care Power* Attorney or Healthcare Power* Attorney or advance* care plan* or advance* directive* or advance* health care plan* or advance* healthcare plan* or advance* medical plan* or hospice* or palliative or terminal care or end-of-life).ab,ti.) AND (exp patient education/ or exp. counseling/ or exp. teaching/ or (discussion* or coaching or navigation* or navigating or learning or awareness or training or conversation* or engag* or promotion* or story or stories or experienc* or sharing or educator* or education* or educating or encourag* or teaching or counseling or information or knowledge or communicat*).ab,ti.) and (exp interviews/ or exp. questionnaires/ or (qualitative or ethnograph* or phenomenol* or grounded theor* or purposive sampl* or hermeneutic* or heuristic* or semiotics or lived experience* or narrat* or life experience* or cluster sample* or action research or observational method* or content analys* or thematic analys* or constant comparative method* or field stud* or theoretical sampl* or discourse analys* or focus group* or ethnological research or ethnomethodolog* or interview* or mixed method* or mixed model* or mixed design* or survey* or questionnaire* or anecdote*).ab,ti.)	Results = 148

Appendix 2

Table 5 Summary of critical appraisal of study quality

Domain	Berry & Planalp	Brighton et al.	Clarke et al.	Foster	Jones et al.	Planalp & Trost	Planalp et al.	Rocque et al.	Seymour et al.
Study purpose: Was purpose or research question stated?	Yes	Yes	Yes	Yes	Yes	Yes	Yes	Yes	Yes
Literature: Was relevant literature reviewed?	Yes	Yes	Yes	Yes	Yes	Yes	Yes	Yes	Yes
Study design: Was a theoretical perspective identified?	Yes	Yes	Yes	Yes	No	Yes	No	Yes	Yes
Sampling: Was the process of purposeful selection described?	No	Yes	Yes	No	Yes	No	No	No	Yes
Was sampling done until redundancy in data was reached?	N.A.	Yes	N.A.	N.A.	N.A.	N.A.	N.A.	N.A.	N.A.
Was informed consent obtained?	Yes	Yes	No	No	Yes	N.A.	N.A.	Yes	N.A.
Data Collection: Was procedural rigor used?	Yes	Yes	N.A.	No	N.A.	Yes	Yes	Yes	Yes
Descriptive clarity: Complete description of site	No	Yes	No	No	Yes	No	No	Yes	Yes
Descriptive clarity: Complete description of participant	Yes	Yes	No	No	Yes	Yes	No	Yes	Yes
Description of role of researcher and relationship with participants	No	Yes	Yes	Yes	No	No	No	Yes	Yes
Identification of assumption and biases of researcher	No	Yes	No	Yes	No	No	No	Yes	No
Analytical rigor: Were data analyses inductive?	No	Yes	N.A.	Yes	Yes	Yes	Yes	Yes	N.A.
Were findings consistent with and reflective of data?	Yes	Yes	Yes	Yes	Yes	Yes	Yes	Yes	Yes
Auditability: Was a decision trail developed?	N.A.	Yes	N.A.	Yes	No	N.A.	Yes	N.A.	No
Was the process of analyzing the data described adequately?	Yes	Yes	No	N.A.	No	Yes	Yes	Yes	Yes
Theoretical connections: Did a meaningful picture emerge?	No	No	Yes	Yes	No	Yes	No	Yes	Yes
Credibility: Do descriptions and interpretations of participants capture the phenomenon?	Yes	Yes	Yes	Yes	No	No	Yes	Yes	Yes
Transferability: Can the findings be transferred to other situations?	Yes	Yes	No	No	No	Yes	Yes	Yes	Yes
Dependability: Was there consistency between data and findings?	No	Yes	Yes	No	No	Yes	Yes	Yes	Yes
Confirmability: Were strategies employed to minimize bias?	No	Yes	Yes	No	No	No	No	Yes	No
Conclusions: Were conclusions appropriate given study findings?	Yes	Yes	Yes	Yes	Yes	Yes	Yes	Yes	Yes
Implications: Were findings meaningful to "laypersons" and communication?	Yes	Yes	No	Yes	Yes	Yes	Yes	Yes	Yes
Total score:	60%	95%	61%	60%	50%	68%	60%	95%	84%

Quality appraisal results and scoring of included studies using McMaster University tool

providing ongoing support to maximize and sustain the impact of the layperson's role.

in study design, data collection, analysis, interpretation, writing of the manuscript, or decision to submit for publication.

Abbreviations
UK: United Kingdom; US: United States

Acknowledgements
This study was presented at the 10th World Research Congress of the European Association for Palliative Care. The abstract is published online in Palliative Medicine (Abstract number P158; https://doi.org/10.1177/0269216318769196).

Funding
This work was supported in part by the National Institutes of Health [K76AG054782] and Department of Veterans Affairs. The funders had no role

Authors' contributions
Study design: HL, CJ, SJ, US, KB, KD, and JJ defined the study question, study question, search aims, and methodology used for identification and analysis of data. Data collection: KD conducted a focused study search and JD, AB, and HL completed study selection. Data analysis: SJ, CJ, US, and KB completed the quality rating for each selected study. JD, AB, and HL completed study extraction. ES, JD, AB, SJ, and HL completed the synthesis of themes. Manuscript preparation: ES, JD, AB, SJ, HL. Critical manuscript revision: CJ, SJ, US, KB, JJ, KD. All authors participated in final revision and have read and approved the manuscript.

Competing interests
The authors have no potential conflicts of interest with respect to the research, authorship and/or publication of this article.

Author details
[1]Internal Medicine Residency, University of Colorado School of Medicine, University of Colorado Anschutz Medical Campus, Aurora, CO, USA. [2]University of Colorado Skaggs School of Pharmacy and Pharmaceutical Sciences, University of Colorado Anschutz Medical Campus, Aurora, CO, USA. [3]VA Eastern Colorado Geriatric Research Education and Clinical Center, Denver, CO, USA. [4]Division of Geriatric Medicine, University of Colorado School of Medicine, University of Colorado Anschutz Medical Campus, 12631 E. 17th Ave, Mail Stop B179, Aurora, CO 80045, USA. [5]Health Sciences Library, University of Colorado Anschutz Medical Campus, Aurora, CO, USA. [6]Division of Hospital Medicine, University of Colorado School of Medicine, Anschutz Medical Campus, Aurora, CO, USA. [7]College of Nursing, University of Colorado Anschutz Medical Campus, Aurora, CO, USA. [8]Division of Cardiovascular Medicine, Sarver Heart Center, University of Arizona, Tucson, AZ, USA.

References
1. Sudore RL, Lum HD, You JJ, Hanson LC, Meier DE, Pantilat SZ, et al. Defining Advance Care Planning for Adults: A consensus definition from a multidisciplinary Delphi panel. J Pain Symptom Manage. 2017;53(5):821–32. e821
2. Brinkman-Stoppelenburg A, Rietjens JA, van der Heide A. The effects of advance care planning on end-of-life care: a systematic review. Palliat Med. 2014;28(8):1000–25.
3. Houben CH, Spruit MA, Groenen MT, Wouters EF, Janssen DJ. Efficacy of advance care planning: a systematic review and meta-analysis. J Am Med Dir Assoc. 2014;15(7):477–89.
4. Institute of Medicine. Dying in America: improving quality and honoring individual preferences near the end of life. Washington, DC: The National Academies Press; 2015. https://doi.org/10.17226/18748.
5. Broadfoot KJ, Candrian C. Relationship-centered care and clinical dialogue: Towards new forms of "care-full" communication. Nat Med J. 2009;1(12):1–2.
6. Sinuff T, Dodek P, You JJ, Barwich D, Tayler C, Downar J, et al. Improving end-of-life communication and decision making: the development of a conceptual framework and quality indicators. J Pain Symptom Manag. 2015; 49(6):1070–80.
7. Sanders C, Seymour J, Clarke A, Gott M, Welton M. Development of a peer education programme for advance end-of-life care planning. Int J Palliat Nurs. 2006;12(5):214. 216-223
8. Calista J, Tjia J. Moving the advance care planning needle with community health workers. Med Care. 2017;55(4):315–8.
9. Fischer SM, Sauaia A, Kutner JS. Patient navigation: a culturally competent strategy to address disparities in palliative care. J Palliat Med. 2007;10(5): 1023–8.
10. Perry E, Swartz J, Brown S, Smith D, Kelly G, Swartz R. Peer mentoring: a culturally sensitive approach to end-of-life planning for long-term dialysis patients. Am J Kidney Dis. 2005;46(1):111–9.
11. Rocque GB, Dionne-Odom JN, Sylvia Huang CH, Niranjan SJ, Williams CP, Jackson BE, et al. Implementation and impact of patient lay navigator-led advance care planning conversations. J Pain Symptom Manag. 2017;53(4): 682–92.
12. Clarke A, Seymour J. "at the foot of a very long ladder": discussing the end of life with older people and informal caregivers. J Pain Symptom Manag. 2010;40(6):857–69.
13. Burbeck R, Candy B, Low J, Rees R. Understanding the role of the volunteer in specialist palliative care: a systematic review and thematic synthesis of qualitative studies. BMC Palliat Care. 2014;13(1):3.
14. Candy B, France R, Low J, Sampson L. Does involving volunteers in the provision of palliative care make a difference to patient and family wellbeing? A systematic review of quantitative and qualitative evidence. Int J Nurs Stud. 2015;52(3):756–68.
15. Connell B, Warner G, Weeks LE. The feasibility of creating partnerships between palliative care volunteers and healthcare providers to support rural frail older adults and their families: an integrative review. Am J Hosp Palliat Care. 2016;34(8):786–94.
16. Downe-Wamboldt B, Ellerton ML. A study of the role of hospice volunteers. Hospice J. 1985;1(4):17–31.
17. Luijkx KG, Schols JM. Volunteers in palliative care make a difference. J Palliat Care. 2009;25(1):30–9.
18. Jack BA, Kirton J, Birakurataki J, Merriman A. 'A bridge to the hospice': the impact of a community volunteer programme in Uganda. Palliat Med. 2011; 25(7):706–15.
19. Germain A, Nolan K, Doyle R, Mason S, Gambles M, Chen H, et al. The use of reflective diaries in end of life training programmes: a study exploring the impact of self-reflection on the participants in a volunteer training programme. BMC Palliat Care. 2016;15:28.
20. Brighton LJ, Koffman J, Robinson V, Khan SA, George R, Burman R, Selman LE. End of life could be on any ward really: a qualitative study of hospital volunteers' end-of-life care training needs and learning preferences. Palliat Med. 2017;9:842–52.
21. Beasley E, Brooker J, Warren N, Fletcher J, Boyle C, Ventura A, Burney S. The lived experience of volunteering in a palliative care biography service. Palliat Suppor Care. 2015;13(5):1417–25.
22. Planalp S, Trost MR. Communication issues at the end of life: reports from hospice volunteers. Health Commun. 2008;23(3):222–33.
23. Tong A, Flemming K, McInnes E, Oliver S, Craig J. Enhancing transparency in reporting the synthesis of qualitative research: ENTREQ. BMC Med Res Methodol. 2012;12:181.
24. Thomas J, Harden A. Methods for the thematic synthesis of qualitative research in systematic reviews. BMC Med Res Methodol. 2008;8:45.
25. Letts L, Wilkins S, Law M, Stewart D, Bosch J, Westmorland M. Guidelines for critical review form: Qualitative studies (Version 2.0) [https://srs-mcmaster.ca/wp-content/uploads/2015/05/Guidelines-for-Critical-Review-Form-Qualitative-Studies.pdf].
26. Moher D, Liberati A, Tetzlaff J, Altman DG, Group P. Preferred reporting items for systematic reviews and meta-analyses: the PRISMA statement. J Clin Epidemiol. 2009;62(10):1006–12.
27. Planalp S, Trost MR, Berry PH. Spiritual feasts: meaningful conversations between hospice volunteers and patients. Am J Hosp Palliat Med. 2011; 28(7):483–6.
28. Foster E. Lessons we learned: stories of volunteer-patient communication in hospice. J Age Ident. 2002;7(4):245–56.
29. Jones P, Heaps K, Rattigan C, Di M-M. Advance care planning in a UK hospice: the experiences of trained volunteers. Eur J Palliat Care. 2015;22(3):144–51.
30. Berry P, Planalp S. Ethical issues for hospice volunteers. Am J Hosp Palliat Med. 2008;25(6):458–62.
31. Litzelman DK, Inui TS, Schmitt-Wendholt KM, Perkins A, Griffin WJ, Cottingham AH, Ivy SS. Clarifying values and preferences for care near the end of life: the role of a new lay workforce. J Community Health. 2017;42(5):926–34.
32. Weeks LE, Macquarrie C, Bryanton O. Hospice palliative care volunteers: a unique care link. J Palliat Care. 2008;24(2):85–93.
33. Gasiorek J, Giles H. Communication, volunteering, and aging: a research agenda. Int J Commun-Us. 2013;7:2659–77.
34. Claxton-Oldfield S, Claxton-Oldfield J. The impact of volunteering in hospice palliative care. Am J Hosp Palliat Med. 2007;24(4):259–63.
35. Clary EG, Snyder M, Ridge RD, Copeland J, Stukas AA, Haugen J, Miene P. Understanding and assessing the motivations of volunteers: a functional approach. J Pers Soc Psychol. 1998;74(6):1516–30.
36. Clarke A, Sanders C, Seymour J, Gott M, Welton M. Evaluating a peer education program for advance end-of-life care planning for older adults: the peer educators' perspective. Int J Disabil Human Dev. 2009;8(1):33–41.
37. Seymour JE, Almack K, Kennedy S, Froggatt K. Peer education for advance care planning: volunteers' perspectives on training and community engagement activities. Health Expect. 2013;16(1):43–55.

13

How do professionals assess the quality of life of children with advanced cancer receiving palliative care, and what are their recommendations for improvement?

Josianne Avoine-Blondin[1,2], Véronique Parent[2], Léonor Fasse[3,4], Clémentine Lopez[4,5,7], Nago Humbert[1,6,8], Michel Duval[1,6,8] and Serge Sultan[1,6,8*] (iD)

Abstract

Background: It is known that information regarding the quality of life of a patient is central to pediatric palliative care. This information allows professionals to adapt the care and support provided to children and their families. Previous studies have documented the major areas to be investigated in order to assess the quality of life, although it is not yet known what operational criteria or piece of information should be used in the context of pediatric palliative care. The present study aims to: 1) Identify signs of quality of life and evaluation methods currently used by professionals to assess the quality of life of children with cancer receiving palliative care. 2) Collect recommendations from professionals to improve the evaluation of quality of life in this context.

Methods: We selected a qualitative research design and applied an inductive thematic content analysis to the verbal material. Participants included 20 members of the Department of Hematology-Oncology at CHU Sainte-Justine from various professions (e.g. physicians, nurses, psychosocial staff) who had cared for at least one child with cancer receiving palliative care in the last year.

Results: Professionals did not have access to pre-established criteria or to a defined procedure to assess the quality of life of children they followed in the context of PPC. They reported basing their assessment on the child's non-verbal cues, relational availability and elements of his/her environment. These cues are typically collected through observation, interpretation and by asking the child, his/her parents, and other members of the care. To improve the assessment of quality of life professionals recommended optimizing interdisciplinary communication, involving the child and the family in the evaluation process, increasing training to palliative care in hematology/oncology, and developing formalized measurement tools.

Conclusion: The formulation of explicit criteria to assess the quality of life in this context, along with detailed recommendations provided by professionals, support the development of systematic measurement strategy. Such a strategy would contribute to the development of common care goals and further facilitate communication between professionals and with the family.

Keywords: Pediatric palliative care, Quality of life, Measurement, Pediatric cancer, Qualitative study

* Correspondence: serge.sultan@umontreal.ca
[1]Centre de Psycho-Oncologie, CHU Sainte-Justine, Montréal, QC H3T 1C5, Canada
[6]Université de Montréal, Montréal, QC, Canada
Full list of author information is available at the end of the article

Background

Cancer is responsible for 20 to 30% of cases of children in palliative care [1–3]. Pediatric palliative care (PPC) consists of active and comprehensive care designed to prevent and alleviate suffering and improve the quality of life (QoL) of children and their families (e.g., [4–6]).

QoL is therefore at the heart of palliative care and is generally described as multidimensional and subjective [6, 7]. The physical, emotional and social aspects of QoL are the most frequently studied [8, 9]. In the specific context of PPC in oncology, recent studies of children with advanced cancer and their parents have revealed that the physical well-being of children is an inherent part of their QoL. Losses and symptoms caused by the disease on the child's overall functioning are of great importance in this respect (e.g., [10]). In addition, more and more studies have highlighted the positive components of QoL, such as maintaining a child's sense of normalcy and everyday pleasures (e.g., [11–14]). Importantly, spiritual dimensions have recently been studied in children and include such themes as maintaining hope and finding meaning in life (e.g., [11, 15]). In an earlier study on professionals who accompanied children in palliative care, we found unique positive dimensions to define the child's QoL such as having fun and focusing on the present moment, feeling valued and appreciated, maintaining a sense of control and feeling that life goes on [16].

In oncology, care is focused on both children's survival and on their overall comfort. Assessing QoL is thus particularly important as it contributes to therapeutic decisions and is useful in improving patients' overall care (e. g., [4, 17, 18]). Several measuring tools have been developed in recent decades to assess the QoL in pediatric oncology [19–21]. However, these strategies rely heavily on coding or reporting the presence or absence of symptoms or complaints [22]. These are usually scales where the child (self-reported version) or his/her parents (proxy version) are the primary respondents [23, 24], but because these tools are focused on periods of curative treatment, they miss important topics that are specific to children with PPC.

In fact, a systematic review of the literature was recently carried out to determine whether the existing measures of QoL could be applied to this population in palliative care. The results indicate that none of the existing measures in oncology would meet the criteria for adequate use in PPC [19]. The PedsQL 4.0 for instance, which is the most widely used tool for measuring QoL in oncology, has been shown to bear shortcomings for this population as a result of inappropriate items that do not take into account the physical limitations of children in palliative care [25]. Measures of QoL do not always incorporate a temporality that is fitting for PPC, where it is recommended to focus on shorter periods of time (e.g. daily assessment) to increase the evaluator's sensitivity to the variability of the child's status over time [16].

In summary, the current tools do not specifically assess the QoL of children with advanced cancer who receive PPC as they do for young patients during treatment or in after-care [19, 25–27]. It has been recommended by different authors that QoL measures be developed to reflect the reality of children with a life-threatening disease [19, 26]. A tool was recently developed on the basis of areas of QoL that had been identified previously [26], but the measure is lengthy (57–65 items per version).

Considering the central importance of QoL as a target in PPC, it is noteworthy that no adequate, accurate and valid instrument is available to date. Although we may expect that professionals use their own judgments to assess the QoL, we do not know what information they use in clinical practice or how they proceed to form an opinion about the QoL of a child. One strategy to address this issue is to obtain input from professionals who have experience with these children. We need to identify how professionals evaluate the QoL of children and what are their suggestions for improving this evaluation [28].

The aim of the study is to explore and describe how professionals evaluate the QoL of the children with advanced cancer receiving PPC and what they recommend to optimize the evaluation of QoL in this area. The specific objectives are 1) to identify which signs or cues and evaluation methods are used by professionals in hematology-oncology to evaluate the QoL of children with advanced cancer receiving PPC and 2) to collect recommendations of professionals to further optimize this evaluation.

Methods

The present study focuses on the second part of an interview taken by professionals in hematology-oncology as part of a study to define the domains of QoL in PPC [16]. The present study is based on an inductive qualitative research method within a descriptive constructivist epistemology [29, 30].

Participants

The participants were 20 health professionals: 3 hematologist-oncologists, 1 psychiatrist, 5 nursing staff members, 2 clinical fellows, 1 nutritionist, 1 art therapist, 1 psychologist, 3 occupational therapists, and 3 physiotherapists. All were selected on the basis of the following criteria: they had to be a member of the Department of Hematology-Oncology of our hospital, have cared for at least one child (≤ 18 years) with advanced cancer receiving PPC, and speak French.

Recruitment

The study received ethical approval from the CHU Sainte-Justine Research Ethics Committee (3547) and the University of Sherbrooke Research Ethics Committee (2013–1245). Data were collected by using maximum variation sampling recruitment strategy from professionals with diverse roles [31]. The selection of participants was based on the comprehensive list of members of the department ($N = 103$). To include different professions and avoid bias of a priori selection, a random selection was made each week to select three professionals across three different professions (physicians, nurses, other professionals). A total of 28 professionals were contacted, among whom 2 participated to a pre-test to refine interview strategies. Among the remaining 26, 23 met the inclusion criteria and 3 refused to participate (participation rate: 20/23 87% for the present analysis). The recruitment was stopped when saturation was attained across these three groups of professions. Written informed consent was collected from the participants during the initial interview. The recruitment and the interviews with participants were conducted by the first author (JAB).

Data collection

Data collection took place from March 7, 2013 to April 2014. Individual semi-structured interviews (average duration of 1 h) were performed to collect data. The interview guide developed by the research team was inspired by Hinds et al. (2004) (see Additional file 1). The present analysis focuses on verbal material collected in response to questions specifically aimed at signs and evaluation methods used by the professionals to assess the QoL of the children in the context of PPC, and the professionals' recommendations to optimize this assessment. Participants also completed a brief sociodemographic questionnaire. The interviews were audio recorded and transcribed for data processing.

Data analysis

Data were analyzed inductively according to the thematic analysis approach [29, 30]. As outlined in the first report [16], data were analyzed according continual thematization process and a thematization journal were used. That way, each transcript was coded according to the two aims of the present study (aim 1: signs and evaluation approaches of QoL; aim 2: recommendations to optimize the QoL assessment). Two lists of codes were made and the process of code comparison was performed for each of these lists. The first themes were created with the aim of maintaining a low level of inference in order to respect the participants' statements as much as possible. Thematic clusters have thus gradually taken shape and highlighted signs and evaluation methods mentioned by the professionals on the one

hand (aim 1) as well as their recommendations to optimize the assessment of QoL (aim 2) on the other. A synthetic and structured representation of each of the thematic clusters was then constructed according to the two aims of the study. The analysis was carried out by hand using Word to allow greater flexibility in the analysis process. The saturation of data was attainted.

Various recommended methodological strategies were employed during the analysis [32, 33] including the systematic use of reflexive journal, triangulation, discussions and exchanges among researchers and feedback meetings with members of the hematology-oncology department. Also, by using a bottom-up process to identify the themes - which helped include comprehensive categories with higher levels of inference - we were able to ensure better validity of the results, as the emphasis from the outset was placed on the participants' responses rather than on a simple classification.

Results

The results highlight that professionals involved in this study do not have access to pre-established criteria or to a defined procedure that they can rely on. They were rather guided by their observations and clinical judgment.

Aim 1. Description of signs and evaluation methods used by professionals to assess the QoL of the children with advanced cancer receiving PPC.

Thematic analysis produced three themes for signs that inform the professionals about the QoL: (1) non-verbal cues and the relational availability of the child; (2) indicators specific to domains of QoL; and (3) indicators specific to the child's life context.

Non-verbal cues and the relational availability of the child

Non-verbal cues and those linked to the child's relational availability allow professionals to form a basic idea of the child's current overall state. Table 1 presents examples of non-verbal cues and relational availability reported by participants.

" [...] she was suffering and you could tell by the way she was breathing and by the position of her body, in her shoulders, her arms, the fact that she was curled up, the fact that she was tense, that her face was stiff, her breathing more superficial." P11.

" I saw her smile and happy from our exchange, and she made me a little heart [on a paper], you know, she wanted to show that she was happy to feel connected. [...] Otherwise, when she was not doing so well, there was no connection or empathy that could be felt or shared." P4.

Table 1 Examples of non-verbal cues and relational availability to observe the quality of life

Positive	Negative
· Smiles	· Absent gaze
· Laughs	· Avoids eye contact
· Better eye contact	· Frowns
· Bright-eyed	· Body tension and restless breathing
· Relaxed facial features	· Has difficulty calming down
· Relaxed body and breathing rhythm	· Is agitated, screams, cries
· Is awake for longer periods of time	· Self-mutilation
· Responds more to questions	· Is closed off
· Accepts and participates more in care	· Is curled up in bed
· Chats more and shows a desire to interact with the environment	· Appears discouraged
· Is more involved in activities	· Responds to questions sparingly or not at all
· Engages in his/her occupations and plays	· Refuses to see professionals and to receive care
	· Diminished relational availability
	· Irritability
	· Sleeps most of the time

Indicators specific to domains of QoL

QoL is also considered to be the result of an evaluation involving different spheres of the child's life. Professionals refer to previously identified areas in an operationalized way: Physical comfort, Psychological alleviation, Fun and the present moment, Sense of control, Feeling that life goes on, and Meaningful social relationships [16]. For example, in "Fun and the present moment", games are an essential criterion. Additional file 2 includes examples of signs associated with each of the dimensions of QoL.

" We'll split up [the evaluation of QoL]: "Well, there is pain relief, is he okay? Yes perfect. Nutrition? Yes perfect... Does she play? Does she have fun?" In the end, it all revolves around their QoL" P20.

Indicators specific to the child's life context

Finally, most participants also mentioned taking into account signs related to the living context of the child and his/her family. These elements help professionals give meaning to other perceived signs that have been detected in the areas of QoL. The sub-themes of this theme are the individual characteristics of the child, his or her medical and care history, family dynamics, and the characteristics of his or her living environment. These aspects of the child's environment helps contextualize and better understand the child's QoL. Additional file 3 includes description and examples of indicators specific to the child's life context.

Interestingly, part of the professionals' responses focused not only on the signs themselves but on ways of accessing the signs of QoL. Subsequent to the coding work, we classified these evaluation methods into 4 themes: (1) Observation; (2) Direct investigation; (3) Interpretation; and (4) The use of diverse informants.

Observation

All participants referred to the observation approach, which allows professionals to identify non-verbal cues, the child's relational availability, his or her life habits, the presence of visible symptoms or lack thereof, and contextual aspects such as the characteristics of the child's physical environment. The observation examples reported by participants help describe this approach as a process of intentional attention directed towards the child's and family's discourses and daily non-verbal cues.

" I remember once he had celebrated his birthday and when he would talk about it, he was all smiles and, you know, he'd often be more tired and have more difficulty speaking, but when he spoke of events that had made him happy like that, it wasn't even a big activity, really, but he had truly had fun. He would talk about it and smile [...] his eyes would light up." P16.

Direct investigation

Most professionals explained that they also gather information about the child's QoL by asking the child, parents or professionals simple and direct questions. Professionals also refer to their notes and reports on file, as well as tools to assess specific areas of QoL such as physical well-being through pain assessments.

"[...] we would ask him: "Are you in pain?", he was able to answer. So we could have that information [...] he couldn't elaborate on it, but...Simple questions, you know: "Are you hungry? Are you in pain?", he could say yes or no." P1.

Direct investigation is an evaluation method that allows professionals to validate their first clinical impressions based on their observations and to deepen and validate their understanding of the child's well-being and that of those around him/her.

Interpretation

Professionals also described the use of two types of interpretation: interpretation based on self and interpretation based on other. Interpretation in this context is a process through which professionals estimate QoL from a preliminary gathering of cues via observation or direct investigation.

Interpretation based on self
This sub-theme describes the appraisal of the child's QoL based on the professional's own points of reference and understanding. It consists of a normative judgment on the QoL of the child treated with PPC.

" I think that, sometimes, health professionals are misguided to speak, to qualify a good or bad quality of life because for them, it would not be a good quality of life." P14.

Interpretation based on other
In contrast, it is an approach that encourages imagining the child's perspective, putting oneself in his or her place to understand and anticipate his or her own subjective QoL. This process comes from an intentional openness to understanding how the other may feel. Participants mentioned this form of interpretation mainly in cases where direct communication with the child was restricted.

" I try and imagine the child's perspective... What brings them joy, but are no longer able to do, well I imagine that it has a big effect on their quality of life." (P5).

The use of diverse informants
The analysis of the participants' responses highlights that most of the professionals have used the perspective of several informants to document the QoL of the child they cared for. This process allowed them to collect richer and complementary information on the child's QoL.

"[...] when we carry out an evaluation, we look for as much information as possible, but from different people. That means, we'll seek out the perspective of the medical team, of the parents, and if we can ask the child, we'll question the child." P1.

From this perspective, all participants mentioned the specific and individual nature of each child's QoL and several insisted that the best informant is first and foremost the child him/herself. Great importance is also attributed to the opinion of the parents, who often provide a glimpse into the child's inner world. Indeed, their perspective is deemed essential, especially when communication with the child is hampered by a disability or restricted because of his or her young age. Furthermore, the evaluation of QoL is reported to be more precise and accurate when the opinions of other professionals involved with the child's care are collected.

In short, the content of the participants' responses indicates that in clinical practice there is actually no planned and systematized evaluation of QoL. The approach is rather left to the professional's discretion. Figure 1 illustrates

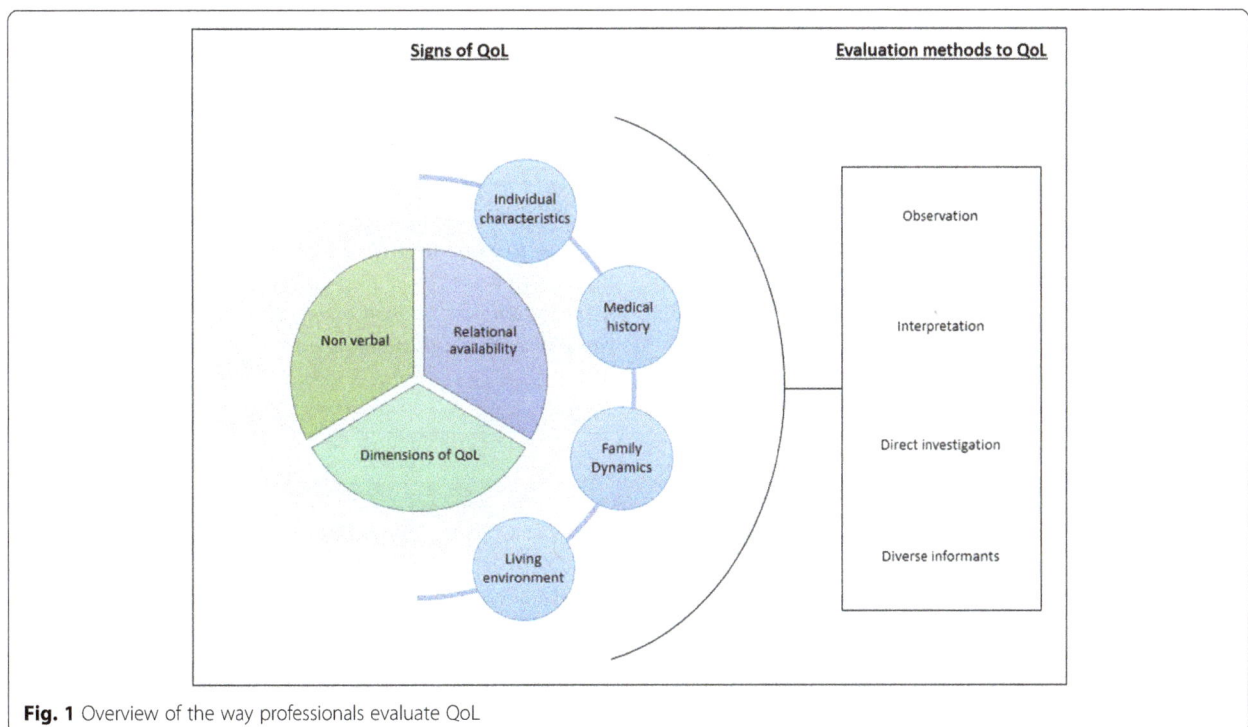

Fig. 1 Overview of the way professionals evaluate QoL

an overview of the signs and ways used by professionals to assess the QoL of children they care for. This underlines that children's QoL evaluation is complex and requires a combination of indicators, as well as a multi-source strategy to allow professionals to form an overall picture of QoL.

Aim 2. Recommendations of professionals to further optimize the evaluation of QoL.

In this part of the interview, the health professionals mentioned several tips to improve the assessment of QoL. These tips are summarized in 4 themes: (1) promote communication among members of the health care team; (2) focus the assessment on the child's needs, the family, and involve them in the assessment process; (3) use of a formal tool to assess the QoL; (4) develop training that is specific to PPC in oncology. Table 2 summarizes the recommendations resulting from the analysis of the content of the participants' responses.

Promote communication among members of the health care team

The professionals suggested that team meetings be held frequently and that the team put together a compilation of key information for the meaningful use of professionals. The involvement of the PPC team is also mentioned as a factor that is conducive to communication, as it helps refocus aims and establish new points of action. It was also recommended that specific moments of exchanges take place, beyond simply discussing file notes.

" What's important is that everyone, even if we have our own perspective, that we manage to put it all together. So even if we do it individually and don't look at the same aspects, in the end, it's helpful because we will not forget the different aspects, but we have to make sure to bring back all these aspects to the team to focus on what the priority should be and ensure that no aspect has been forgotten." P20.

Focus the assessment on the child's needs, the family, and involve them in the assessment process

The involvement of the patient and his or her family, both at the time of the assessment of QoL and in the multidisciplinary meetings, has also been described as a lever that helps create the assessment according to the families' needs, while ensuring the validity of the assessment.

" [...] we need to focus on the family's needs. I may not agree with what the family or what my colleague would like for that child, but if the family says: "This is our priority." Well, that's what we need to focus on. [...] Because if you just come in and say this is how we're going to do things, but that it does not meet their needs, we'd be doing all that for nothing. So even if that's not what we would have prioritized, if the family says: "This is what I want to prioritize.", well that's what we have to do." P20.

Use of a formal tool to assess the QoL

Professionals spontaneously mentioned the value of using an assessment tool that is specific to measuring the QoL of children with PPC, although none had ever used a formal tool or procedure in this context before.

" [...] I think that right now, everyone is sort of using their intuition. And, we don't really have any markers. You go with your intuition and according to the needs you see. [...] we don't have any tools...It's really very intuitive..." P18.

The use of such a tool would provide a common reference point to facilitate communication between patients and professionals, and among professionals of different professions in order to promote agreement and communication.

" I think that it's an aspect that isn't developed enough... it should be part of the basic stuff, just as important as a pain assessment. Relying on something that's already out there or to come up with a new standardized test...so as to be able to quantify it and so that everyone agrees on the same system, on the same way of doing things to go in the same direction and perhaps improve his or her QoL." P2.

Table 2 Professionals recommendations to improve the assessment of QoL

Recommendations	Sub-themes
Promote communication among members of the health care team	· Hold multidisciplinary meetings · Communicate beyond the notes on file · Collect the opinions of a meaningful professional · Involve the palliative care team
Focus the assessment on the child's needs, the family, and involve them in the assessment process	· Be attentive to the needs and desires of the family · Involve them in the assessment process
Use of a formal tool to assess the QoL	· Use standardized tools in the assessment of the dimensions of QoL · Create a formal measure of QoL in PPC in oncology
Develop training that is specific to PPC in oncology	· Become familiar with the context of PPC in oncology through training

Develop training that is specific to PPC in oncology
The use of training that is specific to palliative care and to children with terminal cancer or who are not responding to treatment is a way for professionals to be better informed on the context, its challenges, alternative interventions, and approaches that should be favored in these difficult clinical situations. Indeed, this deeper awareness would help them better understand, evaluate, and improve the QoL of the children and their families.

" I think it needs to be improved perhaps by doing a little more staff training, because I really find that there isn't a lot of training. And as for the health professionals, we are not necessarily certified. [...] it is currently something that is needed, but that we do not have." (P9).

Discussion

This study focuses on signs and evaluation methods of the QoL of children with advanced cancer as reported by professionals, and their recommendations to improve the assessment of QoL. Following the interviews, which we analyzed inductively using a qualitative method, we created a descriptive model that reveals the difficulty of this evaluation in current practices. Our results particularly highlight the importance of collaborative work among the multidisciplinary team members and the need for sharing and collaborating with the children and their family.

Main findings
Signs and evaluation methods to assess the QoL
Based on our findings, the professionals involved in this study do not have access to pre-established criteria or to a defined procedure that they can rely on to assess the QoL of the children they follow in PPC. They are rather guided by their observations and clinical judgment.

With respect to the signs they mentioned, we can draw a parallel within the main areas of QoL (physical, psychological and social) [8, 9]. For example, professionals refer to factors such as pain levels, emotional distress, and whether the child has a supportive network. However, unlike items that are usually listed in the currently available measures of QoL, which are generally focused on deficits [22, 23], professionals reported indicators of QoL that focus on joyful moments, on anchoring oneself in the present moment, and on the pursuit of small daily accomplishments. The emphasis here is on the child's current opportunities, in addition to his or her limitations. The spiritual component of quality of life was not explicitly flagged as an indicator by professionals in the current research. However, the professionals referred to the importance of children feeling that life goes on. A parallel can be drawn between this theme represented by indicators such as the sense of normality

and achievement and those of maintaining hope and finding meaning in life which have been found to characterize the spiritual domain of QoL (e.g., [11, 15]). Importantly, to tap these domains, professionals rely on the collection of non-verbal, relational and contextual cues. This highlights the fact that information sources are varied and should be crosschecked or challenged in order to obtain a picture as complete and reliable as possible of the child's QoL. Furthermore, the level of QoL should be adjusted according to the context, especially when the child is very sick and suffering from severe limitations. The level of QoL should in fact be considered by taking into account the individuality of the child, his or her trajectory of care and the environmental context. The need to take these contextual elements into account makes it indeed difficult to rely on a simple approach through direct assessment that only focus on the traditional dimensions of QoL (e. g., [21, 34, 35]).

The fact that no formal measure is available or used to assess the QoL in PPC leads professionals to adapt to the child's needs according to the priorities they each perceive individually. This can lead to disagreements between different professionals regarding the QoL of a child, as the sharing of relevant information is difficult. This is reflected by the stress put by participants on communication issues. This can be problematic in an interdisciplinary work context where common goals are at the heart of the intervention. These aspects further highlight the importance of communication within teams so that individual perceptions can be shared and disparities identified and resolved [36]. As in assessing pain and emotional distress, the introduction of a formal assessment of QoL - which remains to be developed - could provide a framework for practice that promotes better communication among professionals and with the family [37].

There is a wide variety of information sources that could be used to judge the QoL according to professionals. Yet, having a variety of informants could make it difficult to identify which person should be consulted in order to evaluate the child's QoL (the "best informant") [9, 38, 39], although professionals insist that the child is the best suited to define his/her QoL and that a parent's perspective is essential when communication with the child is impeded. This point of view is consistent with the current assessment procedures in pediatric oncology (e.g., [21, 34, 35]). Importantly, the analysis of the participants' responses emphasizes the importance of their role as informants. This finding provides a new perspective on how to evaluate the QoL by showing that the diversity of their role, as well as the experience professionals acquire with the families, offer a theoretical and complementary understanding to that of the child and his/her family.

Professionals' recommendations to improve the assessment of QoL

In the context of PPC, care must be coordinated among the various parties involved with the child and his/her family to enable personalized care for the child [4]. In line with this principle, communication within the multidisciplinary team is at the forefront of the improvement areas mentioned [36]. Professionals consider that communication within the health care team is essential in order to reach an agreement regarding the child's QoL, beyond the notes that are on file. This recommendation is consistent with the acknowledged principle that interprofessional collaboration allows for the identification of shared areas across different fields, while narrowing the gap in perceptions among team members. Thus, considering that professionals from diverse professions tend to focus their approach on different areas of QoL, holding interdisciplinary meetings is a way of gaining a more complete and shared understanding of the child's QoL. It also helps ensure the coherence of the content of their conversations when discussing care objectives with families [4, 36].

Another recommendation that professionals brought forth is to better include the child and his/her family in order to adequately reflect their needs. This recommendation is consistent with the philosophy of patient-centered care [40], where communication with the child and his/her family allows professionals to better anticipate their actions and to consider the child's and family's values and preferences [4, 41]. It is also a way of limiting attribution biases by professionals and ensuring that individualized assessment are carried out, beyond normative criteria alone [18].

Professionals also recommend receiving training that is specific to PPC. Indeed, it is recognized that the appropriate response to the needs of children in PPC and that of their families requires particular knowledge, skills and techniques [42, 43]. The benefits of receiving training about PPC for health care professionals has been demonstrated [44, 45]. For example, the results of a pre-test post-test study conducted with 50 pediatric clinicians who received training about PPC indicated that following training, participants reported increased confidence levels with respect to their knowledge, skills, and emotional support that they provide to children and their families [45]. It is therefore very likely that PPC-specific training allows professionals to better understand the specific reality of children with advanced cancer, thus ensuring a more accurate assessment of their QoL [44, 45].

Finally, professionals of the present study highlighted the value of creating a measurement tool for QoL that would be adapted to children receiving PPC. This would allow the assessment to be more systematized and objective, as it is currently based on the professionals' relational skills and observations. Several advantages have previously been associated with the use of tools for measuring the QoL of children with cancer: it helps with the sharing of information among team members, improves communication with the child and the family, ensures that more needs are met, and simplifies the recording of data relevant to the child's file [7, 18]. Recent initiatives have developed new strategies [26, 27]. While significant problems of feasibility and recruitment remain, this course of action is nevertheless promising and responds to a current need in the field. Evaluation strategies to be developed should tap the main domains identified in recent research [16].

Strengths and limitations

The limitations of this study mainly concern the sample's composition. 1) This study focused on the signs used by professionals to explore the QoL of children with cancer receiving PPC. The descriptive model therefore does not take into account the points of view of the children and families on QoL. However, it is informative to document professional practices. It should also be noted that the sample comprised professionals working in hematology-oncology, which excludes other clinical contexts that refer to palliative care (e.g., neonatology). 2) The distribution of our sample is also not representative of health care staff in oncology, despite the fact that we tried to include diverse occupations. Indeed, the proportion of physicians is higher than that of nurses. However, it has unlikely led to biases in the presence of certain codes or themes because the data saturation was attained across groups of professions (physicians, nurses, other professionals). 3) As in any qualitative research, self-confirmation bias cannot be ruled out. In order to prevent this problem from occurring, we intentionally used a very open collection procedure as well as methodological safeguards, including the strict upkeep of a journal and the triangulation of the research supervision.

Implications

The present research allows us to discuss the discrepancies between current effective practices and desirable practices as mentioned by professionals. The results of this study therefore suggest the development of a personalized and more systematic evaluation of QoL. We foresee three major implications of the present findings.

First, it is undoubtedly necessary to use several information sources, including child and parents, and signs from different modalities (speech, observation, etc.) to evaluate QoL in the context of PPC, thus approaching a multi-method evaluation that is anchored in the history and current trajectory of the disease.

Second, the assessment must put the child's feelings first and not solely rest on pre-established standards of QoL. An important notion that arises from the present findings is that of the standards or reference levels which the professionals take to compare the actual status of the child. Participants tended to, on the one hand, situate the child's overall QoL according to signs they collect and, on the other hand, to compare this picture to the child's previous and anticipated state with respect to his/her disease. The consequence of this observation is that the approach to assess the QoL in this context should be particularly sensitive to change, for example by focusing on a short temporal perspective such as a day, which is consistent with palliative care practices used with adults [46]. This is coherent with the recommendations of PPC standards, according to which the needs of the child and family evolve through the different stages of the disease. Thus, the assessment of needs should be a continuous, repeated process that occurs on a regular basis according to the evolution of the child's condition [1, 4]. Feasibility and burden are core criteria for a further assessment strategy in this context.

Third, as much of the criteria used are derived from the clinical observations or judgment of professionals, they can be interpreted differently depending on the professional. This result should guide researchers towards an assessment that is validated by the child's and family's perceptions and by different professionals to avoid attribution bias. A proposed solution is to develop simple assessments that would allow sharing information on the central themes of QoL [16, 47].

Conclusion

The results of this qualitative study with 20 professionals in a hematology-oncology department indicate that the assessment of QoL in PPC is currently not formalized and mainly calls for the individual judgment of professionals. Participants reported that the lack of planned or systematized procedures in regard to QoL in their care practices may lead to disagreements on the QoL of the same child in the same situation. To address these issues, professionals recommend interdisciplinary communication, involving the child and his/her family in the assessment process, developing training specific to PPC, and stress the need to create a tool to measure the QoL of children in the context of PPC specifically. Future studies should thus confirm the signs and cues to evaluate the QoL with patients and families, develop a simple and usable tool to assess the QoL. This will allow the sharing of information among professionals, child and family members on the domains relevant to the context of PPC.

Additional files

Additional file 1: Interview Questions. Interview Questions. (PDF 15 kb)

Additional file 2: Signs associated with the dimensions of QoL from the perspective of professionals in hematology-oncology. (PDF 17 kb)

Additional file 3: Description of indicators specific to child's life context. Description of indicators specific to child's life context. (PDF 16 kb)

Abbreviations
PPC: Pediatric palliative care; QoL: Quality of Life

Acknowledgments
The authors are grateful to the Coast-to-Coast Foundation (Canada) for financially supporting this study. Additional funding came from the Sainte-Justine UHC Foundation to the Center of Psycho-Oncology (Dr. Sultan, Montréal, Canada). We thank Gabrielle Ciquier who translated the manuscript into English. We are indebted to the members of the Hematology/Oncology department of the CHU Sainte-Justine (Montréal) who kindly accepted to share their experience and views.

Funding
Funding came from the Sainte-Justine UHC Foundation to the Center of Psycho-Oncology (Dr. Sultan, Montréal, Canada) and from Coast-to-Coast Foundation (Canada) for financially supporting this study.

Authors' contributions
JAB was the primary contributor. She designed the study, collected and analyzed the data and wrote the manuscript. VP co-supervised the project, helped analyze the data and co-wrote the manuscript. LF helped devise the study, interpret the data, and corrected the final manuscript. CL helped devise the study, interpret the data, and corrected the final manuscript. NH helped devise the study and collect the data. MD helped devise the study, collect the data and corrected the final manuscript. SS was the senior author. He secured financial support, co-designed the study, helped collect and interpret the data, and co-wrote the manuscript. All authors read and approved the final manuscript.

Competing interests
The authors declare that they have no competing interests.

Author details
¹Centre de Psycho-Oncologie, CHU Sainte-Justine, Montréal, QC H3T 1C5, Canada. ²Department of Psychology, Université de Sherbrooke, 150, Place Charles-Le Moyne #200, Longueuil, Québec J4K 0A8, Canada. ³Department of Psychology, Université de Bourgogne Franche-Comté, Esplanade Erasme, 21000 Dijon, France. ⁴Hôpital Gustave Roussy, Villejuif, France. ⁵Université Paris Descartes, Paris, France. ⁶Université de Montréal, Montréal, QC, Canada. ⁷Department of child psychiatry, Gustave Roussy, 114, rue Édouard-Vaillant, 94805 Villejuif, France. ⁸Department of Hematology/Oncology, CHU Sainte-Justine, 3175, Chemin de la Côte-Sainte-Catherine, Montréal, Québec H3T 1C5, Canada.

References

1. Children. ETfPCi. Palliative Care for Infants, Children and Young People: The Facts. 2009 [Available from: http://www.fondazionemaruzza.org/wp/wp-content/uploads/2016/10/fatti-eng.pdf. Accessed 17 May 2017.
2. Feudtner C, Kang TI, Hexem KR, Friedrichsdorf SJ, Osenga K, Siden H, et al. Pediatric palliative care patients: a prospective multicenter cohort study. Pediatrics. 2011:1094–101.
3. Widger K, Davies D, Drouin DJ, Beaune L, Daoust L, Farran RP, et al. Pediatric patients receiving palliative care in Canada: results of a multicenter review. Arch Pediatr Adolesc Med. 2007;161(6):597–602.
4. Canadian Hospice Palliative Care Association. Pediatric Hospice Palliative Care: Guiding Principles and Norms of Practice. 2006 [Available from:http://www.chpca.net/media/7841/Pediatric_Norms_of_Practice_March_31_2006_English.pdf. Accessed 8 May 2017.
5. Pui C-H, Gajjar AJ, Kane JR, Qaddoumi IA, Pappo AS. Challenging issues in pediatric oncology. Nat Rev Clin Oncol. 2011;8(9):540–9.
6. Organization. WH. WHO Definition of palliative care for children. 2013 [Available from: http://www.who.int/cancer/palliative/definition/en/. Accessed 24 Apr 2017.
7. Hinds PS, Burghen EA, Haase JE, Phillips CR. Advances in defining, conceptualizing, and measuring quality of life in pediatric patients with cancer. Oncol Nurs Forum. 2006;33(1):23–9.
8. Anthony SJ, Selkirk E, Sung L, Klaassen RJ, Dix D, Scheinemann K, et al. Considering quality of life for children with cancer: a systematic review of patient-reported outcome measures and the development of a conceptual model. Qual Life Res. 2014;23(3):771–89.
9. Pépin A-J, Carret A-S, Sultan S. Quality of life. In: Schneinemann K, Bouffet E, editors. Pediatric neuro-oncology. New York: Springer Science; 2015. p. 277–88.
10. Tomlinson D, Hinds PS, Bartels U, Hendershot E, Sung L. Parent reports of quality of life for pediatric patients with cancer with no realistic chance of cure. J Clin Oncol. 2011;29(6):639–45.
11. Barrera M, D'Agostino N, Gammon J, Spencer L, Baruchel S. Health-related quality of life and enrollment in phase 1 trials in children with incurable cancer. Palliat Support Care. 2005;3(3):191–6.
12. Friedrichsdorf SJ, Postier A, Dreyfus J, Osenga K, Sencer S, Wolfe J. Improved quality of life at end of life related to home-based palliative care in children with cancer. J Palliat Med. 2015;18(2):143–50.
13. Hechler T, Blankenburg M, Friedrichsdorf S, Garske D, Hübner B, Menke A, et al. Parents' perspective on symptoms, quality of life, characteristics of death and end-of-life decisions for children dying from cancer. Klinische Padiatrie. 2008;220(03):166–74.
14. Von Lützau P, Otto M, Hechler T, Metzing S, Wolfe J, Zernikow B. Children dying from cancer: parents' perspectives on symptoms, quality of life, characteristics of death, and end-of-life decisions. J Palliat Care. 2012;28(4):274–81.
15. Kamper R, Van Cleve L, Savedra M. Children with advanced cancer: responses to a spiritual quality of life interview. J Spec Pediatr Nurs. 2010;15(4):301–6.
16. Avoine-Blondin J, Parent V, Lahaye M, Humbert N, Duval M, Sultan S. Identifying domains of quality of life in children with cancer undergoing palliative care: a qualitative study with professionals. Palliat Support Care. 2017;15(5):565–74.
17. Aslakson RA, Dy SM, Wilson RF, Waldfogel J, Zhang A, Isenberg SR, et al. Patient- and caregiver-reported assessment tools for palliative care: summary of the 2017 Agency for Healthcare Research and Quality technical brief. J Pain Symptom Manag. 2017;54:961.
18. Rosenberg AR, Wolfe J. Approaching the third decade of paediatric palliative oncology investigation: historical progress and future directions. Lancet Child Adolesc Health. 2017;1(1):56–67.
19. Coombes LH, Wiseman T, Lucas G, Sangha A, Murtagh FE. Health-related quality-of-life outcome measures in paediatric palliative care: a systematic review of psychometric properties and feasibility of use. Palliat Med. 2016; 30(10):935–49.
20. Eiser C, Morse R. Quality-of-life measures in chronic diseases of childhood. Health Technol Assess. 2001;5(4):1–157.
21. Varni JW, Limbers CA, Burwinkle TM. Impaired health-related quality of life in children and adolescents with chronic conditions: a comparative analysis of 10 disease clusters and 33 disease categories/severities utilizing the PedsQL™ 4.0 generic Core scales. Health Qual Life Outcomes. 2007;5(43):1–15.
22. Davis E, Waters E, Mackinnon A, Reddihough D, Graham HK, Mehmet-Radji O, et al. Paediatric quality of life instruments: a review of the impact of the conceptual framework on outcomes. Dev Med Child Neurol. 2006;48(4):311–8.
23. Cremeens J, Eiser C, Blades M. Characteristics of health-related self-report measures for children aged three to eight years: a review of the literature. Qual Life Res. 2006;15(4):739–54.
24. Hudson BF, Oostendorp LJ, Candy B, Vickerstaff V, Jones L, Lakhanpaul M, et al. The under reporting of recruitment strategies in research with children with life-threatening illnesses: a systematic review. Palliat Med. 2017;31(5):419–36.
25. Huang I-C, Shenkman EA, Madden VL, Vadaparampil S, Quinn G, Knapp CA. Measuring quality of life in pediatric palliative care: challenges and potential solutions. Palliat Med. 2010;24(2):175–82.
26. Cataudella D, Morley TE, Nesin A, Fernandez CV, Johnston DL, Sung L, et al. Development of a quality of life instrument for children with advanced cancer: the pediatric advanced care quality of life scale (PAC-QoL). Pediatr Blood Cancer. 2014;61(10):1840–5.
27. Morley TE, Cataudella D, Fernandez CV, Sung L, Johnston DL, Nesin A, et al. Development of the pediatric advanced care quality of life scale (PAC-QoL): evaluating comprehension of items and response options. Pediatr Blood Cancer. 2014;61(10):1835–9.
28. Krakowski I, Chardot C, Bey P, Guillemin F, Philip T. Coordinated organization of symptoms management and support in all the stages of cancer disease: putting in place pluridisciplinary structures of supportive oncological care. Bull Cancer. 2001;88(3):321–8.
29. Braun V, Clarke V. Using thematic analysis in psychology. Qual Res Psychol. 2006;3(2):77–101.
30. Paillé P, Mucchielli A. L'analyse qualitative en sciences humaines et sociales. 3rd ed. Paris: Armand Colin; 2012.
31. Patton MQ. Qualitative evaluation and research methods. 3rd ed. London: SAGE Publications, inc; 2002.
32. Mays N, Pope C. Qualitative research in health care: assessing quality in qualitative research. BMJ. 2000;320(7226):50–2.
33. Whittemore R, Chase SK, Mandle CL. Validity in qualitative research. Qual Health Res. 2001;11(4):522–37.
34. Collins JJ, Byrnes ME, Dunkel IJ, Lapin J, Nadel T, Thaler HT, et al. The measurement of symptoms in children with cancer. J Pain Symptom Manag. 2000;19(5):363–77.
35. Goodwin DA, Boggs SR, Graham-Pole J. Development and validation of the pediatric oncology quality of life scale. Psychol Assess. 1994;6(4):321.
36. Wilson E, Seymour J. The importance of interdisciplinary communication in the process of anticipatory prescribing. Int J Palliat Nurs. 2017;23(3):129–35.
37. Dabrowski M, Boucher K, Ward JH, Lovell MM, Sandre A, Bloch J, et al. Clinical experience with the NCCN distress thermometer in breast cancer patients. J Natl Compr Cancer Netw. 2007;5(1):104–11.
38. Eiser C, Varni JW. Health-related quality of life and symptom reporting: similarities and differences between children and their parents. Eur J Pediatr. 2013;172(10):1299–304.
39. Jozefiak T. Can we trust in parents' report about their childrens well-being? In: Ben-Arieh A, Casas F, Frones I, Korbin JE, editors. Handbook of child well-being theories, methods and policies in global perspective. Dortmund: Springer; 2014. p. 577–8.
40. Baker A. Crossing the quality chasm: a new health system for the 21st century. BMJ: British Medical Journal. 2001;323(7322):1192.
41. Hays RM, Valentine J, Haynes G, Geyer JR, Villareale N, Mckinstry B, et al. The Seattle pediatric palliative care project: effects on family satisfaction and health-related quality of life. J Palliat Med. 2006;9(3):716–28.
42. American Academy of Pediatrics Committee on Bioethics and Committee on Hospital Care for Children. Palliative Care for Children. Pediatrics. 2000;106(2):351–7.
43. Liben S, Papadatou D, Wolfe J. Paediatric palliative care: challenges and emerging ideas. Lancet. 2008;371(9615):852–64.
44. Barnes K. Staff stress in the children's hospice: causes, effects and coping strategies. Int J Palliat Nurs. 2001;7(5):248–54.
45. Peng N-H, Lee C-H, Lee M-C, Huang L-C, Chang Y-C, DeSwarte-Wallace J. Effectiveness of pediatric palliative care education on pediatric clinicians. West J Nurs Res. 2017;39(12):1624–38.

14

Community readiness and momentum: identifying and including community-driven variables in a mixed-method rural palliative care service siting model

V. A. Crooks[1*], M. Giesbrecht[1], H. Castleden[2], N. Schuurman[1], M. Skinner[3] and A. Williams[4]

Abstract

Background: Health service administrators make decisions regarding how to best use limited resources to have the most significant impact. Service siting models are tools that can help in this capacity. Here we build on our own mixed-method service siting model focused on identifying rural Canadian communities most in need of and ready for palliative care service enhancement through incorporating new community-driven insights.

Methods: We conducted 40 semi-structured interviews with formal and informal palliative care providers from four purposefully selected rural communities across Canada. Communities were selected by running our siting model, which incorporated GIS methods, and then identifying locations suitable as qualitative case studies. Participants were identified using multiple recruitment methods. Interviews were transcribed verbatim and the transcripts were reviewed to identify emerging themes and were coded accordingly. Thematic analysis then ensued.

Results: We previously introduced the inclusion of a 'community readiness' arm in the siting model. This arm is based on five community-driven indicators of palliative care service enhancement readiness and need. The findings from the current analysis underscore the importance of this arm of the model. However, the data also revealed the need to subjectively assess the presence or absence of community awareness and momentum indicators. The interviews point to factors such as educational tools, volunteers, and local acknowledgement of palliative care priorities as reflecting the presence of community awareness and factors such as new employment and volunteer positions, new care spaces, and new projects and programs as reflecting momentum. The diversity of factors found to illustrate these indicators between our pilot study and current national study demonstrate the need for those using our service siting model to look for contextually-relevant signs of their presence.

Conclusion: Although the science behind siting model development is established, few researchers have developed such models in an open way (e.g., documenting every stage of model development, engaging with community members). This mixed-method study has addressed this notable knowledge gap. While we have focused on rural palliative care in Canada, the process by which we have developed and refined our siting model is transferrable and can be applied to address other siting problems.

Keywords: Palliative care, Canada, Rural, Community, Service siting

---

* Correspondence: crooks@sfu.ca
[1]Department of Geography, Simon Fraser University, 8888 University Drive, Burnaby, BC V5A 1S6, Canada
Full list of author information is available at the end of the article

Background

Reflecting a demographic trend witnessed across much of the Global North, Canada is experiencing rapid population aging. According to our last national census, an estimated five million Canadians were 65 years of age or older and this number is expected to double in the next 25 years, reaching over ten million by 2036 [1]. By 2051, about one in four Canadians will be over the age of 65 [1]. This rate of aging, however, is not uniform across the country. Geographically, it is Canada's rural communities that are experiencing the most rapid rates of aging when compared to their urban counterparts [2]. This is largely due to local rural residents 'aging in place', but also to senior in-migration that is occurring in 16% of Canadian rural communities due to factors such as affordability and lifestyle [2, 3]. This rapidly aging rural population is a timely concern with regard to the provision and receipt of palliative care as those aged 65 years and over account for over 75% of the total deaths in Canada each year [4]. Thus, a fast-approaching reality is that health service providers in rural Canadian communities are facing heightened demand for palliative care provision while simultaneously coping with shrinking budgets and in many cases health care restructuring that is affecting service provision [5, 6].

Recognition of the impending growing demand for palliative care has gained attention by provincial, territorial, and municipal governments across Canada [7, 8]. For example, it has been recognized that Canada is facing a scarcity of such services with the gap between demand and service availability continuously expanding [9–12]. Despite this attention, little consideration has been given to the differential geographic, resource, and population contexts that exist between rural and urban service provision and availability [13]. It is within the rural palliative care context that health care decision-makers are faced with the challenge of meeting both immediate and long-term palliative care needs for a relatively small and sparse population dispersed across a vast landscape while at the same time rationing palliative care service allocation due to limited funding and budget allocations [14]. As a result, more rational, systematic and evidence-

informed methods to determine how best to deliver the most effective and efficient care to the greatest number of people are significantly needed. The ability to base such decisions on results generated from evidence-informed, rational, and systematic methods enhances the credibility of such insights and facilitates a more transparent decision-making process. Acknowledging this, policy-makers and administrators are actively seeking such approaches to decision-making that integrate best practices and evidence of effectiveness [15, 16].

Here we offer a novel approach to supporting health service policy-maker and administrator decision-making regarding enhancing palliative care in rural Canadian communities through the development of a mixed-method service siting model tailored to this context. In doing so, we acknowledge that this service-siting approach serves as only one component of a suite of activities or actions that can lead to more equitable palliative care access and provision in rural Canadian communities. We previously ran a pilot study in the Canadian province of British Columbia (BC) that resulted in the creation of a mixed-method siting model [17]. This siting model is summarized in Figure 1. Building from our earlier pilot study, where we developed a preliminary siting model using data focused specifically on BC, here we report on the findings of qualitative interviews conducted with key informants ($n = 40$) in four purposefully selected rural communities across other parts of Canada to assess the appropriateness of the siting model for other rural palliative care service contexts. An important finding of these interviews is that the way in which some of the variables associated with the 'community readiness' component in the existing model, a variable we introduce in greater detail below, need to be altered to be appropriate for a wider range of rural Canadian communities. In this article we examine this finding, justifying a necessary alteration to the siting model using first-hand insights offered by the key informant interview participants. Ultimately, we introduce an important adjustment to the siting model as it was previously reported. In the discussion section we contend that, based on these findings, some aspects of

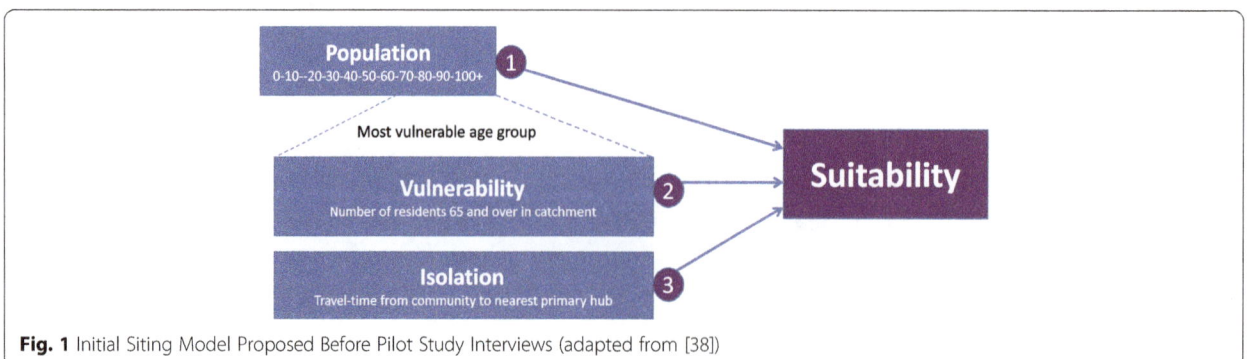

Fig. 1 Initial Siting Model Proposed Before Pilot Study Interviews (adapted from [38])

assessing 'community readiness' for enhancing palliative care in rural areas must be assessed qualitatively or subjectively and in ways that allow for local context to be considered and propose ways for doing this. First, however, in the following sections we provide a brief review on the use of siting models in health care decision making before providing a summary of our pilot study and key findings.

A siting model approach to health care decision-making

Although geographic access does not necessarily equate full health care accessibility, it is a critical prerequisite to enabling equitable care provision [18], including palliative care. As such, a primary concern for decision-makers is determining how to make health care services geographically accessible (e.g., available locally or within a reasonable transit time). Achieving geographic accessibility is particularly problematic in Canada, where rural regions account for approximately 90% of the total land mass and about one third of the total population [19]. Considering this geography, and the existing financial/resource limitations, it is simply not feasible to enhance services in all rural and remote communities [20]. Thus, what is needed is the thoughtful identification of communities that are most suitable for targeting enhancement strategies. A spatial decision support system, or siting model, can assist with this task and can serve as a valuable tool for regional health service planning.

Based on Geographic Information System (GIS) technology, siting models are tools designed to collect, integrate, and model spatial data [21]. Use of such a tool can allow healthcare decision-makers to explore spatial questions, like: where would it be best to site or enhance a specific health service to most effectively serve a dispersed population? The development of siting models provide decision makers with the ability to access relevant data from existing datasets, and sometimes even collect new primary data (as is the case with the current siting model), and model prospective service configurations within and across their regions [14, 22–24]. Thus, siting models hold the potential to provide systematic support to decision-makers as they tackle challenging service siting questions.

While there exists a significant amount of research on the science of siting and model development [23, 25, 26], there are few accounts on the development of specific health service siting models within academic literature [27–30]. The paucity of such published accounts points to the highly privatized use of such models, whereby it is generally those who can afford to pay for such skills and services who are creating and using siting models (e.g., retailers, private hospitals, other corporations). There are, however, some articles and reports that document the development of siting models for use in health services. One such example involves the development of an MRI site in central Newfoundland & Labrador, which is a province in Atlantic Canada [31]. Having no expertise in siting analyses or access to siting model supports, a research team sought to create their own siting model to determine which out of two hospitals would be the most viable host for an MRI. Four variables were considered in their model: access, demand, cost/benefit, and human resources. The findings from their model facilitated the final decision and successful approval for the MRI site development [32]. A second example pertains to the development of a siting model to assist with determining where to site a new acute care hospital in Durham, which is in Northern England [33]. A regional health authority in Durham commissioned a report to characterize the optimal spatial pattern of future hospital development, which was accomplished through considering the adequacy of existing facilities, spatial distribution of potential users, and optimal locations of future services. Relying heavily on spatial statistics, the results of this model recommended a site located within close proximity to another regional health authority.

Despite siting models having been recognized as effective tools for health service decision-makers in various fields, including palliative care, there is little literature for those outside the private realm, who may not be able to afford to commission such projects, to draw from that captures the *rationale* for the inclusion of particular variables in existing models. This limits the transferability of existing models, including the two summarized above, to other contexts. Our research team set out to address this gap by developing a mixed-method siting model that is made freely available, and which offers a sound rationale for the inclusion of each variable and in doing so draws on qualitative insights and existing population-level datasets. As a case study, the focus of our model is on rural palliative care service delivery in Canada. This model can be used by health service administrators to determine which rural communities are most in need of enhancing, and also most ready to enhance, their local palliative care service provision. As we have argued elsewhere, having access to such a tool is an invaluable asset for administrators, decision-makers, and other local community members who are interested in enhancing and expanding upon existing rural palliative care services in Canada [34]. We contend that by sharing details of the development of this model and the rationale for each variable included within, all or part of the model can be assessed for transferability for use in other geographic or health service contexts.

Our pilot study

The analysis presented herein stems from a previously conducted pilot study that aimed to identify communities in rural and remote areas of the province of BC that were most ready to enhance their existing palliative care services [17, 35]. Communities were identified through a siting model that was created to consider palliative care-specific locational factors. Running the model results in identifying communities both ready for and in need of service enhancement in a defined area, but it does not determine the nature of enhancements that are needed nor does it consider cost-based factors as these are outside the scope of the model. Thus, our pilot study created a locational service siting model specific to rural palliative care in BC that ranks communities in terms of their suitability for service enhancement.

Our pilot study began by conducting a spatial analysis to determine the geographic accessibility of existing specialized palliative care services in BC. We did this in order to exclude communities with specialized palliative care on-site. A location analysis model was then developed using GIS, building upon the work of Schuurman et al. [36, 37], to assess the suitability of communities not excluded in this first step to rank their suitability for enhancing palliative care services. This location analysis model involved the following factors: (1) the total population within one-hour of the communities (whereby larger populations were deemed more suitable); (2) the vulnerability of the community, which was calculated as the total population 65 years of age and older within the one-hour area (whereby the larger older populations are more suitable); and (3) the isolation of the community as measured by travel time to the nearest specialized palliative care facility (whereby longer travel times to existing facilities are more suitable). Nineteen communities across rural and remote BC were identified using the GIS location analysis model, providing valuable information regarding which communities are most in need of palliative care service enhancement by ranking them based on the score generated from the four weighted factors [38].

After running the service siting model, the next phase of our pilot research involved conducting interviews with key informants in a cluster of three communities ranked highly by the model to gather information to assist with refining the model and to assess whether or not local experts agreed that they were ready for and in need of palliative care service enhancement. We conducted 31 semi-structured interviews with key informants in the BC communities of Trail, Nelson, and Castlegar. We pursued a number of qualitative analyses that assisted with better understanding the scope of palliative care need in rural BC and the implications of this for our siting model [see 34, 35, 39, 40]. Of relevance to the current article, it became apparent from the interview findings that an important additional factor needed to be added into the siting model: community readiness. As such, specific variables that collectively informed the communities' readiness to enhance palliative care services were identified for inclusion [41]: (1) community awareness, (2) training and education, (3) telemedicine utilization, (4) presence of family doctors, and (5) community momentum. Figure 2 illustrates the revision to the original model and Table 1 provides details on these new variables.

In order to be integrated into the siting model, indicators of each of the identified community readiness variables were developed based on the results of the key informant interviews to be measured as binary yes or no answers for inclusion in the siting model. For example, the *community awareness* variable was considered to be a yes if a hospice society was in operation in the community, which was determined by looking for hospice or palliative care societies in each of the communities using online search engines. The *community momentum* variable was considered to be a yes if a proposal had been developed with the intention of creating a hospice residence in the community, which was determined by contacting and asking local hospice societies. Yes answers received a .20 score and no answers received a 0 score,

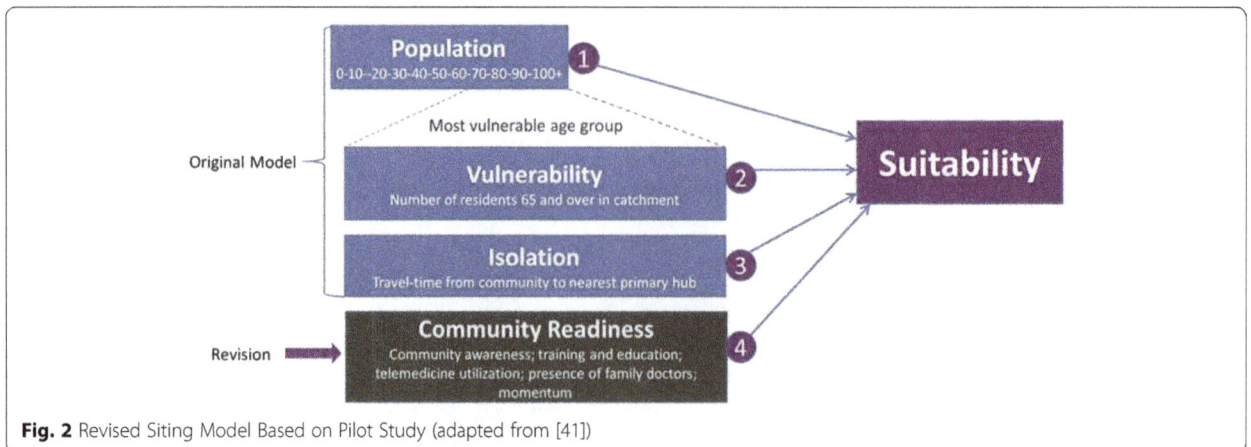

Fig. 2 Revised Siting Model Based on Pilot Study (adapted from [41])

Table 1 Community Readiness Variables and Indicators Added Following Pilot Study (adapted from [41])

Variable	Meaning	Binary Indicator (Y/N)
Community Awareness	Showing evidence that palliative care is a priority issue. Does palliative care have visibility or a 'profile' in the community?	Is there a local hospice society (in that these groups play a major role in local advocacy)?
Training and Education	Strengthening palliative care in rural communities requires providing local education opportunities. Is there a site to host and possibly coordinate such initiatives?	Is there a local college or university campus?
Telemedicine utilization	Telemedicine can increase capacity for providing palliative care in smaller sites. Is the community ready to link to larger centres via telemedicine in order to facilitate information sharing?	Is there regular use of telemedicine at the local hospital?
Presence of family doctors	Family doctors play a vital role in providing palliative care in rural areas. Are there adequate family medicine resources locally to enhance palliative care provision?	Do family doctors practicing locally have an adequate family physician to population ratio?
Momentum	Enhancing palliative care is not an end point, but rather the start of accomplishing larger goals. Has there been demonstration by the community of the desire to increase palliative care capacity?	Has a proposal been put forth to create a local hospice?

which ensured that the maximum score possible for the community readiness arm of the model was 1, which is the same total maximum score for each of the other arms. Readiness scores were tabulated by adding the results of each of the readiness indicators together and adding this score with the previous suitability score in the mixed methods location analysis model. After including the community readiness arm in the model we ran the revised siting model in BC to see if this change made any difference in the suitability rankings assigned to communities [41]. Although the differences were minimal, we believed inclusion of the community readiness variables was of great importance as they offer a 'grounded' perspective, which produces a more refined and robust assessment of a community's suitability and readiness to enhance their palliative care service provision. In the present article we focus once again on these community readiness variables, refining them based on the findings of a new study that has involved applying the siting model across Canada and conducting new key informant interviews in four more rural communities based in other provinces.

Methods

Since completion of the pilot, the research team has now embarked on a national study, which employs the mixed-methods location analysis model across Canada, excluding the province of BC (where it was originally tested), to conduct further model testing and refinement. Based upon the pan-Canadian results, the model showed that 58 communities were identified as highly suitable for enhancing their palliative care services. We next pursued identifying four case study communities from these 58 for further qualitative research. To do this, we narrowed our focus to communities identified in the provinces of Alberta, Manitoba, Ontario, and Newfoundland & Labrador. These provinces were selected based on their geographic and population diversity. For the four

provinces, contextual information about each identified community was garnered (e.g., percent of population employed in agricultural, percent of population self-identified as Aboriginal, etc.) to inform the selection of the qualitative case-study communities that would represent socio-economic and demographic diversity found across Canada while not replicating the profile of those included in the initial BC-based pilot study. It was from this contextual information that the four case-study sites reported on here were purposely selected by our research team: (1) Lloydminster, Alberta/Saskatchewan (an agricultural town with a population of just over 30,000); (2) Thompson, Manitoba (a resource town with a population close to 13,000); (3) Fort Frances, Ontario (a fishing and milling town with almost 8000 residents), and; (4) Happy Valley-Goose Bay, Newfoundland & Labrador (a small town home to a military base with just over 7500 residents).

Following ethics approval from Simon Fraser University and the regional ethics boards for the health authorities that oversee these communities, semi-structured phone interviews were conducted with formal ($n = 34$) and informal ($n = 6$) palliative care providers and administrators across of the four case study communities listed above (10 interviews per community for a total of 40 interviews). Participants were identified through online directories of health service employees, hospice contact information, advertisements in the local paper, and study information that was circulated by some health authorities. Lasting on average 74 min, the interviews inquired into participants' experiences with: palliative care provision; important community characteristics; community health and health care priorities and challenges; community need for palliative care and existing availability; and their perspective on our siting model approach.

All interviews were digitally recorded, transcribed verbatim, and entered into NVivo™ software for data management. Selected transcripts were reviewed by members of the investigative team to identify emerging themes and determine the scope and scale of each. Following this, a coding scheme was developed to capture these themes as well as organize contextual information shared by participants. Thematic analysis ensued on the data set, using investigator triangulation to confirm the assignment of codes to data segments, where emergent patterns in the data were categorized [42]. The emergent patterns were then reviewed, refined, and compared and contrasted to the pilot study findings. It was through this process that the refinement to the community readiness component of the model was identified as a necessary outcome of the interview findings, which is what we report on in the section that follows.

Results

While the pilot study findings pointed to the need to include community readiness as a variable in the siting model, analysis of the data from this new, pan-Canadian, dataset revealed inconsistencies in how to conceptualize this variable. Participants' comments reveal that an inherent challenge exists in accurately pre-determining binary indicators that capture contextually-drive qualitative aspects of the model like community readiness, such as community awareness and momentum. As such, our national study findings indicate that further refinement of the model is necessary to more effectively capture these complex and context-driven factors, breaking them out of the binary ways they were initially summarized in Table 1.

In this section we characterize the breadth of factors that illustrate the presence of community awareness and momentum around building capacity for palliative care in rural Canadian communities from across the four case study communities. Specifically, the interviews point to factors such as educational tools, volunteers, and local acknowledgement of palliative care priorities as reflecting community awareness and factors such as new employment and volunteer positions, new care spaces, and new projects and programs as reflecting momentum. We expand on these factors here in order to assess their scope and demonstrate their relevance to enhancing palliative care in rural communities. In the discussion section that follows we point to the fact that the breadth of factors identified in the current study and our earlier research collectively show that community awareness and momentum variables in the siting model must be assessed subjectively and we consider how this can be done.

Community awareness: Does palliative care have visibility in the community?

During the interviews, it became apparent that participants were aware of local palliative care provision and felt it had a visible presence in each of their four communities. While this may have been confirmed via the original siting model indicator of whether or not there was a local hospice society, other indicators emerged that were equally capable of demonstrating local awareness regarding the importance of palliative care in the community. Specifically, the new indicators that emerged include the presence of: (1) educational tools that promote palliative care awareness and knowledge; (2) community-based palliative care volunteers; and (3) local stakeholder acknowledgement that palliative care is indeed prioritized.

Educational tools that promote local palliative care awareness and knowledge

Review of the transcripts revealed that some community members were actively involved in the development of local palliative care educational tools and training opportunities that aimed to increase awareness about, and visibility of, palliative care. For example, in Happy Valley-Goose Bay, a health care provider described how she, along with two other health workers, developed a palliative care information booklet to disseminate to clients and families. This participant explained how the purpose of the booklet was to make information about palliative care accessible for the local populations by avoiding medical jargon and keeping the information *"as simple and as precise, but true to life, for the palliative care patient and their family so that they'd have an understanding of what was going on."* Some participants described the existence of palliative care training opportunities, such as the development of *"a training session for the nursing staff working on our palliative care beds, so they've actually had some education just recently"* in Lloydminster. Other participants spoke to how they had developed regional interdisciplinary committees to identify gaps in palliative care and develop educational sessions. Furthermore, because many Aboriginal elders die in the hospital in Fort Frances, it was explained that health care administrators have:

> ...made it a priority to train and educate [hospital] staff on cultural competencies and all of that because they recognize that that is needed, so they are working with some First Nations [Aboriginal] organizations to try to develop ... more training and materials around that for their staff.

Such findings demonstrate how community awareness of palliative care operates, and is being further promoted, through the existence of locally developed educational tools and training sessions.

Community-based palliative care volunteers

Across the case study communities it was found that volunteers formally and informally facilitated palliative care provision in their communities, offering various means of support for community members and their families facing a life-limiting illness. Some participants explained that due to their 'close-knit' community culture, in some cases a whole town would informally pull together to ensure families received the care they needed at the end of life. However, in other communities, more formal volunteer groups existed. A participant from Lloydminster described the important role that volunteers play:

My volunteers help with driving people to appointments, doing some running around, friendly visiting...at the hospital we have three palliative care rooms and they're checking, make sure there's coffee and that kind of thing as well as visiting patients and families.

It was often explained that volunteers were mainly responsible for assisting patients with transportation, meals, and emotional/psychosocial support by visiting with patients and their families. The existence of such formal and informal volunteers in the communities demonstrates community awareness about palliative care and the identified need to enhance formal existing services.

Stakeholder acknowledgement that palliative care is a local priority

Although not always in the spotlight, many participants (as local stakeholders in palliative care) described feeling that members of their communities were aware of palliative care and even the need for service enhancement. As this participant from Fort Frances described: "*I think it's [palliative care] one of their big priorities, they are as a community very very good at providing excellent palliative care*", while another explained that "*I think there is an increasing awareness of the need for providing palliative care and what that means.*" Regarding existing conversations on and awareness about the need to enhance local palliative care, this Fort Frances participant stated that:

there is the awareness and there are people coming together to try to provide appropriate palliative care...so the desire and the will is there and people realize that it's something that we have to continue to look at and develop and grow, to meet the needs of the community.

These descriptions highlight local awareness about palliative care and the importance it carries for their communities. Participants also commented on how regional and provincial changes to palliative care policies and programs sometimes created new local awareness of palliative care through conversation among stakeholders. In the case of Thompson, a new advanced care planning strategy led to the development of a new program involving conversations between "*a social worker, or somebody trained, going in and talking to somebody whose still mentally alert...transcribe their conversation about who they are and their life and the things they would like to pass on to their family.*" Taken together, such awareness of the local prioritization of palliative care among stakeholders illustrates one way in which such care is viewed as a priority as well as wider community awareness.

Momentum: Has there been a demonstration by the community of the desire to increase palliative care capacity?

Thematic analysis revealed that community momentum could not be captured through the sole binary indicator of whether or not a proposal for a hospice has been put forward in the community alone. While this factor does capture community momentum, it was found that other factors could similarly depict such desires to increase local palliative care capacity. These additional indicators include the local addition of new: (1) employment or volunteer positions; (2) rooms or spaces dedicated for palliative care; and (3) projects, plans, and programs.

Employment or volunteer positions

Some participants described how recently their communities had seen the addition of new palliative care employment or volunteer positions, which implies that the desire exists to enhance local palliative care services. Particularly in Fort Frances, where a participant described how they recently acquired "*a new nurse practitioner role for palliative care for the whole district...to support other Homecare providers in doing better palliative care.*" It was also mentioned that Fort Frances recently acquired a new palliative care coordinator for their district, which was described by a participant as someone who "*looks quite promising.*" While these new positions are the outcomes of regional priorities and their directives to enhance local palliative care services, other forms of momentum were found to be coming from the communities themselves. For example, in Fort Frances, there had previously been a strong palliative care volunteer group that had "*fizzled out*"; however, at the time of the interviews, a new volunteer coordinator was just assigned and was in the process of seeking out and training a new group of volunteers. She described:

Our volunteers have to go through thirty hours of training before I can actually put them to work... It's like a workshop thing... And then I'm going to be trying to get teaching sessions every couple of months or so somebody will come in and talk about this or that, Alzheimer's or cancer or you know different aspects... But first I need the volunteers to be able to (chuckle) do the workshops.

Although Fort Frances had not put forth a proposal for a new hospice to be created, the findings here depict a community with momentum with members who are actively trying to enhance their palliative care capacity through new employment positions and volunteers.

Rooms or spaces for palliative care

While the creation of a dedicated hospice for palliative care was beyond some rural communities' capabilities, other types of momentum were occurring, particularly in the form of creating new rooms or spaces for palliative care. These rooms and spaces were often found in local hospitals, for example in Lloydminster, where a few participants described how their local hospital recently underwent renovations of three rooms to be set up solely for palliative care patients and their families. This participant stated that *"we've recently added on a palliative care room and renovated the other, like we used to have two palliative care rooms, we now have three and they're linked together."* It was found, however, that for some communities, it was simply not feasible to have dedicated palliative care spaces. Rather, they desired to have more flexible spaces that could accommodate those facing life-limiting illness and their families once the need emerged. This Fort Frances participant explained how they:

> are in the process of arranging for more or less carts so that we can turn any of the three acute care rooms and our two other sites into palliative care rooms. It's a challenge when you only have three acute care rooms and our remote sites to designate one as a palliative care room. So we tend to try and do things a little bit differently and then theoretically any room in our long-term care facility should be able to accommodate palliative care.

Taken together, these findings demonstrate that momentum is occurring in these communities through the creation of more palliative care rooms. However, each community addresses these needs in unique ways, thus reflecting how this indicator of momentum can only be interpreted within the context in which it is occurring.

Projects, plans, and programs

It became apparent that community momentum was being influenced by processes occurring at broader scales, like at the provincial and regional levels. This was found particularly in relation to Fort Frances, where participants described a new strategy that was in place by the Province of Ontario to enhance palliative care capacity. One participant explained the project, called *Advancing Integrative Palliative Care Services Across Ontario,* and how it aims to develop a plan for *"our Local Health Integration Network [LHIN] to say where there are gaps, this is our plan to fill them."* More specifically, another participant explained that:

> the province has asked all of the local health integration networks to come up with palliative care and end of life plans for each one of the fourteen LHINs in the province. There are some LHINs that are further ahead than others...I believe that within our part of northwestern Ontario there is a strong desire to have a strong palliative care infrastructure in place as evidenced by at least our commitment to maintain that palliative care room in the hospital and have some resources at all of our sites to address palliative care service.

Another participant from Fort Frances described how they were in the process of developing working groups to work on various projects, like *"coming up with common definitions and tools for palliative care, looking at caregiver supports, looking at provider education."* At the time of the interviews, this project had just begun and demonstrated a change on the ground through the development of new jobs and volunteer positions in the community, which we discussed previously. As such, Fort Frances is an example of a community with momentum, moving towards enhancing their local palliative care services.

Discussion

In this article we have presented a thematic analysis of 40 interviews conducted with formal and informal palliative care providers from four purposefully selected rural Canadian communities. The goal of these interviews was to gather first-hand insights from people involved in such care provision to identify if and how our existing service-siting model needs to be changed in order to enhance its utility across the diverse community types that make up rural Canada. We developed this model in an earlier pilot study as a way of identifying rural Canadian communities most in need of and most suitable for enhancing their palliative care service provision and conducted initial qualitative interviews about our model in the province of BC. From those pilot interviews we added a 'community readiness' arm to it, as shown in Figure 2 above. Table 1, above, summarizes the variables initially included in this arm of the siting model. The thematic analysis presented here shows that while community readiness remains an important factor in determining the suitability of a rural community for enhancing local palliative care provision, and thus should remain in the model, the way in which two of its associated variables—community awareness and momentum—are assessed must be revised.

Table 2 captures the revisions to the community readiness arm of the siting model informed by the thematic analysis presented herein. The model itself, shown in Figure 2 above, remains the same and the interviews confirmed the importance of including all previously-identified indicators of community readiness in the siting model. However, the way in which the presence or absence of momentum and community awareness are determined based on indicators has been revised using the input provided by the 40 interviewees. The findings show that these two variables cannot be captured using a single binary question as previously proposed by Crooks et al. [41]. Instead, someone applying the model will need to subjectively assess whether or not a community shows locally-relevant evidence of momentum and community awareness. In Table 2 we have provided examples of indicators for both of these variables based on the factors identified in the pilot interviews conducted in BC and the 40 interviews conducted in the current study. These examples, however, must not be thought of as exhaustive in that someone running the model must look for any and all evidence of what they can subjectively interpret as momentum or community awareness regarding palliative care in rural Canadian communities. We encourage those using or running the model to document this process and the sources consulted to justify how they have interpreted the presence or absence of these indicators. Here we have provided an example

of consulting with community members to identify specific indicators. This could certainly be done elsewhere. Other potentially ripe sources of information could include community newspapers and newsletters, provincial health service policy documents, and attending hospital board or administrative meetings.

We noted previously that each of the four arms of the rural palliative care service siting model is assigned a maximum score of 1, and thus population, vulnerability, isolation, and community readiness are weighted equally in the overall suitability score provided. The rationale for this along with discussion regarding how to generate scores for the population, vulnerability, and isolation arms have been introduced elsewhere [14, 38] and are not re-examined here as our sole interest is in the community readiness arm. Following our revision to the indicators used to score each of the five components of community readiness based on the current analysis, as summarized in Table 2 below, three can be scored using binary Y/N questions while the remaining two require subjective assessment. Both the binary and subjective indicators will require obtaining information found online and/or from administrative databases (e.g., family physician practice information) and from local leaders in the palliative care community and so we contend that no new work is introduced by the revision to the siting model proposed here. After this information is gathered and reviewed, the subjectively assessed variables will have a

Table 2 Revised Community Readiness Variables and Indicators

Variable	Meaning	Indicator
Community Awareness	Showing evidence that palliative care is a priority issue. Does palliative care have visibility or a 'profile' in the community?	Subjective Indicator: presence of locally-relevant factors that indicate community awareness can result in 'Yes' for this variable (factors may include: presence of local hospice society; educational tools promoting awareness; presence of community volunteers; stakeholder acknowledgement).
Training and Education	Strengthening palliative care in rural communities requires providing local education opportunities. Is there a site to host and possibly coordinate such initiatives?	Binary Indicator (Y/N): Is there a local college or university campus?
Telemedicine utilization	Telemedicine can increase capacity for providing palliative care in smaller sites. Is the community ready to link to larger centres via telemedicine in order to facilitate information sharing?	Binary Indicator (Y/N): Is there regular use of telemedicine at the local hospital?
Presence of family doctors	Family doctors play a vital role in providing palliative care in rural areas. Are there adequate family medicine resources locally to enhance palliative care provision?	Binary Indicator (Y/N): Do family doctors practicing locally have an adequate family physician to population ratio?
Momentum	Enhancing palliative care is not an end point, but rather the start of accomplishing larger goals. Has there been demonstration by the community of the desire to increase palliative care capacity?	Subjective Indicator: presence of locally-relevant factors that indicate momentum can result in 'Yes' for this variable (factors may include: proposal for local hospice; new employment or volunteer positions; new spaces or places being created; projects and plans implemented at larger scales).

value of .20 entered to indicate that, yes, that indicator is present in the community. Oppositely, a value of 0 will be entered if there is no subjective evidence of its presence. The binary indicators are objectively assessed and .20 is entered to indicate presence while 0 is entered to indicate absence.

Strengths & Limitations

As the Canadian population ages at a rapid rate, growth in future demand for palliative care services cannot be ignored [43]. Here we have not taken a prescriptive approach to articulating how such services can be enhanced to facilitate greater and more responsive access to care. Instead, here we have focused on *where* to deepen service provision by developing a mixed-method service siting model that can assist with identifying which rural Canadian communities are most in need of and most suitable for enhancing their palliative care services. There are increasing calls for greater accountability with regard to health care spending, including in Canada [15, 16], and service siting models are a tool that can support this through making transparent how and why certain decision are made [44, 45]. Through documenting every step of the development and testing of the current model [14, 35, 38, 41], including in the current analysis, we believe that we have facilitated a high level of transparency that can be extended into its use in applied settings to enhance accountability. We also believe that the mixed-methods approach to this siting model that has incorporated qualitative and qualitative data throughout its development, wherein GIS-based location siting models typically rely on administrative data alone, also increases the transparency and accountability for two reasons. First, we have consulted with key stakeholders in several rural communities across Canada to garner their first-hand insights about factors they believe are important regarding the focus of our model to inform its refinement. Second, local consultation is required in using the model to assess the presence or absence of the community readiness variables, and especially those that have subjective indicators, which thereby necessitates local involvement in developing solutions for local needs.

Models of all forms are never perfect as they are based heavily on assumptions. The current siting model is no different. There are also limitations that are worth noting. For example, we equally weight each variable in the community readiness arm of the model as well as each of the four arms included in the model. While we did conduct earlier sensitivity analysis that showed that different weightings of the arm did little to change the overall suitability scores or ranking of communities against one another [41], this has not been done on the community readiness arm of the model. While the current data do not suggest any one community readiness variable to be more important than another, this is an aspect of our design that must be considered by those using the model in real-world settings. The siting model ultimately requires quantitative data to be entered and thus qualitative insights need to be quantified so that communities can be scored. This serves as a limitation in that factors that cannot be quantified cannot be incorporated. With regard to the current interviews, for example, we gleaned important insights about how boundaries and borders can create barriers or facilitators to palliative care service provision and access in rural Canada [46]. We could not link these insights to variables that can be quantitatively assessed and incorporated, and they are thus absent from the model as it is currently constructed. We also acknowledge that our model is focused heavily on formal palliative care provision as it is a service siting model and thus does not consider the full scope of supports that may be needed to facilitate rural-based end of life care more broadly. Finally, on a practical note, we conducted our interviews by phone and thus from a distance and so may have missed conversational nuances in facial expression or tone that would have been caught in person [47]. We were, however, quick to ask for elaboration or clarification in order to overcome this potential limitation as the cost-saving nature of this strategy is what enabled our inclusion of four very distant communities.

Conclusion

Although the science behind siting model development has been documented in academic literature [23, 25, 26], few researchers have developed such models in an open way to address problems of health service siting [27–30]. This mixed-method study has addressed this notable knowledge gap through the detailed documentation of our siting model development, which aims to identify rural Canadian communities most in need of and ready to enhance their palliative care service provision. As we argued in the introduction, this is a needed and timely health service focus given the country's aging population.

Our findings from 40 interviews with formal and informal palliative care providers across four rural Canadian communities demonstrate not only the value in, but also the importance of, incorporating community-driven indicators into service siting models as well as community consultation in the model development process. The findings also show that although the siting model we have developed requires the input of quantitative binary data, community readiness variables, such as momentum and awareness, must first be qualitatively assessed to garner more localized and context-specific information. Efforts to collect such data, for example via consulting with key-stakeholders, will ultimately contribute more 'grounded' knowledge to assist with identifying local needs, and ultimately, developing meaningful local solutions. Thus, our study emphasizes the importance of considering, including, and translating qualitative community-driven variables into quantitative indicators in order to produce more nuanced results that reflect the lived contexts of diverse communities.

While this study has focused on rural palliative care in Canada, the process by which we have developed and refined our siting model is highly transferrable and can be applied to address various other issues, in health services and beyond, within a diverse range of geographic contexts. For instance, our siting model could be adapted internationally for applications in jurisdictions where best practices in rural palliative care decision-making are in demand, such as in the Australian context [48]. GIS-based location service siting models can and do contribute valuable information to decision-makers by demonstrating how the place-based nature of health services can benefit from the visual capabilities of GIS [49]. For example, in our study, the resultant maps and spatial models are tools that can be used to translate numeric rankings into a visual format. This visualization of data holds the potential to assist those in policy to make informed, place-based decisions, while at the same time, facilitate the promotion of rational and transparent decision-making regarding the provision of services, within health care and beyond.

Abbreviations
BC: British Columbia; GIS: Geographic Information Systems

Acknowledgements
We acknowledge the research assistance of Neville Li, who assisted with data coding.

Funding
This study is funded by an Operating Grant awarded by the Canadian Institutes of Health Research (CIHR).

Authors' contributions
VAC and NS lead this study. VAC oversaw data collection and analysis while MG conducted the interviews. VAC and MG conceptualized the current analysis with input from all members of the investigative team. VAC and MG worked on confirming interpretation of the data used in this analysis. HC, NS, MS and AW are all investigators on the grant who provided input in developing research instruments, participant recruitment, and case study community selection. They reviewed data extracts and participated in an initial meeting to determine the scope of this analysis. All authors have reviewed and approved of this article.

Authors' information
VAC holds the Canada Research Chair in Health Service Geographies and a Scholar Award from the Michael Smith Foundation for Health Research. HC holds the Canada Research Chair in Reconciling Relations for Health, Environments, and Communities. MS holds the Canada Research Chair in Rural Aging, Health and Social Care. AW holds the CIHR Research Chair in Gender, Work and Health.

Labrador-Grenfell Health (NFLD), Nunatsiavut Government (NFLD), and the NunatuKavut Research Review Advisory Committee (NFLD). All study participants provided their informed consent.

Competing interests
The authors declare that they have no competing interests.

Author details
[1]Department of Geography, Simon Fraser University, 8888 University Drive, Burnaby, BC V5A 1S6, Canada. [2]Department of Geography and Planning and Department of Public Health Sciences, Queens University, 62 Fifth Field Company Lane, Kingston, ON K7L 3N6, Canada. [3]Trent School of the Environment, Trent University, 1600 West Bank Drive, Peterborough, ON K9L 0G2, Canada. [4]School of Geography & Earth Sciences, McMaster University, 1280 Main Street West, Hamilton, ON L8S 4M1, Canada.

References
1. Canadians in context - aging population [https://www.canada.ca/en/public-health/corporate/publications/chief-public-health-officer-reports-state-public-health-canada/chief-public-health-officer-report-on-state-public-health-canada-2014-public-health-future/changing-demographics.html].
2. Dandy K, Bollman RD. Seniors in rural Canada. In: *Rural and Small Town Canada: Analysis Bulletin.* vol. 7. Statistics Canada: Ottawa; 2008.
3. 2006 Census: Portrait of the Canadian Population in 200, by Age and Sex: Subprovincial population dynamics [https://www12.statcan.gc.ca/census-recensement/2006/as-sa/97-551/p17-eng.cfm].
4. Fact sheet- hospice palliative care in Canada [http://www.chpca.net/media/7622/fact_sheet_hpc_in_canada_may_2012_final.pdf].
5. Canadian Rural Revitalization Foundation. In: Markey S, Breen SP, Lauson A, Gibson R, Ryser L, Mealy R, editors. The state of rural Canada 2015; 2015.
6. Browne A. Issues affecting access to health service in northern, rural and remote regions of Canada. In: Northern Article Series. Prince George, BC: University of Northern British Columbia; 2010.
7. Canada H. Canadian strategy on palliative and end-of-life care: final report. Health Canada: Ottawa; 2007.
8. BC Palliative Care Benefits Program [https://www2.gov.bc.ca/gov/content/health/practitioner-professional-resources/pharmacare/prescribers/plan-p-bc-palliative-care-benefits-program].
9. Canadian Hospice Palliative Care Association. Fact sheet: hospice and palliative care in Canada. Ottawa, ON: Canadian Hospice and Palliative Care Association; 2012.
10. Canadian Hospice Palliative Care Association. Caring for Canadians at end of life: A strategic plan for hospice, palliative, and end-of-life care in Canada to 2015. Ottawa: Canadian Hospice Palliative Care Association; 2009.
11. Romanow RJ. Building on values: the future of health care in Canada. Commission on the Future of Health Care in Canada: Ottawa; 2002.
12. Carstairs S. Still not there: quality end of life care: a progress report. Ottawa; 2005. http://www.chpca.net/media/7883/Still_Not_There_June_2005.pdf.
13. Crooks VA, Schuurman N. Reminder: palliative care is a rural medicine issue. Canadian Journal of Rural Medicine. 2008;13:139–40.
14. Schuurman N, Randall E. A spatial decision support tool for estimating population catchments to aid rural and remote health service allocation planning. Health Informatics Journal. 2011;17(4):277–93.
15. Tunis S. Reflections on science, judgment, and value in evidence-based decision making: a conversation with David Eddy. Health Aff. 2007;26(4):500–15.
16. Kohatsu N, RObinson J, Torner J. Evidence-based public health: an evolving concept. Am J Prev Med. 2004;27(5):417–21.
17. Cinnamon J, Schuurman N, Crooks VA. A method to determine spatial access to specialized palliative care services using GIS. BMC Health Serv Res. 2008;8:140.

18. Glazier R, Gozdyra P, Yeritsyan N. Geographic access to primary care and Hospital Services for Rural and Northern Communities: report to the Ontario Ministry of Health and Long-Term Care. Toronto: Institute for Clinical Evaluative Sciences; 2011.

19. Williams A, Kulig JC. Health and place in rural Canada. In: Kulig JC, Williams a, editors. *Health in rural Canada*. Vancouver: UBC Press; 2012. p. 1–23.

20. Pereira GJ. Palliative care in the hinterlands: a description of existing services and doctors' attitudes. Aust J Rural Health. 2005;13:343–7.

21. Shim J, Wharkentin M, Courtney J, Power D, Sharda R, Carlsson C. Past, present, and future of decision support technology. Decis Support Syst. 2002;33(2):111–26.

22. Gatrell A, M S. Health and health care applications. In: Longley P, Goodchild M, Maguire D, Dhind D, editors. *Geographical Information Systems: Principles, Techniques, Management and Applications 2nd Abridged edition*. New York: John Wlley & Sons; 2005.

23. McLafferty S. GIS and health care. Annu Rev Public Health. 2003;24:25–42.

24. Schuurman N, Fiedler R, Grzybowski S, Grund D. Defining rational hospital catchments for non-urban areas based on travel-time. Int J Health Geogr. 2006;5:43.

25. Ishfaq R, Soz C. Hub location-allocation in intermodal logistic networks. Eur J Oper Res. 2011;210(2):213–30.

26. Bonneu F, Thomas-Agnan C. Spatial point process models for locaiton-allocation problems. Computational Statustics & Data Analysis. 2009;53(8):3070–81.

27. Syam S, Cote M. A location-allocation model for service providers with application to non-for-profit health care organizations. OMEGA – Int J Manag Sci. 2010;38(3–4):157–66.

28. Sahin G, Sural H, Meral S. Locational analysis for regionalization of Turkish red crescent blood services. Comput Oper Res. 2007;34(3):692–704.

29. Harper P, Philips S, Gallaher J. Geographical simulation modelling for the regional planning of oral and maxillofacial surgery across London. Jounral of the Operational Reserach Society. 2005;56(2):134–43.

30. Walsh S, Page P, Gesler WM. Normative models and healthcare planning: network-based simulations within a geographic information systems environment. Health Serv Res. 1997;32(2):243–60.

31. Lo C, Mealey J, Nurse R. Review of MRI siting options for the central region of Newfoundland and Labrador. Newfoundland: central Region; 2009.

32. New MRI Announced for Central Newfoundland [http://www.releases.gov.nl.ca/releases/2009/health/0601n10.htm].

33. Mohan J. Location-allocation models, social science and health service planning: an example from north East England. Soc Sci Med. 1983;17(8):493–9.

34. Castleden H, Crooks VA, Schuurman N, Hanlon N. "It's not necessarily the distance on the map...": using place as an analytic tool to elucidate geographic issues central to rural palliative care. Health & place. 2010;16(2):284–90.

35. Crooks VA, Castleden H, Schuurman N, Hanlon N. Visioning for secondary palliative care service hubs in rural communities: a qualitative case study from British Columbia's interior. BMC palliative care. 2009;8:15.

36. Schuurman N, Bell N, Hameed SM, Simons R. A model for identifying and ranking need for trauma service in non-metropolitan regions based on injury risk and access to services. J Trauma. 2008;65:54–62.

37. Schuurman N, Crooks VA, Amram O. A protocol for determining differences in consistency and depth of palliative care service provision across community sites. Health & social care in the community. 2010;18(5):537–48.

38. Cinnamon J, Schuurman N, Crooks VA. Assessing the suitability of host communities for secondary palliative care hubs: a location analysis model. Health & place. 2009;15:822–30.

39. Castleden H, Crooks VA, Hanlon N, Schuurman N. Providers' perceptions of aboriginal palliative care in British Columbia's rural interior. Health & social care in the community. 2010;18(5):483–91.

40. Crooks VA, Castleden H, Hanlon N, Schuurman N. 'Heated political dynamics exist ...': examining the politics of palliative care in rural British Columbia, Canada. Palliat Med. 2011;25(1):26–35.

41. Crooks VA, Schuurman N, Cinnamon J, Castleden H, Johnston R. Refining a location analysis model using a mixed-method approach: community readiness as a key factor in siting rural palliative care services. Journal of Mixed Methods Research. 2011;5(1):77–95.

42. Ayres L. Thematic analysis. In: given LM, editor. vol. 1&2 *The Sage Encyclopedia of Qualitative Research Methods*. Thousand Oaks: Sage Publications; 2008. p. 867–8.

43. Carstairs S, MacDonald ML. THE PRISMA symposium 2: lessons from beyond Europe. Reflections on the evolution of palliative care research and policy in Canada. J Pain Symptom Manag. 2011;42(4):501–4.

44. Newton M, Scott-Findlay S. Taking stock of current societal, political and academic stakeholders in the Canadian healthcare knowledge translation agenda. Implementation science : IS. 2007;2:32.

45. Andersen E, Shepherd M, Salisbury C. Taking of the suit: engaging the community in primary health care decision-making. Health Expect. 2006;9:70–80.

46. Giesbrecht M, Crooks VA, Castleden H, Schuurman N, Skinner MW, Williams A. Palliating inside the lines: the effects of borders and boundaries on palliative care in rural Canada. Soc Sci Med. 2016;168:273–82.

47. Novick G. Is there a bias against telephone interviews in qualitative research? Res Nurs health. 2008;(4):391–8.

48. Mills J, Rosenberg JP, McInerney F. Building community capacity for end of life: an investigation of community capacity and its implications for health-promoting palliative care in the Australian Capital Territory. Critical Public Health. 25:218–30.

49. Jacquez GM. Spatial analysis in epidemiology: nascent science or a failure of GIS? J Geogr Syst. 2000;2:91–7.

15

The interaction of socioeconomic status with place of death: a qualitative analysis of physician experiences

Joshua Wales[*], Allison M. Kurahashi and Amna Husain

Abstract

Background: Home is a preferred place of death for many people; however, access to a home death may not be equitable. The impact of socioeconomic status on one's ability to die at home has been documented, yet there remains little literature exploring mechanisms that contribute to this disparity. By exploring the experiences and insights of physicians who provide end-of-life care in the home, this study aims to identify the factors perceived to influence patients' likelihood of home death and describe the mechanisms by which they interact with socioeconomic status.

Methods: In this exploratory qualitative study, we conducted interviews with 9 physicians who provide home-based care at a specialized palliative care centre. Participants were asked about their experiences caring for patients at the end of life, focusing on factors believed to impact likelihood of home death with an emphasis on socioeconomic status, and opportunities for intervention. We relied on participants' perceptions of SES, rather than objective measures. We used an inductive content analysis to identify and describe factors that physicians perceive to influence a patient's likelihood of dying at home.

Results: Factors identified by physicians were organized into three categories: patient characteristics, physical environment and support network. Patient preference for home death was seen as a necessary factor. If this was established, participants suggested that having a strong support network to supplement professional care was critical to achieving home death. Finally, safe and sustainable housing were also felt to improve likelihood of home death. Higher SES was perceived to increase the likelihood of a desired home death by affording access to more resources within each of the categories. This included better health and health care understanding, a higher capacity for advocacy, a more stable home environment, and more caregiver support.

Conclusions: SES was not perceived to be an isolated factor impacting likelihood of home death, but rather a means to address shortfalls in the three identified categories. Identifying the factors that influence ability is the first step in ensuring home death is accessible to all patients who desire it, regardless of socioeconomic status.

Keywords: Palliative care, Social class, House calls, Socioeconomic factors, Healthcare disparities, Place of death

* Correspondence: Joshua.wales@sinaihealthsystem.ca
The Temmy Latner Centre for Palliative Care, Sinai Health System, 60 Murray Street, 4th Floor, Box 13, Toronto, ON M5T 3L9, Canada

Background

Home has emerged as the preferred place of death for most patients [1–3] and as a cost-effective alternative to institutionalized death [4]. Studies have shown that access to home death is influenced by a number of personal factors, including age [5, 6], sex [5], education [7], disease type [8, 9], marital status or cohabitation [6, 10–12], preferred place of death [13], ethnicity [8, 10], informal support networks [6, 14], and cultural affiliations [8]. Access to care in the home has also been associated with home death. Previous studies investigating the availability and utilization of home care and home visits found that patients were more likely to die at home or out of acute care if they lived in an area with more home hospice providers [10], received home care in the last 6 months of life [15], or received more nursing and personal support worker visits [6, 16, 17].

Associations between socioeconomic status (SES) and place of death in the literature are inconsistent. Several studies found that rates of home death are lower for patients defined as lower SES or low income [10, 12, 17–24]. Conversely, other studies did not find a significant association between place of death and socioeconomic status based on perceived or actual income level [11, 25–29], deprivation score [30], or education level [31].

Previous studies that have identified SES-dependent differences in rates of home death have hypothesized factors to explain these disparities: patient or family capacity to provide adequate care at home [18, 22], level of access to care services [20, 22], personal preferences [22], care-related costs [18], control over monetary resources [23], and ability to secure local supports [20]. Few studies, however, have directly explored the mechanisms by which these determinants – including SES – result in disparities of home death rates. A more complete understanding of these socioeconomic determinants of home death may provide some insight into the inconsistent findings in the literature and help to address SES-related inequities that may exist in accessing home death.

This exploratory study aims to identify the key factors perceived to influence likelihood of home death and define the mechanisms by which they interact with SES. The findings presented here are based on the experiences of physicians who provide home-based palliative care in an urban Canadian context. In future research, we will use the factors identified in this study to refine the research question and capture the perspectives of patients, families and other healthcare providers. They may also highlight areas of opportunity for policy and practice development to mitigate potential disparities within a home-based palliative care context.

Methods

Study design

Working within a Qualitative Description framework [32], the investigators used inductive qualitative content analysis [33] to describe the factors that may influence the likelihood of home death and describe how these factors interact with patient socioeconomic status. Qualitative description studies aim to provide a comprehensive summary of a phenomenon that can be used as an entry point for further study [32]. Our data were informed by physician's perceptions of their patients' SES and did not employ empiric indices of patients' socioeconomic statuses. At the time of recruitment, the principal investigator (JW) was completing his residency and was known to participants as a colleague and student. He currently practices as a staff physician at the centre. The study coordinator (AK) has experience conducting research interviews but is not a clinician. She was known by all participants. The study protocol was approved by the local Research Ethics Board. The methods and findings are described according to the consolidated criteria for reporting qualitative research (COREQ) guidelines [34].

Population

We interviewed physicians whose clinical practice is focused on providing palliative care services to individuals at home. Physicians providing home-based palliative care may be well placed to comment on the determinants of home death. First, they can compare between their experiences and interactions with different patients and patient support networks, which occur in a home environment. Second, their experiences leading goals of care discussions can inform insights into the decision-making processes around place of death. Finally, they can root their perceptions about patient SES in their experiences discussing financial capacity with patients when planning care services.

In order to generate a deep understanding of the factors perceived within a home-based palliative care context, we recruited physicians from a single palliative care centre in Toronto, Ontario. The centre is one of the largest home palliative care programs in Canada, and offers 24/7 physician support to patients with life-limiting illness in their homes. Seventeen physicians dedicate an average of 13 full time equivalents (FTEs) to home care practice. Physicians have had a focused practice in palliative care at the centre ranging from 1.5 to 20 years. The area served by the palliative care centre has nearly equal distribution between income quartiles [16] but incudes neighbourhood clusters of both low- and high-income households [35]. The catchment area is divided into smaller zones, which are serviced by one or two physicians each. Because each zone has a distinct socioeconomic and cultural make-up, some physicians may service areas with a higher density of low-income households than other physicians.

In 2016, the centre recorded 12,551 encounters (physician calls or home visits) with patients. Both types of encounters are necessary to provide palliative care in patients' homes. On average, there were 80.5 encounters per physician FTE per month, and each patient experienced an average of 5.9 encounters.

Sample size and recruitment

The principal investigator sent an email invitation to participate in the study to all physicians practicing with the palliative care centre who provide home-visits. Interested physicians contacted the study coordinator to schedule an interview. Of the 17 physicians contacted, 9 participated in the study. Four physicians were not responsive, three had scheduling conflicts, and one declined as they felt their experiences would not contribute to understanding the research question. Participants were made aware of JW's role in the study and the safeguards that were used to preserve privacy during the consenting process.

Data collection

The semi-structured interview guide was created and refined by JW and AK through a process of evaluating each question's relevance to the overall study aim. The final interview guide (Appendix 1) consisted of a mix of open ended and quantitative questions. An interview preamble informed patients that the researchers were interested in the experiences of home-care palliative physicians and the factors they believe to influence a patient's ability to die at home. Participants were not given definitions for the terms "high" and "low" socioeconomic status, nor patient economic data. Earlier questions probed physicians' general experiences and factors believed to influence the likelihood of home death. Later questions targeted factors related to socioeconomic status, discrepancies resulting from SES, and strategies to address these discrepancies. Individual or telephone interviews were conducted during February 2016. AK conducted all interviews in order to protect participant confidentiality and reduce potential response bias that may have presented if the principal investigator had conducted the interviews.

Data analysis

All interviews were audio recorded, professionally transcribed verbatim and de-identified to maintain participant privacy. AK compared completed transcripts to audio recordings to verify accuracy. Based on AK's field notes, the researchers periodically met to discuss emerging concepts, noting ones that were new or redundant

with earlier interviews. Based on these reviews, greater focus was placed on questions probing socioeconomic status and caregiver support levels after the first 6 interviews were completed. Three more interviews were conducted, but no new concepts emerged. Two reviewers (JW & AK) independently open-coded the first three interview transcripts using NVivo version 10 software, generating detailed, non-hierarchical lists of codes. The reviewers then met to compare and refine their list of open codes (64 codes). At this time, duplicate codes were merged and the resulting 37 codes were defined and organized into five categories: Patient Factors, Caregiver Factors, System Factors, Socioeconomic Factors and Strategies to decrease disparity. The reviewers independently coded all nine interview transcripts according to this coding framework, applying all relevant codes to capture interactions between factors. The reviewers met again to compare their application of codes. Any discrepancies were resolved through discussion. Data within each category were reviewed and grouped into sub-categories [33], which represent key factors. The researchers used visual schemata to conceptualize the relationships between factors within and between categories. Factors were continually compared against the primary data to ensure accurate representation. This iterative process of categorization and comparison was continued until no new factors emerged. Because the consistency of concepts across interviews demonstrated the stability of the coding framework (i.e. no new codes were added), and because no new factors were emerging from ongoing data abstraction, the researchers agreed that saturation had been reached [33, 36–38], and that no additional interviews were required. If, following analysis, saturation had not been reached, efforts would have been made to schedule interviews with those physicians who previously had scheduling conflicts. Given JW's position at the palliative care centre, efforts were made to recognize his own personal clinical experiences, and how they informed the analysis of the data. Any conclusions drawn were discussed with the study coordinator and examined against the data to ensure they were not unduly coloured by biases derived from his clinical experience.

Counts and percentages were calculated for Yes/No questions. Median and range were calculated for the question asking about percentage of patient population felt to be of lower SES.

Results

Participant responses to quantitative questions are presented in Table 1. All participants indicated that they had cared for patients they would consider to be of lower SES. When describing their current practice, participants indicated that on average, approximately 30%

Table 1 Participant quantitative responses

Participant	Q5: Have you ever cared for patients you would consider to be of lower socioeconomic status? (Yes or No)	Q6: What percentage of your current patent population would you consider to be of lower socioeconomic status? (%)	Q7: Do you feel that there is a difference in a patient's ability to die at home depending on if they are of lower or higher socioeconomic status? (Yes or No)
1	Yes	30	Yes
2	Yes	38	Yes
3	Yes	33	Yes
4	Yes	5–10	Yes
5	Yes	90	Yes
6	Yes	10–20	No
7	Yes	90	Yes
8	Yes	20	Yes
9	Yes	20–25	Yes

of their patients (range 7.5–90%) could be considered to be of lower socioeconomic status, reflecting the different areas served by each physician. All but one participant (89%) indicated that they believed socioeconomic status had an impact on a patient's ability to die at home.

During the 20–40 min interviews, physicians described several factors that they perceived to impact ability to die at home. These factors were grouped into three categories: patient characteristics, physical environment, and support network (Table 2). While a higher perceived SES was not identified as a primary determinant of a successful home death, it was consistently noted to strengthen the other key categories that were identified. Below, we describe each factor, how they are perceived to interact with SES, and possible strategies to decrease disparities in accessing home death.

Patient characteristics

Two patient characteristics were believed to influence a patient's ability to die at home: their preferences about place of death, and their ability to navigate the health care system. These factors were informed by perceptions of a patient's background, culture and character traits as

well as their physical, emotional or mental state that were felt to impact their likelihood of dying at home.

Patient preference was seen as a key determinant of place of death. Physicians reported that patient preference for home death was often determined by emotional factors, such as patient and caregiver discomfort, fear, or anxiety. These emotions were mainly centred around fear of coping poorly, perceived or actual burden on caregivers, and the potential lasting impact of home death on family members.

"There are some people for whom it's not a number of hours or amount of money issue, they just don't feel comfortable dying at home"… "When given the choice of palliative care unit or home, and somebody doesn't want to put their family through something, it doesn't matter if they can hire caregivers or not... because it's the emotional aspect of dying at home. Sometimes I've been told, you know, if I die here so-and-so won't be able to sleep here anymore." (Participant 1)

Many respondents attributed patient fear about home death to poor illness understanding, which was associated

Table 2 Identified categories and factors

Category	Definition	Factors
Patient Characteristics	Characteristics related to a patient's background, culture and character traits, as well as their physical, emotional or mental state were believed to influence their ability to die at home. These were described by 8/9 participants.	1. Patient preferences about place of death 2. Patient ability to navigate the health care system
Physical Environment	A patient's physical environment refers to the location (home or housing) where they will receive palliative care. Characteristics pertaining to the physical environment were believed to influence likelihood of dying at home. This was described by 8/9 participants.	1. Environment suitability to accommodate care 2. Environment stability 3. Environment safety
Support Network	The support network includes any individual who provided care or assistance to the patient during their end-of-life care trajectory. Having more support was equated with a greater likelihood of dying at home. This was described by 9/9 participants.	1. Caregiver availability and ability to organize and coordinate services 2. Ability to supplement care needs with paid-caregiving services 3. Health care provider advocacy for patient needs

with perceived lower levels of education, language barriers or lack of access to resources.

> "If [patients] don't really understand or know what to expect, then they're easily anxious and thus call a lot or go to hospital a lot because they just don't feel comfortable being at home, even though, probably, some aspects of that care can be done quite adequately at home. They just can't deal with that." (Participant 5)

Beyond preference, participants noted that patients required the ability to navigate the health care system, advocate for their health care needs, and assemble a support network. Participants felt that ability to advocate was influenced by a patient's level of education, socioeconomic status, and understanding of their disease trajectory.

> "I think the other factor, too, is whether they have somebody advocating for them, so whether they are able to know who to talk to and how to access care... Those who may not have English as the first language or those who are new, don't know who to turn to or who to ask... They don't know if they should be asking or can ask." (Participant 3)

Physical environment

Factors relating to a patient's physical environment primarily pertained to the suitability, stability and safety of their housing for meeting the needs of patients and caregivers at the end of life. A physical environment was perceived to be suitable to support home death if it was able to accommodate medical equipment and care providers, had access to the basic amenities (e.g. toilet, shower), and was free of hazards (e.g. bedbugs, vermin, mould).

> "Sometimes a place is so small or cluttered that you can't put a hospital bed in, or sometimes there are vermin in the dwelling, so [also] physical factors of them not being able to get from one place to the other, not having access to the washroom or a shower." (Participant 1)

Participants felt that patients living without access to reliable or subsidized housing were less likely to die out of an institutionalized setting.

> "It's not a widespread problem but for the people who don't have access to housing, it is a big problem" (Participant 9)

Socioeconomic status was perceived to impact these factors, insofar as poverty was associated with less suitable and more precarious housing.

The safety of the home environment also influenced the ability or willingness of providers to care for patients at home. The safety concerns described were typically associated with lower-income situations, and included residing in neighbourhoods with run down buildings, a higher prevalence of mental health issues, and substance abuse issues.

> "The other piece is safety. In a lot of these places, can we have things like opioids and controlled substances in a place where if they're alone they need to keep the door unlocked and so who is going to go in and potentially affect them... And then not only myself as a physician but the nursing staff, the safety and a lot of these places unfortunately are deemed unsafe." (Participant 3)

These perceived and actual concerns for personal safety may preclude providers from participating in a patient's after hours care.

> "One of the barriers, especially in my area is a lot of those areas are what we call 'no go' zones at night. So, if someone calls after hours or when it's dark, a doctor is not going to go out to see them because it's unsafe." (Participant 5)

Some physicians acknowledged that what constituted a suitable environment for home death can be subjective. When describing patients living in less-suitable environments, some participants appeared to remain objective when evaluating whether a patient might be able to die there.

> "In some cases you don't impose your sense of what a good home is, and I may not be willing to live in that kind of environment.... You can't impose– That's not how I would want to live or want to care for someone. I guess we kind of have insight about what we think we might need, so the running water and the shower and room to turn and manoeuvre and all the things that we think the person might need as they get sicker." (Participant 6)

Other physicians suggested that care provider bias about a patient's environment might impact where that patient ultimately dies.

> "The sad thing is that it's so integrated into how I think about patients now, almost right from the get

go. I will have a sense of 'is this going to work or is it not'. And it's not like I would say it's absolutely not going to work if the patient has very limited finances, but it's something that we address much more quickly in the visits. I almost wonder: do we end up steering the patient away from an anticipated home death because we can tell [that it will be difficult to provide end of life care]." (Participant 2)

Support networks

Support networks included any individuals who provided care or assistance to the patient during their end-of-life care trajectory. Participants highlighted three support-related factors that improved a patient's likelihood of dying at home: having family caregivers who are available and able to organize and coordinate services, being able to supplement care needs with paid-caregiving services, and having health care providers who would advocate for patient needs.

"I would say if the family and the patient, but mainly the family, are committed to making it happen at home, and they have enough numbers, possibly more than one committed family member to share the load, then I think it's possible." (Participant 2)

Like the physician above, all respondents highlighted the presence of a caregiver as the most significant factor in achieving a home death, if that is what the patient desires. Physicians noted the key role of caregivers as advocates who organized and coordinated service delivery. Socioeconomic status was perceived to influence caregiver support in two ways. Frist, participants believed that family members who are unable to take time off work for economic reasons are less available to be primary caregivers.

"I think one of the real kind of hidden ways in which socioeconomics comes into play, is when caregivers need to work in order to keep the food on the table and the rent and the hydro paid and all that... So I would love to see a situation where we supported caregivers financially to do caregiving." (Participant 9)

Second, participants felt that caregivers' abilities to advocate were associated with education level, language skills, and familiarity with the health care system. Caregiver emotional factors were also significant; discomfort with home death, or inability to cope with the demands placed on caregivers were frequently cited reasons for transitioning to an institutional setting.

Patients that were perceived to have more financial resources were frequently able to compensate for a lack of informal caregiver support by purchasing private care. This ability to afford private services was consistently described as the primary means by which socioeconomic status impacts home death.

"People with a lower socioeconomic status can't afford to pay for private health because [the home care services organization] cannot provide all the support that's required"… "I have met people who have higher…assets, and they're using those assets to pay for private care, and it makes it possible for them to stay in home because they can, essentially, purchase all of the care that they need that they would get in the palliative care unit." (Participant 1)

Finally, participants perceived health care providers as more likely to take on the responsibility for advocacy when caring for lower SES populations, noting that some clinicians go "above and beyond their duties" to get patients what they need. One explanation provided as to why clinicians were more likely to take on this responsibility for lower SES patients was recognition of the significant difference advocacy could make to patient outcomes in this population.

"In some cases if [patients] have lower socioeconomic statuses and you have people in the health care field that will advocate for you-…It's almost like you may be empathized with a little bit more because [you] have less" (Participant 5)

Strategies to decrease disparities

Participants identified increasing access to home-based support services, including home care support, personal support workers or other specialized care, as a strategy that might address SES-based disparities in patients' abilities to die at home. As a part of this support, participants felt that it would be beneficial to have a designated provider for assessing, advocating and coordinating services for lower SES patients, instead of considering this to be an extra task, above and beyond one's current duties.

"Maybe even something simple, like making it part of someone's job to do those things, to look at how much money do [the patients] have? How can the system benefit [the patient] the most and advocate for them. But not make it part of [the provider's] job so that they're going above and beyond…. But make it part of someone's job to do that, would probably be the best way [to address discrepancies]" (Participant 5)

Participants also identified enhancing support for caregivers as a strategy to improve a patient's chances of dying at home. Providing income support for necessities like food and housing was hypothesized to relieve financial and time burden, thus providing caregivers more flexibility to engage as primary caregivers at end of life."-

> Somehow providing support for their housing, for food, for being off work, and then more directly, patient care, providing more support for those people who can't afford the extra help, but do need extra help" (Participant 4)

Discussion

The aim of this study was to identify the key factors perceived to influence likelihood of home death, and describe the mechanisms by which they may interact with SES. Physicians in our study identified multiple factors that were perceived to influence the likelihood of home death. These factors emerged within three main categories: patient characteristics, physical environment, and support networks. Participants indicated that stability within each category was necessary for home death, and that strengths in one could supplement weaknesses in another. For example, a patient's ability to advocate for themselves can bolster their support system by maximizing publicly funded home support. Conversely, some deficits were too large to be compensated for by strength in other categories; for example, if a patient characteristic, such as anxiety, decreases the desire to stay at home, neither an optimal physical environment, nor a robust support system would compensate for this.

Our findings suggest that, while SES is not a primary factor in determining likelihood for home death, it may influence the other main categories of determinants. Higher SES may strengthen support networks, contribute to a more stable home environment, and increase patient comfort with home death. This finding may partially explain why some studies evaluating SES on a population level did not find SES to be a significant predictor of home death [11, 25–31]; our findings suggest that the interaction between SES and other determinants such as social support or preference for place of death is complex, and thus may be obscured in population-level studies. That SES was not identified as an independent key factor of home death in our study may also result from its examination within a home-palliative care setting. In a 2015 systematic review of patients receiving specialized home care, Chen found that receiving specialist care may decrease socioeconomic inequities in access to preferred home death [39]. Similarly, Barclay found that receiving home-hospice palliative care within a continuous care model was able to eliminate

disparities in the rates of transfer from home between patients classified as low or high income [40].

Preference for home death [11], and awareness of dying and realistic coping attitudes [41] have been cited as predictors of home death. Our participants indirectly linked SES to preference by way of illness understanding: Patients perceived to have less education, language barriers or lack of access to resources were believed to have poorer illness understanding, and therefore experienced greater discomfort with dying in the home. These findings are consistent with literature that has identified socioeconomic determinants that increase rates of preference for home death, including identifying as non-Hispanic white race [42], greater education level, greater income levels, greater awareness of advanced directives [43], and more supportive living arrangements [44]. These findings can be contrasted with earlier studies, which found that immigrant or direct descendants express a higher preference for home death [45] and a higher likelihood of dying at home [24]. Building on our findings, further research is needed to more completely characterize how socioeconomic factors influence preference for home death.

Finally, support systems comprised of informal caregivers and supplemented with paid-services and dedicated health care providers were felt to improve a patient's likelihood of home death. In Canada, informal caregivers play a significant role in the provision of home care [46–48], and have been found to be predictors of home death [11, 12, 14, 27]. De Conno (1996) found that family support was a greater predictor of home death than either financial or housing conditions [27], reflecting the value of caregiver support described by our participants. Our findings further characterize the link between SES and support networks: higher SES may improve an informal caregiver's capacity to support the patient by decreasing financial pressures, thus allowing more time for caregiving, and by compensating for gaps in informal caregiver support through greater access to paid supports. This is supported by literature. In Canada, 43% of caregivers indicated that caregiving duties disrupted their normal work routine [49]. Studies have also shown social support networks in lower SES families to have access to fewer resources, thus limiting informal caregiver capacity to provide adequate care [50, 51]. Meanwhile, caregivers with more job flexibility and disposable income are able to provide more care themselves and require fewer home care services [16]. These same caregivers may be better able to advocate for needed services [17, 20]. Finally, the economic burden that families incur while supporting home death, even within publicly funded health systems, can be significant [11, 21, 52, 53]. As Rossi et al. note in their Italian survey of family and caregivers of patients dying of cancer, a large proportion of families exhaust almost all of their savings in providing care at the end of life [54], suggesting that families with greater financial resources would face fewer barriers to home death.

Areas of potential intervention

Strengthening support networks to facilitate home death was a primary focus of our participants, which is supported by the literature. Barclay et al. demonstrated that providing more intensive, continuous home palliative care decreased socioeconomic disparities in incidence of home death [40]. Likewise, Yamagishi et al. (2012) proposed that improving 24-h support at home is required to make home death more accessible [55].

Participants noted that a focus on caregivers, through emotional support, education, and financial assistance could also improve support network robustness, thereby contributing to improved patient state of mind. This complements the findings of Milberg et al. (2014), who found that patients who felt less supported by family had higher degrees of stress, anxiety, and increased worries about personal and financial security [56].

Better education of patients and caregivers, both around illness understanding as well as the structure of the medical system, is also a potential area of intervention. There have been documented difficulties with health literacy and physician communication in lower SES populations [57], so these populations should be especially prioritized.

Limitations

We recognize that physicians' perspectives may not capture the everyday realities of patients and their families at the end of life. Indeed, physicians may perceive their low SES patients as being more dependent, less responsible and less rational than higher SES patients [58], which may manifest as lack of empathy, compassion and respect for patients resulting in poor utilization of medical services [59]. Monnickendam et al. (2007) also found that social consciousness of physicians was low, and any helping behaviours were largely detached from systemic poverty-related issues [60]. As well, our findings may not be representative of the experiences of health care providers from different disciplines and settings [18, 61, 62]. While our physician participants largely appeared to demonstrate both empathic responses to patients of lower SES, and cogent analyses of the structural impacts of poverty and the systems-level policies that may improve a patient's agency over place of death, it is important to keep in mind potential biases they may bring to this discourse.

Furthermore, we relied on a physician's perception of their patients' socioeconomic statuses, the accuracy of

which was not validated. Indeed, participants perceived a wide variation in the socioeconomic make-up of their practices, ranging from 7.5–90%. This may be partly explained by the wide geographic disparities within the city of Toronto, but may also indicate physicians' inaccurate perceptions of the socioeconomic status of their patients. Given that socioeconomic status was perceived to impact place of death, this finding illustrates potential benefit of implementing a formalized poverty screening tool, such as the one described by Brcic et al. [63]. The physicians who participated in this study provide care to patients in their homes, which may have informed their perception of their patients' SES. Previous studies have documented that visiting patients in their home can provide additional insight into the gaps patients may face in their care [64].

The generalizability of our findings may be limited due to the fact that our study was based within a publically funded health care system where patients have access to home care and specialized palliative care services, regardless of socioeconomic status. Results may not be as applicable, therefore, in jurisdictions where primary health care is not universally available.

Future research

While our exploratory data suggest relationships and dependencies among the broad categories that we identified, further research with a larger and more diverse group of informants is necessary to generate a clearer model of home death.

Our respondents did not comment at length on the factors that shape preference for place of death. They did, however, note that emotional stressors do have a significant impact on patient and family comfort with home death. Further study of the determinants of patient preference would assist in addressing any modifiable factors that may arise from socioeconomic disparity.

Conclusions

Our study provides preliminary insights into the key factors that influence home death, and defines the mechanisms by which they and socioeconomic status interact. These findings were informed by the perceptions of home palliative care physicians in an urban setting in Toronto, Canada. Our participants noted three categories of factors that affect a successful home death: patient characteristics, physical environment, and support networks. While socioeconomic status was not seen by physicians as the primary determinant of a patient's ability to die a home, a higher SES was perceived to interact with these three categories of factors by strengthening support networks, optimizing physical home environments, and increasing patient comfort with home death. Possible areas of intervention to increase access to home death focused on better support for patients and families through increased resources and advocacy. Increasing the agency of those who prefer home death in an equitable way is a public policy imperative and should be prioritized by clinicians and policy-makers.

Abbreviations
FTE: Full time equivalent; SES: Socio-economic status

Funding
This research was supported by the Temmy Latner Centre for Palliative Care.

Authors' contributions
JW, AH and AMK contributed to the conceptualization of this study. JW and AMK participated in the development of data collection tools, data analysis, data interpretation, preparation and editing of the manuscript. AMK completed data collection. All authors have read and approved the final manuscript.

Authors' information
Dr. Joshua Wales is a community palliative care physician at the Temmy Latner Centre for Palliative care. Allison Kurahashi is the Senior Educational Research Coordinator at the Temmy Latner Centre for Palliative Care. Dr. Amna Husain is an Associate Professor in the Department of Family and Community Medicine at the University of Toronto, and Research Lead and palliative care physician at the Temmy Latner Centre for Palliative Care.

Competing interests
The authors declare that they have no competing interests.

References
1. Agar M, Currow DC, Shelby-James TM, et al. Preference for place of care and place of death in palliative care: are these different questions? Palliat Med. 2008;22(7):787–95. https://doi.org/10.1177/0269216308092287.
2. Gomes B, Higginson IJ, Calanzani N, et al. Preferences for place of death if faced with advanced cancer: a population survey in England, Flanders, Germany, Italy, the Netherlands, Portugal and Spain. Ann Oncol. 2012;23(8): 2006–15. https://doi.org/10.1093/annonc/mdr602.
3. Higginson IJ, Sen-Gupta GJ. Place of care in advanced cancer: a qualitative systematic literature review of patient preferences. J Palliat Med. 2000;3(3): 287–300. https://doi.org/10.1089/jpm.2000.3.287.
4. Zimmer JG, Groth-Juncker A, McCusker J. Effects of a physician-led home care team on terminal care. J Am Geriatr Soc. 1984;32(4):288–92. https://doi.org/10.1111/j.1532-5415.1984.tb02023.x.
5. Burge F, Lawson B, Johnston G. Trends in the place of death of cancer patients, 1992-1997. CMAJ. 2003;168(3):265–70. [published Online First: 2003/02/05]
6. Gomes B, Higginson IJ. Factors influencing death at home in terminally ill patients with cancer: systematic review. Br Med J. 2006;332(February):515–8. https://doi.org/10.1136/bmj.38740.614954.55

7. Weitzen S, Teno JM, Fennell M, et al. Factors associated with site of death: a national study of where people die. Med Care. 2003;41(2):323–35. https://doi.org/10.1097/01.MLR.0000044913.37084.27.
8. Bruera E, Sweeney C, Russell N, et al. Place of death of Houston area residents with cancer over a two-year period. J Pain Symptom Manag. 2003; 26(1):637–43. [published Online First: 2003/07/10]
9. Cárdenas-Turanzas M, Carrillo MT, Tovalín-Ahumada H, et al. Factors associated with place of death of cancer patients in the Mexico City metropolitan area. Support Care Cancer. 2007;15(3):243–9. https://doi.org/10.1007/s00520-006-0152-4.
10. Gallo WT, Baker MJ, Bradley EH. Factors associated with home versus institutional death among cancer patients in Connecticut. J Am Geriatr Soc. 2001;49(6):771–7. https://doi.org/10.1046/j.1532-5415.2001.49154.x.
11. Guerriere DN, Husain A, Marshall D, et al. Predictors of place of death for those in receipt of home-based palliative Care Services in Ontario, Canada. J Palliat Care. 2015;31(2):76–88.
12. Houttekier D, Cohen J, Bilsen J, et al. Determinants of the place of death in the Brussels metropolitan region. J Pain Symptom Manag. 2009;37(6):996–1005. https://doi.org/10.1016/j.jpainsymman.2008.05.014.
13. Karlsen S, Addington-Hall J. How do cancer patients who die at home differ from those who die elsewhere? Palliat Med. 1998;12(4):279–86. https://doi.org/10.1191/026921698673427657.
14. Aoun S, Kristjanson LJ, Currow D, et al. Terminally-ill people living alone without a caregiver: an Australian national scoping study of palliative care needs. Palliat Med. 2007;21(1):29–34. https://doi.org/10.1177/0269216306073198. [published Online First: 2006/12/16]
15. Barbera L, Sussman J, Viola R, et al. Factors associated with end-of-life health service use in patients dying of Cancer. Healthc Policy. 2010;5(3):e125–43. https://doi.org/10.12927/hcpol.2013.21644.
16. Cai J, Guerriere DN, Zhao H, et al. Socioeconomic differences in and predictors of home-based palliative care health service use in Ontario, Canada. Int J Environ Res Public Health. 2017;14(7) https://doi.org/10.3390/ijerph14070802. [published Online First: 2017/07/19]
17. Howell D, Abernathy T, Cockerill R, et al. Predictors of home care expenditures and death at home for Cancer patients in an integrated comprehensive palliative home care pilot program. Healthc Policy. 2011;6(3): 73–92. https://doi.org/10.12927/hcpol.2011.22179.
18. Burge FI, Lawson B, Johnston G. Home visits by family physicians during the end-of-life: does patient income or residence play a role? BMC Palliat Care. 2005;4(1):1. https://doi.org/10.1186/1472-684X-4-1.
19. Decker SL, Higginson IJ. A tale of two cities: factors affecting place of cancer death in London and New York. Eur J Pub Health. 2007;17(3):285–90. https://doi.org/10.1093/eurpub/ckl243.
20. Grande G, Addington-Hall J, Todd C. Place of death and access to home care services: are certain patient groups at a disadvantage? Soc Sci Med. 1998;47(5):565–79. https://doi.org/10.1016/S0277-9536(98)00115-4.
21. Higginson IJ, Costantini M. Dying with cancer, living well with advanced cancer. Eur J Cancer. 2008;44(10):1414–24. https://doi.org/10.1016/j.ejca.2008.02.024.
22. Higginson IJ, Jarman B, Astin P, et al. Do social factors affect where patients die: an analysis of 10 years of cancer deaths in England. J Public Health Med. 1999;21(1):22–8. https://doi.org/10.1093/pubmed/21.1.22.
23. McCusker J. Where cancer patients die: an epidemiologic study. Public Health Rep (Washington, DC : 1974). 1983;98(2):170–6.
24. Motiwala SS, Croxford R, Guerriere DN, et al. Predictors of place of death for seniors in Ontario: a population-based cohort analysis. Can J Aging. 2006; 25(4):363–71. https://doi.org/10.1353/cja.2007.0019.
25. Fukui S, Kawagoe H, Masako S, et al. Determinants of the place of death among terminally ill cancer patients under home hospice care in Japan. Palliat Med. 2003;17(5):445–53. https://doi.org/10.1191/0269216303pm782oa. [published Online First: 2003/07/29]
26. Fukui S, Fukui N, Kawagoe H. Predictors of place of death for Japanese patients with advanced-stage malignant disease in home care settings: a nationwide survey. Cancer. 2004;101(2):421–9. https://doi.org/10.1002/cncr.20383. [published Online First: 2004/07/09]
27. De Conno F, Caraceni A, Groff L, et al. Effect of home care on the place of death of advanced cancer patients. Eur J Cancer (Oxford, England : 1990). 1996;32(7):1142–7.

28. Cantwell P, Turco S, Brenneis C, et al. Predictors of home death in palliative care cancer patients. J Palliat Care. 2000;16(1):23–8. [published Online First: 2000/05/10]

29. Fukui S, Fujita J, Tsujimura M, et al. Predictors of home death of home palliative cancer care patients: a cross-sectional nationwide survey. Int J Nurs Stud. 2011;48(11):1393–400. https://doi.org/10.1016/j.ijnurstu.2011.05.001. [published Online First: 2011/05/31]

30. Masucci L, Guerriere DN, Cheng R, et al. Determinants of place of death for recipients of home-based palliative care. J Palliat Care. 2010;26(4):279–86. [published Online First: 2011/01/28]

31. Alonso-Babarro A, Bruera E, Varela-Cerdeira M, et al. Can this patient be discharged home? Factors associated with at-home death among patients with cancer. J Clin Oncol. 2011;29(9):1159–67. https://doi.org/10.1200/JCO.2010.31.6752. [published Online First: 2011/02/24]

32. Sandelowski M. What's in a name? Qualitative description revisited. Res Nurs Health. 2009;23(4):334–40. https://doi.org/10.1002/nur.20362.

33. Elo S, Kyngas H. The qualitative content analysis process. J Adv Nurs. 2008; 62(1):107–15. https://doi.org/10.1111/j.1365-2648.2007.04569.x. [published Online First: 2008/03/21]

34. Tong A, Sainsbury P, Craig J. Consolidated criteria for reporting qualitative research (COREQ): a 32-item checklist for interviews and focus groups. Int J Qual Health Care. 2007;19(6):349–57. https://doi.org/10.1093/intqhc/mzm042. [published Online First: 2007/09/18]

35. Social Policy Analysis & Research. Profile of low income in the city of Toronto. Toronto Demographics. Toronto: City of Toronto; 2011.

36. Hennink MM, Kaiser BN, Marconi VC. Code saturation versus meaning saturation: how many interviews are enough? Qual Health Res. 2017;27(4):591–608. https://doi.org/10.1177/1049732316665344. [published Online First: 2016/09/28]

37. Kerr C, Nixon A, Wild D. Assessing and demonstrating data saturation in qualitative inquiry supporting patient-reported outcomes research. Expert Rev Pharmacoecon Outcomes Res. 2010;10(3):269–81. https://doi.org/10.1586/erp.10.30. [published Online First: 2010/06/16]

38. M. Morse J, Barrett M, Mayan M, et al. Verification strategies for establishing reliability and validity in qualitative research. Int J Qual Methods 2002;1(2):13–22. doi: https://doi.org/10.1177/160940690200100202.

39. Chen H, Nicolson DJ, Macleod U, et al. Does the use of specialist palliative care services modify the effect of socioeconomic status on place of death? A systematic review. Palliat Med. 2015; https://doi.org/10.1177/0269216315602590.

40. Barclay JS, Kuchibhatla M, Tulsky JA, et al. Association of hospice patients' income and care level with place of death. JAMA Intern Med. 2013;173(6):450–6. https://doi.org/10.1001/jamainternmed.2013.2773. [published Online First: 2013/02/20]

41. Hinton J. Which patients with terminal cancer are admitted from home care? Palliat Med. 1994;8(3):197–210. https://doi.org/10.1177/026921639400800303. [published Online First: 1994/01/01]

42. Barnato AE, Anthony DL, Skinner J, et al. Racial and ethnic differences in preferences for end-of-life treatment. J Gen Intern Med. 2009;24(6):695–701. https://doi.org/10.1007/s11606-009-0952-6. [published Online First: 2009/04/24]

43. Foreman LM, Hunt RW, Luke CG, et al. Factors predictive of preferred place of death in the general population of South Australia. Palliat Med. 2006; 20(4):447–53. https://doi.org/10.1191/0269216306pm1149oa. [published Online First: 2006/08/01]

44. Iecovich E, Carmel S, Bachner YG. Where they want to die: correlates of elderly persons' preferences for death site. Soc Work Public Health. 2009; 24(6):527–42. https://doi.org/10.1080/19371910802679341. [published Online First: 2009/10/13]

45. Schou-Andersen M, Ullersted MP, Jensen AB, et al. Factors associated with preference for dying at home among terminally ill patients with cancer. Scand J Caring Sci. 2016;30(3):466–76. https://doi.org/10.1111/scs.12265. [published Online First: 2015/09/24]

46. Donner G, Fooks C, McReynolds J, et al. Bringing care home. Toronto: Ministry of Health and Long Germ Care; 2015.

47. Sinha M, Bleakney A. Spotlight on Canadians: results from the General Social Survey. Receiving care at home. Ottawa: Statistics Canada; 2014.

48. Um S-g, Lightman N. Ensuring healthy aging for all: home care access for diverse senior populations in the GTA. Toronto: Wellesley Institute; 2016.

49. Sinha M. Spotlight on Canadians: results from the General Social Survey. Portrait of caregivers, 2012. Ottawa: Statistics Canada; 2013.

50. Lewis JM, DiGiacomo M, Currow DC, et al. Social capital in a lower socioeconomic palliative care population: a qualitative investigation of individual, community and civic networks and relations. BMC Palliat Care. 2014;13(1):30. https://doi.org/10.1186/1472-684X-13-30.

51. The Change Foundation. A profile of family caregivers in Ontario. Toronto: The Change Foundation; 2016.

52. Chochinov HM, Janson K. Dying to pay: the cost of end of life care. J Palliat Care. 1998;14(4):5–15.

53. Hanratty B, Jacoby A, Whitehead M. Socioeconomic differences in service use, payment and receipt of illness-related benefits in the last year of life: findings from the British household panel survey. Palliat Med. 2008;22(3):248–55. https://doi.org/10.1177/0269216307087140.

54. Rossi PG, Beccaro M, Miccinesi G, et al. Dying of cancer in Italy: impact on family and caregiver. The Italian survey of dying of Cancer. J Epidemiol Community Health. 2007;61(6):547–54. https://doi.org/10.1136/jech.2005.045138.

55. Yamagishi A, Morita T, Miyashita M, et al. Preferred place of care and place of death of the general public and cancer patients in Japan. Support Care Cancer. 2012;20(10):2575–82. https://doi.org/10.1007/s00520-011-1373-8.

56. Milberg A, Wåhlberg R, Krevers B. Patients' sense of support within the family in the palliative care context: what are the influencing factors? Psychooncology. 2014;23(12):1340–9. https://doi.org/10.1002/pon.3564.

57. Lewis JM, DiGiacomo M, Currow DC, et al. Dying in the margins: understanding palliative care and socioeconomic deprivation in the developed world. J Pain Symptom Manag. 2011;42(1):105–18. https://doi.org/10.1016/j.jpainsymman.2010.10.265.

58. van Ryn M, Burke J. The effect of patient race and socio-economic status on physicians' perceptions of patients. Soc Sci Med. 2000;50(6):813–28. https://doi.org/10.1016/S0277-9536(99)00338-X.

59. Stewart M, Reutter L, Makwarimba E, et al. Determinants of health-service use by low-income people. Can J Nurs Res. 2005;37(3):104–31. [published Online First: 2005/11/05]

60. Monnickendam M, Monnickendam SM, Katz C, et al. Health care for the poor—an exploration of primary-care physicians' perceptions of poor patients and of their helping behaviors. Soc Sci Med. 2007;64(7):1463–74. https://doi.org/10.1016/j.socscimed.2006.11.033.

61. Dumont S, Jacobs P, Turcotte V, et al. Palliative care costs in Canada: a descriptive comparison of studies of urban and rural patients near end of life. Palliat Med. 2015;29(10):908–17. https://doi.org/10.1177/0269216315583620. [published Online First: 2015/06/05]

62. Goodridge D, Lawson J, Rennie D, et al. Rural/urban differences in health care utilization and place of death for persons with respiratory illness in the last year of life. Rural Remote Health. 2010;10(2):1349. [published Online First: 2010/05/05]

63. Brcic V, Eberdt C, Kaczorowski J. Development of a tool to identify poverty in a family practice setting: a pilot study. Int J Family Med. 2011;2011:812182. https://doi.org/10.1155/2011/812182. [published Online First: 2012/02/09]

64. Hervada-Page M, Fayock KS, Sifri R, et al. The home visit experience: a medical student's perspective. Care Manag J. 2007;8(4):206–10. [published Online First: 2008/02/02]

16

Symptom management, nutrition and hydration at end-of-life: a qualitative exploration of patients', carers' and health professionals' experiences and further research questions

Jessica Baillie[1]*[ID], Despina Anagnostou[2], Stephanie Sivell[2], Jordan Van Godwin[3], Anthony Byrne[2] and Annmarie Nelson[2]

Abstract

Background: Symptom management is an essential aspect of palliative and end-of-life care, but evidence suggests that patients' symptoms may not always be relieved, causing significant harm to patients and magnifying their relatives' distress. A growing body of evidence focuses on symptom management at the end-of-life, but research funding for palliative care remains disproportionately low. It is therefore crucial that research funding is targeted at areas of importance to patients and relatives. The Palliative and end-of-life care Priority Setting Partnership (PeolcPSP) undertook a UK-wide free-text survey to establish research priorities within palliative and end-of-life care and disseminated its results in 2015. Much of the data were related more broadly to personal perceptions and experiences rather than specific research questions. The aim of this article is to report on a supplementary analysis exploring the experiences and questions of PeolcPSP survey respondents regarding symptoms, hydration and nutrition.

Methods: The PeolcPSP data (n = 1403) were coded by a team of qualitative researchers in a supplementary analysis. There were 190 responses that related to symptoms, nutrition and hydration. The data were analysed thematically using Braun and Clarke's approach.

Results: Five themes were identified: pain, breathlessness, agitation, nutrition and hydration. The majority of responses related to symptoms that were sub-optimally managed, in particular pain. Nutrition and hydration were of significant concern, particularly for carers. Overall, respondents consistently asked about the most effective, evidence-based methods for managing symptoms and suggested areas where further research is necessary.

Conclusions: This study highlights the perceptions and experiences of patients, families and professionals within palliative care, highlighting the need for improved care, communication and further research to establish which treatments are most effective within a palliative care population. This is essential to reduce harm and distress for patients and families.

Keywords: Symptom assessment, Pain management, Nutritional status, Dehydration, Palliative care, Terminal care, Qualitative research

* Correspondence: BaillieJ2@cf.ac.uk
[1]School of Healthcare Sciences, Cardiff University, Cardiff, UK
Full list of author information is available at the end of the article

Background

The World Health Organisation estimates that 20 million people need palliative care around the world each year [1]. In high income countries, such as the United Kingdom (UK), 69–82% of people who die need palliative care [2]. Furthermore, a recent analysis suggests that by 2040, 87. 6% of dying people will need palliative care [3]. The palliative care approach aims to improve the "quality of life of patients and their families facing the problem associated with life-threatening illness" [4]. Access to specialist palliative care has been found to increase likelihood of dying in the preferred place of care, is economically more effective and reduces symptom burden [5].

Management of symptoms, including pain, is an essential aspect of palliative care, along with psychological, spiritual and social support [4]. A recent systematic review of 143 studies of people with malignant and non-malignant conditions, identified that the following symptoms had 50% or more prevalence: pain, fatigue, anorexia, dyspnoea and worry [6]. Management of symptoms is considered a priority by relatives of people at the end of their lives [7], however patients' symptoms may not always be relieved at the end-of-life [8]. Bereaved relatives have reported traumatic experiences of patients' symptoms not being effectively managed [9, 10].

There is a growing body of evidence considering interventions to manage symptoms including (not limited to) pain, dyspnoea, vomiting, xerostomia, fatigue and agitation for patients with malignant and non-malignant palliative conditions [11–15]. Furthermore, clinical guidelines from the National Institute for Health and Care Excellence (NICE) outline pathways for managing different symptoms for adults in the last days of life: anxiety, delirium and agitation; breathlessness and noisy secretions; nausea and vomiting; supporting hydration [16]. Government policy highlights the need for appropriate and prompt management of symptoms at the end-of-life, to reduce distress for patients and their relatives [17].

In a recent editorial, Higginson [18] highlighted the need for further palliative care research and better utilisation of existing research, following the Neuberger Report [19]. Researchers have raised concerns about the small proportion of research funding allocated to palliative care, particularly in comparison to cancer research [18]. Furthermore, evidence suggests that the research priorities of researchers may not align with those of patients [20, 21], potentially leading to wasted research investment but also patients' needs not being met [22]. Therefore, Marie Curie and key stakeholder organisations established the Palliative and End of life Care Priority Setting Partnership (PeolcPSP), facilitated by the James Lind Alliance. Surveys with free-text responses have been used successfully within palliative care research to gain detailed insights into patients' and families' perspectives [23, 24]. Patients, current and bereaved carers, healthcare professionals, volunteers and members of the public were surveyed about their unanswered questions relating to palliative and end-of-life care. The top 10 research priorities were identified following the James Lind Alliance process, which focused on interventions [25, 26].

Supplementary analysis allows "a more in-depth investigation of an emergent issue or aspect of the data which was not addressed in the primary study" ([27], p.8). The PeolcPSP survey solicited free-text responses, which generated qualitative accounts of respondents' perspectives and experiences. Following completion of the James Lind Alliance protocol, it was evident that a supplementary analysis would enable analysis of the data set as a whole, including rich data exploring respondents' experiences that were not associated with interventional treatments.

The aim of this article is to report on a supplementary analysis of the experiences and questions of PeolcPSP survey respondents regarding symptoms, hydration and nutrition.

Methods

This article has been written according to the Standards for Reporting Qualitative Research (Additional file 1) [28].

PeolcPSP study design and data collection

The PeolcPSP survey, designed by members of the PeolcPSP team, asked respondents to write responses to two questions (Table 1), identify which category best described them and state where they lived in the UK. The survey ran from December 2013 until May 2014, and was available via a Survey Monkey link widely advertised and in paper format in Marie Curie hospices and nursing services. In total, 1403 completed responses were received. Each individually completed survey was downloaded into NVivo 10 (QSR International Pty Ltd. 2012) as a PDF file from Survey Monkey (San Mateo, California, USA). The paper responses were typed into a word document, checked for accuracy and uploaded onto NVivo 10 (QSR International Pty Ltd. 2012).

Supplementary data analysis

An initial coding framework for the supplementary analysis was inductively developed by AN from 200 responses and tested on 50 responses. All 1403 responses were then coded

Table 1 Survey questions

Q. What questions do you have about care, support and treatment of people who are in the last few years of their lives that could help them to live as well as possible? This could also include question(s) about care and support for current carers or families.

Q. What questions do you have about care, support and treatment of people for those rapidly approaching the end of their lives? This could also include question(s) about care and support for current or bereaved carers or families looking after someone at the end of life.

in NVivo 10 (QSR International Pty Ltd. 2012) by a team of qualitative researchers (JB, DA, SS, JVG) using the coding framework, which was adapted as coding progressed to reflect the breadth of the data [29]. The research team (JB, DA, SS, JVG, AB and AN) met weekly during the study period to discuss the coding of the data, whether additional codes had been added to the framework, and – rarely – to resolve any discrepancies through discussion. In total, 190 responses (14%) related to symptoms, nutrition and hydration.

The data relating to symptoms and nutrition/hydration were then analysed thematically by two researchers (JB and DA). Thematic analysis, using Braun and Clarke's approach, [30] was chosen as it is a flexible approach that can provide a detailed and complex interpretation of the data. This involved:

1. familiarisation with the data through reading and rereading (as described above);
2. generating initial codes using NVivo that described features of the data (as described above);
3. searching for themes and grouping codes into potential themes;
4. reviewing and refining themes;
5. defining and naming themes;
6. producing the written report outlining the themes and final analysis [30].

Respondents

In total, 190 individual responses related to symptoms and nutrition/hydration. Respondents could choose multiple categories that they felt best described them, e.g., bereaved carer and professional. Therefore, as outlined in Table 2, respondents identified as patients (n = 8),

Table 2 Survey Respondents

Respondent (Reporting ID)	Responses relating to symptoms
I am in the last few years of my life (Patient)	8
I am a carer or family member or partner or friend of someone in the last few years of their life (Current carer)	24
I am a bereaved carer or family member or friend (Bereaved Carer)	60
I am a professional working with people in the last few years of life (Professional)	89
I am a volunteer working with people in the last few years of life (Volunteer)	4
I am a member of the public who has an interest in the subject (Member of Public)	27
Other	23
Total	n = 235 Individual responses: n = 190

current carers (n = 24), bereaved carers (n = 60), professionals (n = 89), volunteers (n = 4), members of the public (n = 27) and people who selected "other" (n = 23). Forty respondents identified in more than one category; the volunteers (n = 4) all identified as current or bereaved carers. Fourteen healthcare professionals identified in multiple categories as: a patient (n = 1), patient and current carer (n = 1), bereaved carer (n = 7), current carer (n = 4), and a bereaved and current carer (n = 1). Of the 12 respondents who selected "other", 10 identified as a current or bereaved carer. Nine of the current carers also reported as being bereaved.

Ethical considerations

Respondents were asked to consent to their participation in the PeolcPSP survey, following a written explanation of the study. The responses were stored on a secure server, only accessible to the research team. Respondents were not asked for identifiable personal information, but responses were anonymised at the point of analysis if respondents included information that could identify them in their responses. Ethical approval was deemed not necessary for the PeolcPSP survey and supplementary analysis by the study sponsor.

Rigour

The integrity of the supplementary analysis was promoted in three ways. The analysis included the perspectives of multiple groups of respondents, including patients, carers and healthcare professionals, thus increasing the credibility of the study [31]. The data were coded by multiple researchers and the data relating to symptoms were analysed by two researchers (JB and DA), enhancing the trustworthiness of the study findings [32, 33]. Furthermore, the researchers – experienced healthcare professionals or health service researchers - recognised their impact on the research process and sought to be reflexive [34], which was again aided through co-coding and analysis of the data.

Results

Overall, this study identifies that respondents perceive there to be scope and need for improvement in symptom management for individuals at the end-of-life. The following themes and subthemes were identified (see Fig. 1) and are discussed in turn: pain (assessment, management and place of care); breathing difficulties (management and respiratory secretions); terminal agitation (assessment and sedation); nutrition (determining need and enteral feeding); and hydration (thirst, risk, artificial hydration and Liverpool Care Pathway).

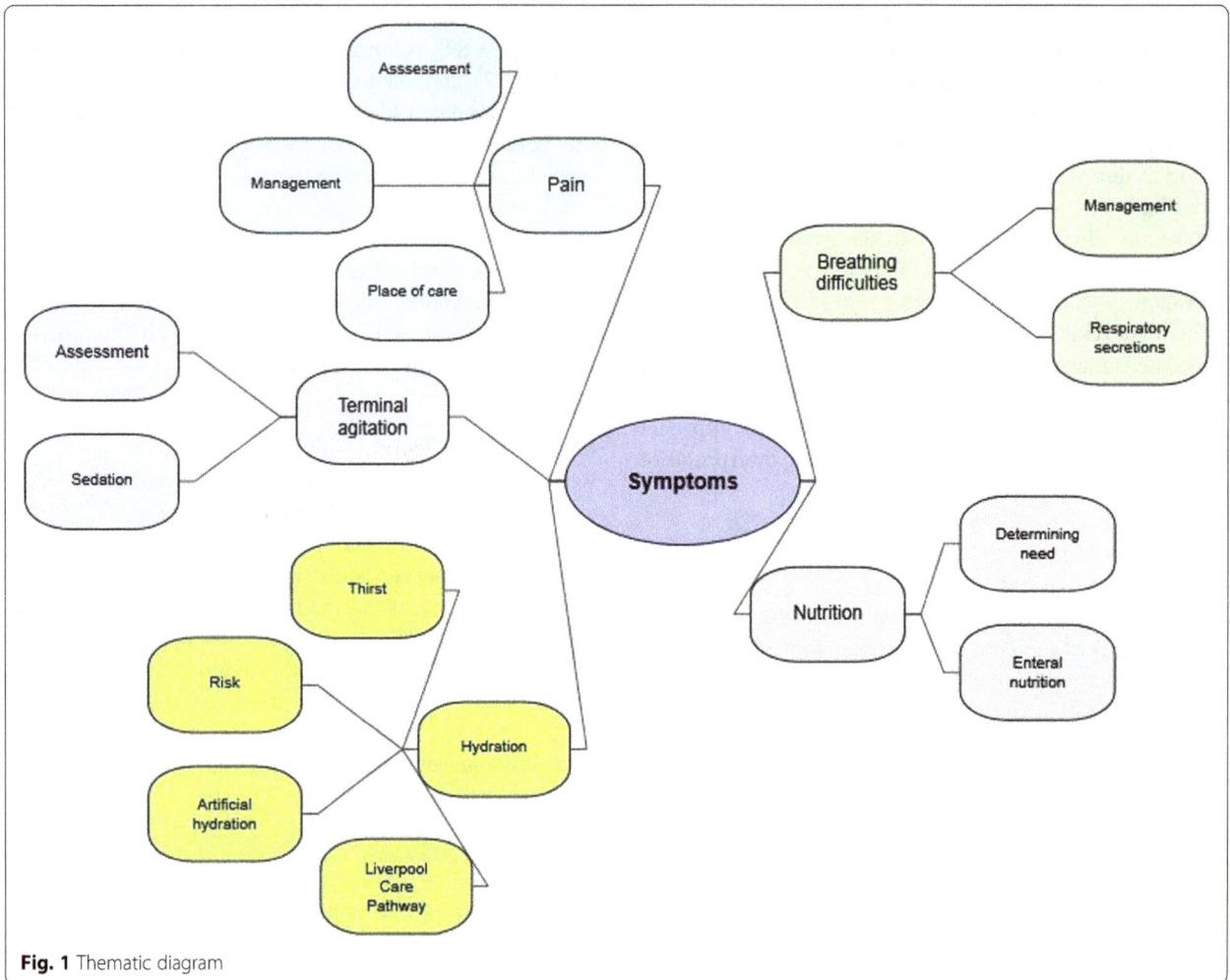

Fig. 1 Thematic diagram

Pain

Pain was the symptom most discussed by respondents. Interestingly, few responses came from people identifying as being in the last few years of life. Primarily responses were from healthcare professionals and current or bereaved carers. Respondents discussed pain assessment, management and the impact of place of care.

Assessment

The need for effective pain assessment was highlighted as an important issue by bereaved carers and healthcare professionals. Of note, carers questioned how they would know if their relative (the patient) was in pain, which was viewed as particularly problematic if the patient had a degree of cognitive impairment or were unable to express themselves verbally. Multiple responses related to dementia and concern about how pain can be assessed in patients with this diagnosis:

"How to tell when someone in the very end stages of dementia is in pain and or distress" (R855 - Other - My husband died last year)

Respondents questioned whether methods for assessing pain in people unable to communicate verbally, or with cognitive impairment, were adequate and evidence-based. One healthcare professional, whose son had died from a brain tumour, called for more appropriate methods of assessing pain in people unable to verbally communicate, recognising that pain is a subjective experience:

"How can we assess pain in people who are semi-conscious or under high doses of drugs?...I realise pain can be subjective, but it would be worth looking to develop better pain tools for those who are unable to communicate (either due to level of consciousness, impact of drugs, or due to the condition such as MND or stroke." (R1064 - Bereaved Carer; Professional)

Management

Healthcare professional competencies Respondents questioned whether healthcare professionals would be competent and confident to effectively manage their relative's pain. Respondents highlighted that pain management was a central aspect of palliative care and their primary concern for people at the end-of-life was that they were pain free. Carer respondents sought reassurance that healthcare professionals would manage their dying relatives' pain appropriately and ensure they were comfortable:

> "How do I know that my relative will be pain free at the end of life, will he/she be properly cared for by professional people" (R1376 – Current Carer)

However, others – primarily bereaved carers - shared their upsetting experiences of their relatives being in pain at the end of their lives. The use of evocative language in the quote below conveys the respondent's deep feelings about their experience:

> "Mummy said to me that why was she suffering so when she had been so good all her life and was this the medieval age as she was being tortured?" (R339 – Bereaved Carer)

Several respondents reflected on the reticence of healthcare professionals to prescribe or administer adequate analgesia as a particular barrier to achieving pain control. While one respondent described nurses refusing to give morphine to their dying relative, another queried why healthcare professionals were seemingly wary of administering analgesia:

> "why is it that people who are delegated tasks e.g. pain control are often frightened to do their job - with drugs often late or ineffective?" (R272 – Member of Public)

One bereaved carer described a General Practitioner refusing to prescribe analgesia for their dying mother:

> "she was restless, unable to settle and clutching at her chest which made me think she was in a lot of pain. Eventually the staff agreed to call out the on-call GP, who came quickly but said he couldn't give her a pain killing injection as it might kill her, although she was clearly dying; in fact she did die within an hour or two of his visit." (R812 – Bereaved Carer)

Models of care Respondents offered recommendations for how to improve pain management. A member of the public suggested measures to ensure appropriate, timely pain management for patients. One suggestion included the use of technology such as Skype to enable a healthcare professional to assess a patient without the need for a home visit or the patient attending a clinic:

> "pain control needs to be faster, more comprehensive, run by skype, run by experts who can actually prescribe, by people who are not frightened to prescribe and make people comfortable - why is this often not the case?" (R272 – Member of Public)

Managing non-malignant pain Many respondents questioned the most effective ways of managing pain for patients with non-malignant conditions, including motorneurone disease, Parkinson's and heart failure. For example, a carer asked:

> "What sort of help works best - control of pain and other symptoms, ensuring no restlessness or distress? What is best for those with dementia or heart trouble or other conditions?" (R409 – Current Carer, Bereaved Carer)

Place of care
Respondents felt strongly that place of care affected the likelihood of adequate pain management. In terms of hospital care, there was concern that pain relief was not planned for, and patients would not be prescribed adequate levels of analgesia by non-palliative care professionals. A bereaved carer questioned whether non-palliative care professionals need more support to care for patients who are reaching the end of their lives:

> "Pain and symptom control is so important, however it is not always delivered in a timely way in hospital. Why do junior doctors find it difficult to prescribe the analgesia in the doses prescribed by the hospice? Do they need more support?" (R1049 – Bereaved Carer, Member of Public)

Conversely, there was unease from other respondents that individuals being cared for at home would not receive effective pain management:

> "Support is just not there for people in the last weeks of life for whom medication at home is not adequate to control pain." (R801 – Bereaved Carer)

Much of the worry about pain management at home related to out-of-hours care provision and whether patients could quickly access analgesia when required;

these concerns were reiterated by a palliative care nurse and a patient:

> "Why does it still take so long to get someone to come and give pain relief etc. out of hours? The patients should be able to get pain relief etc. very quickly." (R998 - Other - I am a Marie Curie Nurse)

> "how do I deal with things such as nausea, tooth problems and debilitating pain, which can strike at any time (but typically do strike at weekends/pubic holidays)?" (R1165 – Patient)

Place of care was an important issue for carers who lived with feelings of guilt if they were unable to fulfil their relative's end-of-life wishes. One bereaved carer discussed her feeling of failure that she could not manage her late mother's pain at home:

> "I would have liked her to be able to die at home, that was what she wanted, but I wasn't sure if I could manage her pain and whether getting the Hospice at Home care team there when needed would be feasible. I know I let her down over this." (R398 – Current Carer, Bereaved Carer)

Breathing difficulties

Breathing difficulties as a symptom was mentioned less frequently than pain, but was a consistent concern for respondents, who were primarily bereaved/current carers and healthcare professionals. Respondents discussed management of breathing difficulties and respiratory secretions.

Management

Respondents questioned the best treatment for breathlessness and discussed the most appropriate time for treatment to commence. One respondent asked when pulmonary rehabilitation should be started for patients with Chronic Obstructive Pulmonary Disease (COPD):

> "Not all COPD patients have access to pulmonary rehabilitation despite NICE guidelines, and there is potential to improve their understanding, exercise tolerance and overall progression if targeted at the right time. But when is this?" (R75 - Professional)

Another respondent questioned how support for people with respiratory problems can be improved and whether intervention for breathlessness improves quality of life:

> "We currently have no way of measuring if we are having any impact on a patient's quality of life following input from a physiotherapist, or medical input to manage breathlessness. It would also be beneficial to know if we were able to see patients like this slightly earlier in the disease process, whether we could improve their quality of life for longer." (R75 - Professional)

Respiratory secretions

Respondents asked a series of questions related to terminal respiratory secretions, primarily suggesting that this symptom is poorly managed and asking the reasons for this:

> "Why is symptom control of respiratory secretions so poorly managed?" (R1235 – Patient, Current Carer, Professional, Member of the public)

Professionals recognised that this symptom is also upsetting for families:

> "Why do we not have effective treatment for the management of respiratory secretions? This problem causes distress for many families who care for and are therefore dealing with this distressing symptom." (R822 - Professional)

Terminal agitation

Respondents queried how agitation is best assessed and managed through the use of sedation. One respondent argued for a change in the diagnosis and subsequent treatment of "terminal agitation" through recognising it as "hyperactive delirium":

> "Terminal agitation is a term that has little meaning. Hyperactive delirium at the end of life is a more accurate description. The difference is important since the former is traditionally treated with midazolam while the latter sets in train an assessment and management of the cause and, if drugs are needed, non-sedative haloperidol becomes first choice. An evaluation of end of life hyperactive delirium is long overdue." (R907 - Professional)

Assessment

Several respondents recognised the need for appropriate identification and assessment of terminal agitation, questioning whether biochemical markers can be used to properly diagnose this condition:

"Are there biochemical markers that can help ascertain patients with terminal agitation?" (R1331 - Professional)

Sedation
The majority of responses in the agitation theme focused on management, specifically sedation. Carers discussed their negative experiences where sedatives were either not prescribed, or were not effective for their relative. Healthcare professional respondents questioned which sedative was most effective for agitated patients at the end-of-life, and how to ensure adequate doses of sedation are prescribed:

"What is the most effective way to use sedation (e.g. during terminal restlessness) - in order to get the balance right between not giving too much but at the same time giving enough to ease distress." (R578 - Other - I am a professional now working in another speciality but worked in palliative care between 1997 and 2003)

While respondents recognised the need to treat agitation, there was apprehension about the effect of sedation on the patient. Respondents were worried that carers were not given sufficient information about sedation, which could cause distress. There was also concern that sedation could make communication between the patient and relative difficult, cause nightmares, and hasten death, prompting one respondent to enquire about the effect on the person who has been sedated:

"When people are sedated, are they really unaware of pain/what is being done to them/voices of those they love/extraneous noise from adjacent patients and ward activity? Or are they trapped in a situation where they are aware but cannot tell us? How do we know? How do we know when a person is unconscious rather than sedated?" (R320 – Current Carer, Professional)

Nutrition
Nutrition was discussed in terms of the longer palliative phase and respondents highlighted the importance of determining patients' nutritional needs and the role of enteral nutrition.

Determining need
Several respondents indicated that further research was required to determine the nutritional needs of people towards the end of their lives. They suggested that identifying nutritional markers would enable healthcare

professionals to identify when patients' nutritional needs are changing. One healthcare professional felt a stronger evidence base would enable carers to feel reassured if the person at the end of their life reduced their dietary intake:

"I have had so many experiences of relatives and professional carers distressed because their loved one/service user hasn't eaten properly. It would be great to be able to re-assure them from the strong position of empirical evidence that their relative is not distressed." (R1320 - Professional)

Enteral nutrition
There were many responses from healthcare professionals querying the role of enteral nutrition for people at the end-of-life. Respondents felt a stronger evidence base was needed regarding if and when enteral nutrition should be administered. Others discussed patients' information needs and decision-making, including support given to patients to commence and withdraw nutritional support:

"How realistic is the information given to patients regarding PEG feeds... Are they made fully aware that feeding would naturally diminish as the patient deteriorates and that it is therefore not appropriate to be giving 2000 calories in the last weeks/days of life." (R349 – Professional)

Responses from bereaved carers discussed distressing experiences of enteral nutrition, which highlighted poor communication and lack of respect for patient autonomy. One respondent discussed her father, who had a living will refusing artificial nutrition, being repeatedly asked about having enteral nutrition during the last 4 weeks of his life:

"We found it very hard, because the feeding tube was mentioned again and again, and it was difficult to constantly having to defend his and our decision. The question is: How can health care professionals be persuaded that it is ok not to want a feeding tube and that this is down to patient choice and often better for the patient." (R687 – Bereaved Carer)

Hydration
Responses to hydration focused on the last few days of life and considered thirst, risk, the role of intravenous and subcutaneous fluids, and bereaved carers sharing their experiences of hydration and the Liverpool Care Pathway (LCP).

Thirst

Several respondents were concerned about patients being thirsty at the end of their lives. One bereaved carer asked whether it is "cruel" not to hydrate patients, while another questioned whether individuals experience a dry mouth or thirst:

> "We say that people who do not want to drink at the end of life do not experience thirst, just dry mouth. How do we know?" (R320 – Current Carer, Professional)

Risk

Conversely, respondents recognised the risks associated with patients drinking if they have dysphagia. A healthcare professional, who also identified as a bereaved carer, highlighted inconsistent practice, which demonstrated the need for communication between patients, carers and healthcare professionals:

> "How to balance providing fluids to those who are dying who cannot swallow safely or easily? The practice of maintaining hydration/nutrition seems variable and inconsistent across patients/hospitals. How can the withdrawal of these be done in a sensitive and consensual way for person, family and medical/caring staff?" (R329 – Bereaved Carer, Professional, Member of Public)

Artificial hydration

Following on from these concerns about patients being unable to swallow and thus experiencing thirst, respondents asked about the role of intravenous and subcutaneous fluids. Healthcare professionals questioned whether administration of fluids makes patients more comfortable:

> "In the last few days of life families often worry about their loved ones not being given fluids, as a result they are often prescribed subcutaneous fluids. Does this really make the patient more comfortable or not?" (R12 - Professional)

Respondents recognised the concerns of carers and called for further research to identify the support needs of carers when managing artificial hydration for a dying person:

> "I think families of dying patients would benefit from research on ways to support them in coming to terms with the withdrawal of IV drips and hydration in the last days of life. I'm convinced this is the source of

much dissatisfaction with end of life care." (R275 – Bereaved Carer)

Another respondent suggested that research is needed to holistically evaluate the role of intravenous fluids for dying patients:

> "What are the advantages and disadvantages (physical, social, psychological) of parenteral hydration towards end of life - balancing appropriate hydration with the body's natural ceasing of normal function (also bearing in mind the distress that can be caused when a body cannot cope with increased hydration; the potential for medical 'kit' acting as barrier between patient and loved ones towards end of life etc)." (R578 - Other - I am a professional now working in another speciality but worked in palliative care between 1997 and 2003.)

Liverpool Care Pathway

Hydration was an emotive subject for bereaved carers, who shared distressing stories of relatives' deaths, revealing their guilt, anger and sorrow about the Liverpool Care Pathway (LCP). One individual recalled her mother's death and her residual feelings of guilt that, following the Neuberger Report [19], her mother died feeling thirsty:

> "My mother died of breast cancer in the hospice in [names town]. My questions would have been about the Liverpool pathway - it still haunts me whether we did the right thing, and now that it has been stopped, I live with a terrible feeling of guilt that my suspicions were right. It felt wrong to stop fluids but the doctor told me she would effectively drown if they were continued. My mother kept trying to speak to me but was too weak, and I couldn't make out what she was saying. I am so afraid that she was asking for water." (R398 – Current Carer, Bereaved Carer)

One respondent spoke in even stronger terms about the LCP and described their relative as being "put to death":

> "We as a family have not been able to grieve for our mother who was taken away from us, she was put to death on the LCP and nothing was explained, we were told this is what's going to happen now!! There was no dignity watching my mother gasp for breath over 4 days, she was denied food and water, why was this." (R502 – Current Carer, Other - I watched my mother suffer for 4 days on the LCP)

While one respondent questioned how oral fluids could be stopped without an assessment from a speech and language therapist, other respondents asked why their relatives were not given artificial hydration when they could no longer swallow. A bereaved carer asked why the LCP denied artificial hydration, which resulted in them "begging" healthcare professionals for help, highlighting the importance of appropriate communication and engagement with carers at the end-of-life:

> "My mother was refused a drip in her final days. As an effect of her brain tumour, she ceased to be able to swallow on 26th December... she was incredibly thirsty and dehydrated but was - despite me begging for help - refused IV fluids even though they would have made her more comfortable. It appears that the Liverpool Pathway specifically denies fluids as part of end of life 'care'" (R422 – Bereaved Carer)

Discussion

Undertaking a supplementary analysis of the PeolcPSP data provided a rich insight into the perspectives of 190 patients, carers and healthcare professionals from across the UK. The findings overwhelmingly highlighted that patients, carers, healthcare professionals and members of the public view symptom management as an essential aspect of palliative and end-of-life care. These findings, when located in the broader healthcare context, prompt consideration of evidence-based symptom management, place of care, and specialist/generalist palliative care.

Evidence-based symptom management

Despite continuing advances in the field of palliative care, symptoms such as pain and breathlessness remain at the forefront of the concerns of clinicians, patients and families [11]. Poorly controlled symptoms have been documented in patients with malignant and non-malignant conditions [35–37], which was reflected in this supplementary analysis.

Bereaved carers in this supplementary analysis expressed concern that pain was under recognised in people unable to verbally communicate, including people with dementia. A recent meta-analysis identified multiple pain assessment tools for patients with dementia, but there was insufficient information on their validity [38]. Furthermore, several non-verbal pain assessment tools have been developed, although a review concluded these tools do not determine level of pain and further research is needed to test the tools with different patient populations [39]. Notably, this supplementary analysis highlights that some carers perceive that the patient's pain is not being assessed, suggesting that healthcare professionals may not be assessing pain in people with dementia or who are non-verbal, or they are not communicating their assessment to carers. A recent qualitative case study identified that pain assessment tools

were not used in practice with patients with dementia, nor were carers included in the pain assessment process [38]. They propose a new decision support tool for hospital-based healthcare professionals to assess pain in patients with dementia [38]. This supplementary analysis highlighted that carers want to know how to assess if their relative is in pain, and further consideration is therefore needed of carers' role in pain assessment.

This supplementary analysis identified some carers' concerns that doctors were under-prescribing analgesia, resulting in the patient experiencing pain. Specifically, respondents questioned the wariness of some doctors to prescribe analgesia for their dying relatives, including one respondent who reported a GP's concerns that he would hasten the death of her mother. Conversely, the Neuberger Report into the LCP highlighted that some carers suspected that the administration of opioids had hastened the death of their relatives [19]. Doctors' reluctance in prescribing and administering strong analgesics at the end-of-life, due to fear of hastening patient death, has been documented [40]. A recent systematic review of the influence of opioids on survival of advanced cancer patients, showed that there is no evidence associating the use of opioids for symptom control in advanced disease with patient survival [41]. Recently, the British Medical Association (BMA) released guidelines for doctors about the use of analgesia for pain management at the end-of-life, aiming to improve analgesic use [42]. They reiterated that there is insufficient evidence that appropriately prescribed analgesia hastens death but reiterated doctors' concerns about this.

Unfortunately, many respondents highlighted poor experiences of care where carers' perceptions were that their relatives were denied food and drinks towards the end of their lives. Eating and drinking is an area that resonates with families due to its familiarity; families may see nutrition and hydration as a basic form of nurturing for their dying relative [43]. Responses in this survey related to the now-withdrawn LCP; the Neuberger Report similarly raised concerns about withholding nutrition and hydration [19]. Guidelines outlining hydration and nutrition at the end-of-life were subsequently developed by the Royal College of Nursing (RCN) [44]; General Medical Council (GMC) guidelines to support decision making were published in 2010 [43]. The impact of these guidelines on practice is unknown at present.

Healthcare professional respondents asserted the need to determine patients' nutrition and hydration needs at the end-of-life, including whether patients' nutritional needs diminish as disease progresses, and whether patients feel the sensation of thirst (rather than dry mouth). Respondents argue that establishing answers to these questions would enable healthcare professionals to reassure carers, reducing distress. A recent literature review identified that carers experienced greater distress than patients at reduced nutrition and water intake, leading to attempts at "force feeding" (p. 919) and pressuring their relatives to eat and drink, hoping this would increase survival and quality of life [45]. Artificial hydration and nutrition were viewed positively by these carers [45]. Conversely, this supplementary analysis revealed that some respondents were frustrated when artificial hydration was encouraged against the patient's or family's wishes. The Department of Health reports that there remains insufficient high quality evidence regarding assisted nutrition and hydration for patients at the end-of-life [46].

This supplementary analysis demonstrated the necessity for further research into symptom, nutrition and hydration assessment and management. While research was specifically mentioned by healthcare professionals and one carer, other carers asked questions that research may answer. High quality randomised controlled trials (RCT) are critical to test interventions in palliative care, ultimately informing clinical care [47]. Currently, the prevalence and impact of symptoms at the end-of-life are underestimated [48, 49]. Recent RCTs demonstrate the feasibility and necessity for high quality, phase three clinical trials for improving symptom control in this patient population [50–53]. Studies conducted to date have shown that care can be improved [53, 54], patients have a substantial burden of symptoms [49], and that the toxicity and harm of some interventions not underpinned by high quality evidence is underestimated [52, 55]. It is therefore imperative for palliative care to engage further with high quality research.

Place of care

Respondents had concerns about place of care and whether symptoms, in particular pain, would be better managed in hospital or at home. A large UK survey identified that members of the public associated pain relief with hospital and only 27% of respondents thought they would be pain-free at home at the end of their lives. [54] This was despite 78% of respondents expressing a wish to die at home [56]. A recent systematic review identified that family caregivers viewed hospital as an unsuitable location for palliative care [57]. However, distressing symptoms made home care difficult and, over time, led to hospital being viewed as the preferable option [57]. The Neuberger Report highlighted the concerns of carers that their relatives did not receive adequate and appropriate analgesia in hospital settings at the end of their lives [19]. The recent VOICES survey in England reported that bereaved individuals considered pain management in the last 3 months of life to be more effective in the hospice environment and least effective at home [10]. There are thus conflicting views about which location of care is associated with perceived

improvement in symptom management. This was further reflected in this supplementary analysis, which highlighted that respondents were unhappy with pain relief in both home and hospital. Researchers have attempted to establish whether home or hospital is associated with improved symptom control, although results are inconclusive [58]. However, one Cochrane systematic review identified a small, but statistically significant improvement in symptom burden in patients who received specialist palliative care at home [59].

Research consistently concludes that home is the preferred place of care at the end of life for a majority of people with both malignant and non-malignant conditions [60–62], and their carers [57]. Symptoms are one aspect of complex decisions about place of care and this supplementary analysis emphasised that management of symptoms – particularly pain – is a central concern for patients, carers, healthcare professionals and members of the public. It is crucial that high quality evidence around symptom management is established and utilised [19], to ensure that patients' symptoms are effectively managed, regardless of care location.

Non-specialist palliative care

Respondents reported dissatisfaction with symptom management by non-specialist palliative care healthcare professionals and questioned whether there was a need for enhanced support to manage symptoms for people with advanced disease. Many patients may not be identified as having palliative care needs, and will therefore not be referred to specialist palliative care teams or specialist palliative care settings at the end-of-life [63]. It is therefore important for increased knowledge transfer of symptom management to both generalists and specialists [64]. A recent review of the current evidence of pharmacological and non-pharmacological interventions for symptom management, produced guidelines for the management of multiple symptoms, aiming to support generalists in the provision of comfort care [65]. Furthermore, in the UK, the NICE pathway outlines symptom management for adults in the last days of life [16].

Recommendations

Further high quality research for symptom management, including RCTs, is needed and crucially needs to be utilised, to ensure patients' symptoms are managed across care locations. Furthermore, the role of assisted nutrition and hydration for patients at the end-of-life requires investigation, including patients' and families' perspectives. The role of carers in assessing their relatives' pain needs to be considered, in particular educational support for carers if they are to adopt this role. Finally, the impact of guidelines and responsibilities from the RCN and GMC regarding end-of-life care requires evaluation.

Limitations

While the researchers were unable to clarify respondents' reports, or illicit further in-depth information as would be standard in a qualitative interview, the respondents focused on areas of interest to them, without influence from the researchers. Although the researchers were unable to confirm the identity of respondents, due to the anonymous nature of the data, the detailed responses were congruent with individuals who had experience of the phenomena they described. Overwhelmingly respondents identified as being healthcare professionals and current or bereaved carers, with only eight patient respondents who mentioned symptom control. However, the focus of carers' and healthcare professionals' responses was the patient and ensuring their symptoms were managed effectively.

Conclusions

The article has reported on a supplementary analysis of the experiences and questions of the PeolcPSP survey respondents regarding symptoms, hydration and nutrition. Concerns about uncontrolled symptoms and quality of care have been identified from across the respondent groups. Robust, high-quality research investigating the best interventions and medications to manage symptoms will reduce distress for both patients and families, and reduce possible harm of current treatments. Management of symptoms should be equitable across different care settings, to enable patients to remain and die in their preferred place of care. Finally, and possibly unexpectedly, a proportion of healthcare professionals both identified themselves and responded as clinicians, and patients or carers. Palliative care is everybody's business and the results of this supplementary analysis highlight the need for urgent efforts to improve patient care, sustained by a solid research evidence base.

Abbreviations

BMA: British Medical Association; COPD: Chronic obstructive pulmonary disease; GMC: General Medical Council; LCP: Liverpool Care Pathway; NICE: National Institute for Health and Care Excellence; PeolcPSP: Palliative and end-of-life care Priority Setting Partnership; RCN: Royal College of Nursing; RCT: Randomised controlled trial; UK: United Kingdom

Acknowledgements

Our thanks go to all of our respondents, to everyone who helped disseminate the survey, to the ESRC, Katherine Cowan, Dr. Sabine Best and the PeolcPSP steering group for their support for this supplementary project.

Funding

This work was supported by Marie Curie core grant funding to the Marie Curie Palliative Care Research Centre, Cardiff University, grant reference number MCCC-FCO-11-C.

Authors' contributions

AN conceived, designed and oversaw the project, coded the data, and contributed to the drafting of the paper. JB and DA coded and analysed the data, and drafted the paper. SS, JVG and AB coded the data and contributed to the drafting of the paper. All authors read and approved the final manuscript.

Competing interests

The authors declare that they have no competing interests.

Author details

[1]School of Healthcare Sciences, Cardiff University, Cardiff, UK. [2]Marie Curie Palliative Care Research Centre, Division of Population Medicine, School of Medicine, Cardiff University, Cardiff, UK. [3]DECIPHer, School of Social Sciences, Cardiff University, Cardiff, UK.

References

1. World Health Organization. Global atlas of palliative care at the end of life. http://www.who.int/nmh/Global_Atlas_of_Palliative_Care.pdf; 2014.
2. Murtagh F, Bausewein C, Verne J, Groeneveld E, Kaloki Y, Higginson I. How many people need palliative care? A study developing and comparing methods for population-based estimates. Palliat Med. 2014;28(1):49–58.
3. Etkind S, Bone A, Gomes B, Lovell N, Evans C, Higginson I, et al. How many people will need palliative care in 2040? Past trends, future projections and implications for services. BMC Med. 2017;15(1):102.
4. World Health Organization. WHO definition of palliative care. http://www.who.int/cancer/palliative/definition/en/; 2017.
5. Dixon J, King D, Matosevic T, Clark M, Knapp M. Equity in the provision of palliative care in the UK: review of evidence. Personal Social Services Research Unit; London School of Economics and Political Science. http://www.pssru.ac.uk/archive/pdf/4962.pdf; 2015.
6. Moens K, Higginson I, Harding R. Are there differences in the prevalence of palliative care-related problems in people living with advanced cancer and eight non-cancer conditions? A systematic review. J Pain Symptom Manag. 2014;48(4):660–77.
7. Stajduhar K, Funk L, Cohen S, Williams A, Bidgood D, Allan D, et al. Bereaved family members' assessments of the quality of end-of-life care: what is important? J Palliat Care. 2011;27(4):261–9.
8. Solano J, Gomes B, Higginson I. A comparison of symptom prevalence in far advanced cancer, AIDS, heart disease, chronic obstructive pulmonary disease and renal disease. J Pain Symptom Manag. 2006;31(1):58–69.
9. Gallagher R, Krawczyk M. Family members' perceptions of end-of-life care across diverse locations of care. BMC Palliat Care. 2013;12:25.
10. Office for National Statistics. National survey of bereaved people (VOICES): England, 2015. https://www.ons.gov.uk/peoplepopulationandcommunity/healthandsocialcare/healthcaresystem/bulletins/nationalsurveyofbereavedpeoplevoices/england2015#main-points. 2015.

11. Lorenz KA, Lynn J, Dy SM, Shugarman LR, Wilkinson A, Mularski RA, et al. Evidence for improving palliative care at the end of life: a systematic review. Ann Intern Med. 2008;148(2):147–59.

12. Dy S. Evidence-based approaches to pain in advanced cancer. Cancer J. 2010;16(5):500–6.

13. Gilbertson-White S, Aouizerat B, Jahan T, Miaskowski C. A review of the literature on multiple symptoms, their predictors, and associated outcomes in patients with advanced cancer. Palliat Support Care. 2011;9(1):81–102.

14. von Gunten C. Interventions to manage symptoms at the end of life. J Palliat Med. 2005;8(Suppl 1):S88–94.

15. Wilkie D, Ezenwa M. Pain and symptom management in palliative care and at end of life. Nurs Outlook. 2012;60(6):357–64.

16. National Institute for Health and Care Excellence. Managing symptoms for an adult in the last days of life. https://www.nice.org.uk/guidance/ng31; 2017.

17. Welsh Government. Palliative and end of life care delivery plan. http://gov. wales/docs/dhss/publications/170327end-of-lifeen.pdf; 2017.

18. Higginson IJ. Research challenges in palliative and end of life care. BMJ Support Palliat Care. 2016;6(1):2–4.

19. Neuberger J. More care, less pathway: a review of the Liverpool Care Pathway. https://www.gov.uk/government/uploads/system/uploads/attachment_data/file/212450/Liverpool_Care_Pathway.pdf; 2013.

20. Crowe S, Fenton M, Hall M, Cowan K, Chalmers I. Patients', clinicians' and the research communities' priorities for treatment research: there is an important mismatch. Res Involv Engagem. 2015;1:2.

21. Tallon D, Chard J, Dieppe P. Relation between agendas of the research community and the research consumer. Lancet. 2000;355:2037–40.

22. Chalmers I, Bracken M, Djulbegovic B, Garattini S, Grant J, Gülmezoglu A, et al. How to increase value and reduce waste when research priorities are set. Lancet. 2014;383:156–65.

23. Bowyer A, Finlay I, Baillie J, Byrne A, McCarthy JS, C, Snow V, et al. Gaining an accurate reflection of the reality of palliative care through the use of free-text feedback in questionnaires: the AFTER study. BMJ Support Palliat Care. 2016.doi:https://doi.org/10.1136/bmjspcare-2015-000920.

24. Sampson C, Finlay I, Byrne A, Snow V, Nelson A. The practice of palliative care from the perspective of patients and carers. BMJ Support Palliat Care. 2014;4:291–8.

25. Cowan K, Oliver S. The James Lind alliance guidebook. http://www.jlaguidebook.org/pdfguidebook/guidebook.pdf. 2013.

26. Palliative and end of life care Priority Setting Partnership. Palliative and end of life care Priority Setting Partnership (PeolcPSP): putting patients, carers and clinicians at the heart of palliative and end of life care research. https://palliativecarepsp.files.wordpress.com/2015/01/peolcpsp_final_report.pdf; 2015.

27. Heaton J. Secondary analysis of qualitative data: a review of the literature. University of York: Ref: R000222918; 2000.

28. O'Brien B, Harris I, Beckman T, Reed D, Cook D. Standards for reporting qualitative research: a synthesis of recommendations. Acad Med. 2014;89(9):1245–51.

29. Nelson A. Beyond the questions: shared experiences of palliative and end of life care. https://www.mariecurie.org.uk/globalassets/media/documents/research/publications/beyond-the-questions-esrc-report.pdf; 2016.

30. Braun V, Clarke V. Using thematic analysis in psychology. Qual Res Psychol. 2006;3:77–101.

31. Denscombe M. The good research guide for small-scale social research projects. 4th ed. Maidenhead: Open University Press; 2010.

32. Armstrong D, Gosling A, Weinman J, Marteau T. The place of inter-rater reliability in qualitative research: an empirical study. Sociology. 1997;31(3):597–606.

33. Barbour R. Checklists for improving rigour in qualitative research: a case of the tail wagging the dog? Br Med J. 2001;322:1115.

34. Koch T. Establishing rigour in qualitative research: the decision trail. J Adv Nurs. 1994;19(5):976–86.

35. Puntillo KA, Arai S, Cohen NH, Gropper MA, Neuhaus J, Paul SM, et al. Symptoms experienced by intensive care unit patients at high risk of dying. Crit Care Med. 2010;38(11):2155.

36. Hui D, dos Santos R, Chisholm GB, Bruera E. Symptom expression in the last seven days of life among cancer patients admitted to acute palliative care units. J Pain Symptom Manag. 2015;50(4):488–94.

37. Clark K, Connolly A, Clapham S, Quinsey K, Eagar K, Currow DC. Physical symptoms at the time of dying was diagnosed: a consecutive cohort study to describe the prevalence and intensity of problems experienced by imminently dying palliative care patients by diagnosis and place of care. J Palliat Med. 2016;19(12):1288–95.

38. Closs S, Dowding D, Allcock N, Hulme C, Keady J, Sampson E, et al. Towards improved decision support in the assessment and management of pain for people with dementia in hospital: a systematic meta-review and observational study. Health services and delivery research. 2016;No.430.

39. McGuire D, Kaiser K, Haisfield-Wolfe M, Iyamu F. Pain assessment in non-communicative adult palliative care patients. Nurs Clin N Am. 2016;51(3):397–431.

40. Gardiner C, Gott M, Ingleton C, Hughes P, Winslow M, Bennett M. Attitudes of health care professionals to opioid prescribing in end-of-life care: a qualitative focus group study. J Pain Symptom Manag. 2012;44(2):206–14.

41. Lopez-Saca J, Guzman J, Centero C. A systematic review of the in uence of opioids on advanced cancer patient survival. Curr Opin Support Palliat Care. 2013;7(4):431–7.

42. British Medical Association. Improving analgesic use to support pain management at the end of life. https://www.bma.org.uk/-/media/files/pdfs/collective%20voice/policy%20research/public%20and%20population%20health/analgesics-end-of-life.pdf?la=en; 2017.

43. General Medical Council. Treatment and care towards the end of life: good practice in decision making. http://www.gmc-uk.org/static/documents/content/Treatment_and_care_towards_the_end_of_life_-_English_1015.pdf; 2010.

44. Royal Collge of Nursing. Getting it right every time: nutrition and hydration at the end of life. http://rcneolnutritionhydration.org.uk/; 2015.

45. del Rio M, Shand B, Bonati P, Palma A, Maldonado A, Taboada P, et al. Hydration and nutrition at the end of life: a systematic review of emotional impact, perceptions, and decision-making among patients, family, and health care staff. Psycho-Oncology. 2012;21:913–21.

46. Department of Health. One chance to get it right: one year on report. https://www.gov.uk/government/uploads/system/uploads/attachment_data/file/450391/One_chance_-_one_year_on_acc.pdf; 2015.

47. Johnson M, Ekstrom M, Currow D. In response to C Walshe, 'The state of play'. Palliat Med. 2017; https://doi.org/10.1177/0269216317710424.

48. Homsi J, Walsh D, Rivera N, Rybicki LA, Nelson KA, LeGrand SB, et al. Symptom evaluation in palliative medicine: patient report vs systematic assessment. Support Care Cancer. 2006;14(5):444.

49. Pidgeon T, Johnson CE, Currow D, Yates P, Banfield M, Lester L, et al. A survey of patients' experience of pain and other symptoms while receiving care from palliative care services. BMJ Support Palliat Care. 2016;6(3):315–22.

50. Abernethy AP, Currow DC, Frith P, Fazekas BS, McHugh A, Bui C. Randomised, double blind, placebo controlled crossover trial of sustained release morphine for the management of refractory dyspnoea. BMJ. 2003;327(7414):523–8.

51. Johnson MJ, Kanaan M, Richardson G, Nabb S, Torgerson D, English A, et al. A randomised controlled trial of three or one breathing technique training sessions for breathlessness in people with malignant lung disease. BMC Med. 2015;13(1):213.

52. Hardy J, Quinn S, Fazekas B, Plummer J, Eckermann S, Agar M, et al. Randomized, double-blind, placebo-controlled study to assess the efficacy and toxicity of subcutaneous ketamine in the management of cancer pain. J Clin Oncol. 2012;30(29):3611–7.

53. Higginson IJ, Bausewein C, Reilly CC, Gao W, Gysels M, Dzingina M, et al. An integrated palliative and respiratory care service for patients with advanced disease and refractory breathlessness: a randomised controlled trial. Lancet Respir Med. 2014;2(12):979–87.

54. Agar MR, Lawlor PG, Quinn S, et al. Efficacy of oral risperidone, haloperidol, or placebo for symptoms of delirium among patients in palliative care: a randomized clinical trial. JAMA Intern Med. 2017;177(1):34–42.

55. Boland JW, Allgar V, Boland EG, Oviasu O, Agar M, Currow DC, et al. Opioids, benzodiazepines, anti-cholinergic load and clinical outcomes in patients with advanced cancer. BMJ Support Palliat Care. 2017;7(Suppl 1):A1–2.

56. Sue Ryder. A time and a place: what people want at the end of life. https://www.sueryder.org/~/media/files/about-us/a-time-and-a-place-sue-ryder.ashx; 2013.

57. Woodman C, Baillie J, Sivell S. The preferences and perspectives of family caregivers towards place of care for their relatives at the end-of-life. A systematic review and thematic synthesis of the qualitative evidence. BMJ Support Palliat Care. 2016;6(4):418–29.

58. Higginson I, Sarmento V, Calanzani N, Benalia H, Gomes B. Dying at home - is it better: a narrative appraisal of the state of the science. Palliat Med. 2013;27(10):918–24.

59. Gomes B, Calanzani N, Curiale V, McCrone P, Higginson I. Effectiveness and cost-effectiveness of home palliative care services for adults with advanced illness and their caregivers. Cochrane Database Syst Rev. 2013;6:CD007760.

60. Gomes B, Calanzani N, Gysels M, Hall S, Higginson I. Heterogeneity and changes in preferences for dying at home: a systematic review. BMC Palliat Care. 2013;12:7.
61. Higginson I, Sen-Gupta G. Place of care in advanced cancer: a qualitative systematic literature review of patient preferences. J Palliat Med. 2000;3:287–300.
62. Murtagh F, Bausewein C, Petkova H, Sleeman K, Dodd R, Gysels M, et al. Understanding place of death for patients with non malignant conditions: a systematic literature review. Final report. NIHR service delivery and organisation programme: national institute for health research. 2012;http://www.netscc.ac.uk/hsdr/files/project/SDO_FR_08-1813-257_V01.pdf.
63. Harrison N, Cavers D, Campbell C, Murray S. Are UK primary care teams formally identifying patients for palliative care before they die? Br J Gen Pract. 2012;62(598):e344–e52.
64. Quill T, Abernethy A. Generalist plus specialist palliative care — creating a more sustainable model. N Engl J Med. 2013;368(13):1173–5.
65. Blinderman C, Billings J. Comfort care for patients dying in the hospital. N Engl J Med. 2015;373(26):2549–61.

Permissions

List of Contributors

Christy Noble
Medical Education Unit, Gold Coast Health, Level 2 PED Building, 1 Hospital Boulevard, Southport, QLD 4215, Australia
School of Pharmacy, University of Queensland, Brisbane, QLD, Australia

Christy Noble and Andrew Teodorczuk
School of Medicine, Griffith University, Griffith, QLD, Australia

Laurie Grealish
School of Nursing and Midwifery and Menzies Health Institute Queensland, Griffith University, Griffith, Queensland, Australia

Laurie Grealish, Brenton Shanahan and Balaji Hiremagular
Gold Coast Health, Griffith, QLD, Australia

Jodie Morris
Myton Hospices, Coventry, UK

Sarah Yardley
Central and North West London NHS Foundation Trust, London, UK
Marie Curie Research Department, University College London, London, UK

Sandra Martins Pereira, Joana Araújo and Pablo Hernández-Marrero
Instituto de Bioética, Universidade Católica Portuguesa, Rua Diogo Botelho, 1327 4169-005 Porto, Portugal
UNESCO Chair in Bioethics Instituto de Bioética, Universidade Católica Portuguesa, Porto, Portugal
CEGE: Centro de Estudos em Gestão e Economia Research Centre in Management and Economics Católica Porto Business School, Universidade Católica Portuguesa, Porto, Portugal

Hanna T. Klop, Anneke L. Francke and Bregje D. Onwuteaka-Philipsen
Amsterdam Public Health Research Institute (APH), Department of Public and Occupational Health, Expertise Centre for Palliative Care, VU University Medical Center, 1007 MB Amsterdam, The Netherlands

Anke J. E. de Veer and Anneke L. Francke
Netherlands Institute for Health Services Research (NIVEL), 3500 BN Utrecht, Netherlands

Sophie I. van Dongen and Judith A. C. Rietjens
Department of Public Health, Erasmus University Medical Center, 3000 CA Rotterdam, Netherlands

Ruth Piers
Department of Geriatric Medicine, Ghent University Hospital, Ghent, Belgium

Ruth Piers and Lieve Van den Block
End-of-life Care Research Group, Vrije Universiteit Brussel (VUB) and Ghent University, Laarbeeklaan 103, 1090 Brussels, Belgium

Gwenda Albers and Wouter Van Mechelen
Flanders Federation for Palliative Care, Vilvoorde, Belgium

Jan De Lepeleire
Department of Public Health and Primary Care, ACHG, KU Leuven, Leuven, Belgium

Jan Steyaert
Department of Sociology, University of Antwerp, Antwerp, Belgium
Flemish Expertise Centre on Dementia Care, Antwerp, Belgium

Els Steeman
Academic Centre for Nursing and Midwifery, KULeuven, Leuven, Belgium

Let Dillen
Department of Geriatric Medicine, Ghent University Hospital, Ghent, Belgium

Matthias Vogl and Reiner Leidl
Helmholtz Zentrum Munich, German Research Center for Environmental Health, Institute of Health Economics and Health Care Management, Munich, Germany

Joni Gilissen and Lieve Van den Block
Department of Family Medicine and Chronic Care, Vrije Universiteit Brussel (VUB), Laarbeeklaan 103, 1090 Brussels, Belgium

Burkhard Dasch
Department of Anesthesiology, Intensive Care Medicine, Palliative Care Medicine and Pain Management, Berufsgenossenschaftliches Universitätsklinikum Bergmannsheil gGmbH Bochum, Medical Faculty of Ruhr University Bochum, Bürkle-de-la-Camp-Platz 1, 44789 Bochum, Germany

Claudia Bausewein and Berend Feddersen
Department of Palliative Medicine, Munich University Hospital, Ludwig-Maximilians-University Munich, Munich, Germany

Shirley Chambers, Ann Bonner and Patsy Yates
Faculty of Health, Queensland University of Technology, Brisbane, Australia

Shirley Chambers, Patsy Yates and Ann Bonner
National Health and Medical Research Council, Centre for Research Excellence in End of Life Care, Brisbane, Australia

Helen Healy, Adrian Kark, Sharad Ratanjee and Ann Bonner
Kidney Health Service, Metro North Hospital and Health Service, Queensland Health, Brisbane, Australia

Helen Healy, Wendy E. Hoy, Geoffrey Mitchell and Ann Bonner
National Health and Medical Research Council, Chronic Kidney Disease Centre for Research Excellence, Brisbane, Australia

Helen Healy, Wendy E. Hoy and Geoffrey Mitchell
Faculty of Medicine, University of Queensland, Brisbane, Australia

Carol Douglas
Palliative Care Service, Royal Brisbane and Women's Hospital, Queensland Health, Brisbane, Australia

Patsy Yates
Centre for Palliative Care Research and Education, Queensland Health, Brisbane, Australia

Anne Black, Tamsin McGlinchey, Maureen Gambles and Catriona Rachel Mayland Palliative Care Institute Liverpool, Cancer Research Centre, University of Liverpool, 200 London Road, Liverpool L3 9TA, UK

John Ellershaw
Royal Liverpool and Broadgreen University Hospitals NHS Trust, Prescot Street, Liverpool L7 8XP,UK

Josie Dixon and Martin Knapp
Personal Social Services Research Unit (PSSRU), London School of Economics and Political Science (LSE), Houghton Street, London WC2A 2AE, UK

Tao Wang, Alex Molassiotis, Betty Pui Man Chung and Jing-Yu Tan
School of Nursing, The Hong Kong Polytechnic University, Hung Hom, Hong Kong

Jing-Yu Tan
College of Nursing and Midwifery, Charles Darwin University, Darwin, Australia

Shaouli Shahid
Centre for Aboriginal Studies (CAS), Curtin University, Kent Street, Bentley, WA 6102, Australia

Shaouli Shahid, Emma V. Taylor, Shelley Cheetham, John A. Woods and Sandra C. Thompson
Western Australian Centre for Rural Health (WACRH), School of Population and Global Health, The University of Western Australia, Geraldton, WA 6530, Australia

Shelley Cheetham
School of Nursing, Midwifery and Paramedicine, Curtin University, Kent Street, Perth, WA 6102, Australia

Samar M. Aoun
Palliative Care Unit, School of Psychology and Public Health, La Trobe University, Melbourne 3086, Australia
Institute for Health Research, Notre Dame University, Fremantle, WA 6160, Australia

Ludwig-Maximilians-Universitaet Munich, Munich School of Management, Institute of Health Economics and Health Care Management & Munich Centre of Health Sciences, Munich, Germany

Eva Schildmann, Farina Hodiamont, Helen Kalies and Claudia Bausewein
Munich University Hospital, Department of Palliative Medicine, Ludwig-Maixmilians-Universitaet Munich, Marchioninistr. 15, 81377 Munich, Germany

Bernd Oliver Maier
St. Josephs-Hospital, Department of Palliative Medicine and Interdisciplinary Oncology, Wiesbaden, Germany

Marcus Schlemmer and Susanne Roller
Krankenhaus Barmherzige Brüder Munich, Department of Palliative Medicine, Munich, Germany

Elizabeth Somes
Internal Medicine Residency, University of Colorado School of Medicine, University of Colorado Anschutz Medical Campus, Aurora, CO, USA

Joanna Dukes
University of Colorado Skaggs School of Pharmacy and Pharmaceutical Sciences, University of Colorado Anschutz Medical Campus, Aurora, CO, USA

Hillary D. Lum
VA Eastern Colorado Geriatric Research Education and Clinical Center, Denver, CO, USA

Adreanne Brungardt, Sarah Jordan and Hillary D. Lum
Division of Geriatric Medicine, University of Colorado School of Medicine, University of Colorado Anschutz Medical Campus, 12631 E. 17th Ave, Mail Stop B179, Aurora, CO 80045, USA

Kristen DeSanto
Health Sciences Library, University of Colorado Anschutz Medical Campus, Aurora, CO, USA

Christine D. Jones
Division of Hospital Medicine, University of Colorado School of Medicine, Anschutz Medical Campus, Aurora, CO, USA

Urvi Jhaveri Sanghvi and Jacqueline Jones
College of Nursing, University of Colorado Anschutz Medical Campus, Aurora, CO, USA

Khadijah Breathett
Division of Cardiovascular Medicine, Sarver Heart Center, University of Arizona, Tucson, AZ, USA

Josianne Avoine-Blondin, Nago Humbert, Michel Duval and Serge Sultan
Centre de Psycho-Oncologie, CHU Sainte-Justine, Montréal, QC H3T 1C5, Canada

Josianne Avoine-Blondin and Véronique Parent
Department of Psychology, Université de Sherbrooke, 150, Place Charles-Le Moyne #200, Longueuil, Québec J4K 0A8, Canada

Léonor Fasse
Department of Psychology, Université de Bourgogne Franche-Comté, Esplanade Erasme, 21000 Dijon, France

Léonor Fasse and Clémentine Lopez
Hôpital Gustave Roussy, Villejuif, France

Clémentine Lopez
Université Paris Descartes, Paris, France

Nago Humbert, Michel Duval and Serge Sultan
Université de Montréal, Montréal, QC, Canada

Clémentine Lopez
Department of child psychiatry, Gustave Roussy, 114, rue Édouard-Vaillant, 94805 Villejuif, France

Nago Humbert, Michel Duval and Serge Sultan
Department of Hematology/Oncology, CHU Sainte-Justine, 3175, Chemin de la Côte-Sainte-Catherine, Montréal, Québec H3T 1C5, Canada

V. A. Crooks, M. Giesbrecht and N. Schuurman
Department of Geography, Simon Fraser University, 8888 University Drive, 1, and Burnaby, BC V5A 1S6, Canada

H. Castleden
Department of Geography and Planning and Department of Public Health Sciences, Queens University, 62 Fifth Field Company Lane, Kingston, ON K7L 3N6, Canada

M. Skinner
Trent School of the Environment, Trent University, 1600 West Bank Drive, Peterborough, ON K9L 0G2, Canada

A. Williams
School of Geography & Earth Sciences, McMaster University, 1280 Main Street West, Hamilton, ON L8S 4M1, Canada

Joshua Wales, Allison M. Kurahashi and Amna Husain
The Temmy Latner Centre for Palliative Care, Sinai Health System, 60 Murray Street, 4th Floor, Toronto, ON M5T 3L9, Canada

Jessica Baillie
School of Healthcare Sciences, Cardiff University, Cardiff, UK

Jordan Van Godwin
DECIPHer, School of Social Sciences, Cardiff University, Cardiff, UK

Despina Anagnostou, Stephanie Sivell, Anthony Byrne and Annmarie Nelson
Marie Curie Palliative Care Research Centre, Division of Population Medicine, School of Medicine, Cardiff University, Cardiff, UK

Index